Deco for Divers

A Diver's Guide to Decompression Theory and Physiology

Mark Powell

An AquaPress Book
Published by AquaPress Ltd
25 Farriers Way
Temple Farm Industrial Estate
Southend-on-Sea
Essex SS2 5RY
United Kingdom

First Published 2008
AquaPress and the AquaPress Logo are Trademarks of AquaPress Ltd.

A CIP catalogue record for this book is available from the British Library.

Diving is an inherently dangerous sport. The information contained in this book is supplied merely for the convenience of the reader and should not be used as the sole source of information. This book is not a substitute for proper training by a recognized diver training agency. The author and publisher have made every effort to ensure that the information in this book is correct at time of going to press. However, they accept no liability or responsibility for any loss, damage, accident, injury or inconvenience sustained by any person using this book or following advice presented in it. Any and all such liability is disclaimed.

For information on all other AquaPress titles visit www.aquapress.co.uk

ISBN 13: 978-1-905492-07-7
ISBN 10: 1-905492-07-3

Foreword

This is a truly remarkable book which covers all the various theories of decompression and ascents for divers in a most readable and understanding manner. The elimination of the mathematics and jargon means that any diver should easily understand the basis for the diverse decompression procedure.

The author has been able to be very objective and not select any one of these many methods used by tables and dive computers as being necessarily the best. The ability to read and compare all of these in one place allows the diver to make up his or her own mind as to which is indeed the safest. Mark Powell is to be congratulated for writing this excellent book and making decompression and ascent so understandable for any diver. He shows an excellent understanding of the many different methods with clear explanations and figures.

As a technical diver, he uses many of these methods for safe ascents himself and the clarity of his presentation is far superior to the complex books and papers in this field today. There is no other comprehensive book on decompression to my knowledge which is so easy to read and understand by the average recreational or technical diver.

Every diver can benefit from this knowledge and I certainly recommend the International Divers Alert Network and Undersea and Hyperbaric Medical Society to include this title in their book lists.

Peter B. Bennett, Ph.D., D.Sc.
Executive Director, UHMS
Emeritus Professor of Anesthesiology,
Duke University Medical Center
Founder & 1st President, DAN

Contents

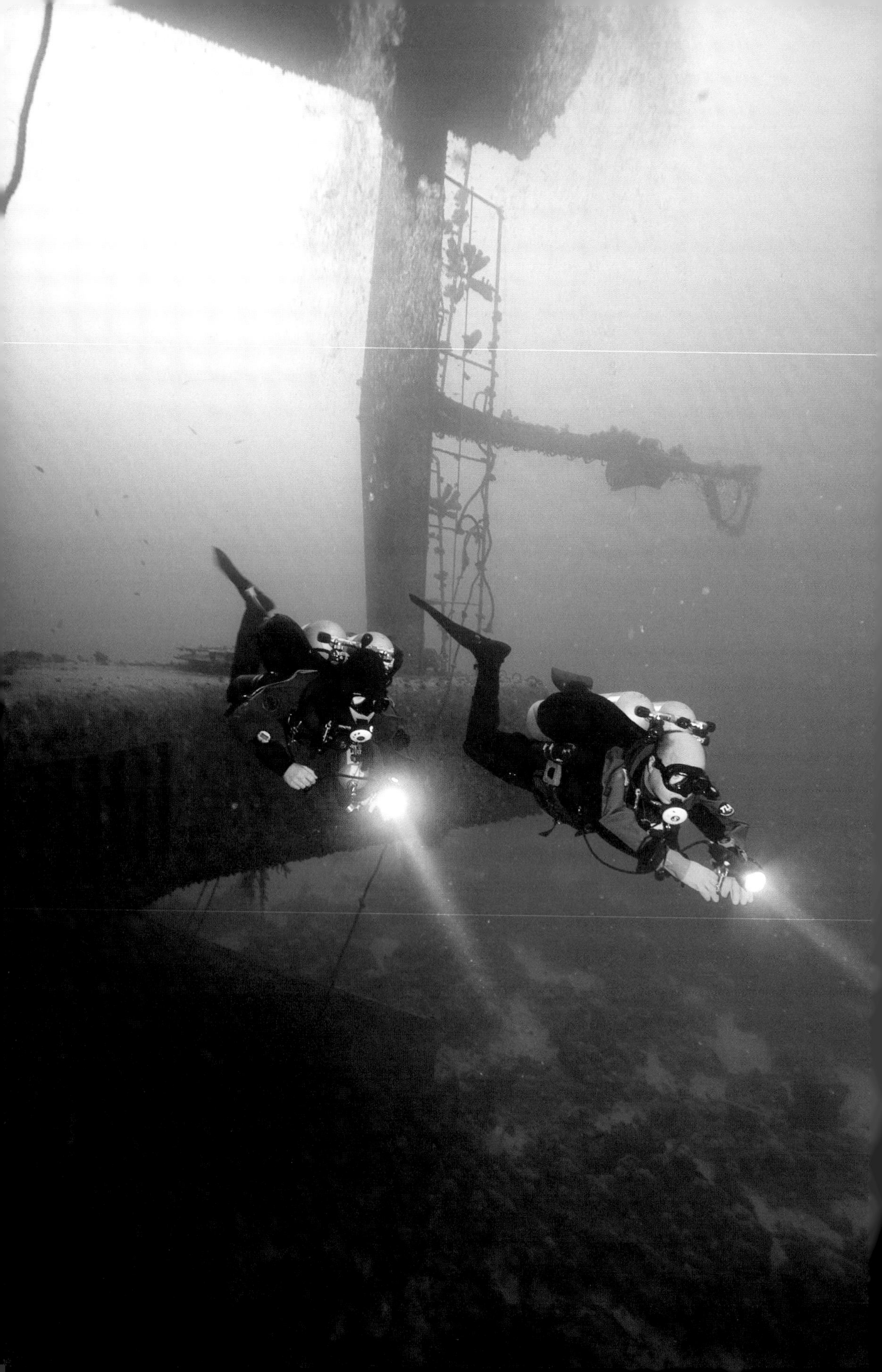

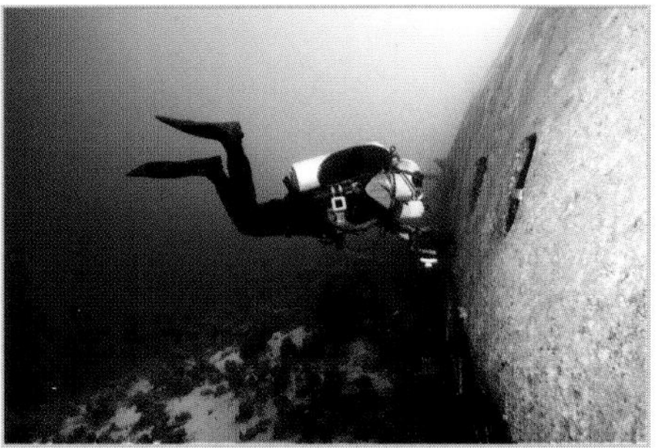

This book is aimed at divers who are interested in finding out a little more about the physiology and concepts underlying decompression

Introduction

This book was written to provide an accessible source of information on decompression theory. It is aimed at divers who are interested in finding out a little more about the physiology and concepts of decompression. The idea initially took root when I first started trying to learn more about decompression theory in order to satisfy my own interest. There were a number of sources of introductory information giving the basics of decompression theory. Some of these are very good introductions to the subject and are well explained. However I found that if I wanted to find out any more about any aspect of the theory there was a shortage of follow-on information. The only option was to jump into the original source articles, research papers or conference proceedings. Often the original source material was highly detailed with each paper looking at great depth into a single aspect of the individual concepts. A further hindrance was that many of these original papers were published in quite obscure journals or as research reports. Journals such as the Undersea and Hyperbaric Medicine Journal or the Aviation, Space and Environmental Medicine Journal can only be found in specific research or university libraries. Many of the papers written by decompression researchers working for the British, US and other navys were published as internal research notes and were not available in even the most comprehensive libraries. I was frustrated by this gap between the introductory texts and the source material. What I wanted was an intermediate overview that went into more detail but wasn't written for academics or researchers. Unfortunately there was no such text available.

When I became a technical diving instructor I started teaching other people about decompression theory. I tried to give an overview of decompression theory at this intermediate level to give my students a better understanding of what was happening during decompression dives. This was always very popular amongst divers who, like me, had always wanted to understand more about the concepts and models underlying decompression theory. I was always being asked if I could recommend a good book which covered this area but as before,

Left: A pair of divers explore a Red Sea wreck

there was no such text available. Over time I started giving out notes for the decompression theory portion of my courses and these notes started building. Initially they were just a few pages but the notes became more and more comprehensive and started to cover more and more areas. Eventually they grew into this book.

As I wrote this book I could have started almost every sentence with 'current thinking is' or 'we currently believe'. There are many theories as to the causes and mechanics of decompression but very few known facts.

"There is a false sense of security amongst recreational divers that decompression is a well understood science and that decompression illness can easily be avoided if you stick to your decompression tables."

This confidence is not shared by many decompression researchers. They realise that there is so much we still don't understand.

As we will see during the course of the book there are a number of quite different theories on various aspects of decompression theory. Not all of these theories can be correct. One of the major problems in giving a definitive explanation is that there is very little scientific evidence behind many of the theories. This problem of insufficient evidence can be seen where there are directly competing theories on a single issue. It is possible to find a paper on one aspect of decompression theory which is directly contradicted by another paper. Which one is correct? This problem is not unique to decompression research but is exacerbated by the fact that many studies are performed on test groups that are too small to be considered statistically significant. Tests are often conducted in less than ideal experimental conditions with test subjects being given control of the experiment and asked for a subjective view of the results. This leads to the situation where you can get contradictory results and often interested parties leap on the result that backs up their point of view without acknowledging other points of view.

Despite all the issues I have raised above, recreational diving is a very safe activity compared to other activities. Millions of dives are carried out each year using current decompression models with a very small incidence of decompression illness.

Many of the early advances in the field of decompression theory were driven by navy research scientists or medical officers. Haldane's development of the dissolved gas model through to Workman's development of the M-value idea was driven by military interest. In the 1960s and 1970s the discovery of oil reserves in deep water led to a significant interest in developing new diving techniques for deeper and longer dives. During this period the major oil exploration companies invested heavily in decompression research. With the increased use of remotely operated vehicles (ROVs) the interest in decompression research in the oil companies was greatly reduced. With the reduction in research in the military and commercial sectors the funding for decompression research has also been greatly reduced.

The increase in popularity of technical diving has raised the interest in decompression theory when pushed beyond the limits of recreational diving. Technical diving involves diving deeper than recreational limits for extended periods of time and using mixed gases other than air. Technical diving is pushing the boundaries of many aspects of diving and decompression theory is one such area. With the reduction in research on the military and commercial sectors it is becoming increasingly common for the needs of technical divers to drive decompression research.

Technical divers who are extending recreational diving concepts to technical diving decompression may be taking a much higher risk. Applying concepts tried and tested in the recreational diving range can produce unexpected or incorrect results when applied outside of their intended range. Decompression ideas that are valid within the recreational diving range are not necessarily valid beyond this range.

As an analogy we can consider a post natal clinic which measures the length/height of babies from birth to 6 months old. With enough measurements we can calculate an average height for ages from birth to 6 months. From this data we can extrapolate to 1 year, 2 years or more. However this extrapolation becomes increasingly inaccurate as the age is increased. The rate of growth slows down and then stops as we become older and so the relationship between age and height that applies from birth to 6 months becomes increasingly unreliable as we get older. Blindly extrapolating the data will result in a prediction that by age 21 we will be approximately 4m tall. Diving in the recreational range can be thought of as analogous to age 0 to 6 months in that we have plenty of data points for this range and can use these to accurately predict what will happen in this range. As we increase the depth and start to go into decompression diving then we are extrapolating past the 6 months point and so our predictions will start to become less reliable. In this range traditional methods of predicting decompression may still provide useable dive profiles but they are based on less than ideal assumptions. As we dive deeper and longer and move into the range of extreme technical dives then decompression predictions based on traditional recreational models can be compared to the predictions of a 4m tall, 21 year old.

Adopting the latest fashion in decompression theory still doesn't mean that the technical diver is free from risk. Divers who download one of the latest PC planning tools from the internet; use it to plan a dive and just blindly follow the plan it gives them are gambling with their health and more on the assumption that this piece of software is correct.

"Blindly following a set of tables, PC planning program or any other form of decompression planning without understanding some of the principles of decompression theory can be highly dangerous."

As I have explained I am a diver and a technical diving instructor. I am not a doctor or a decompression researcher. As such there is no original research or thoughts in this book. All I have tried to do is to bring together and explain the ideas and theories that have been proposed by others. In doing this I have necessarily had to summarise some of the core ideas. In some cases this process has taken an aspect of decompression theory which spans many articles and conference proceedings and summarises it in just a couple of paragraphs. In this case it is inevitable that much has to be left out and many of the ideas and explanations must be simplified. I have tried to simplify things to the point where they can easily be understood without loosing the key point.

In chapter one we start with a thorough review of the history and development of decompression theory. This chapter gives details on the life and work of some of the early researchers in this area as well as detailing the discoveries they are responsible for. Starting with Robert Boyle's experiments with a vacuum pump which provided the first documented occurrence of decompression sickness, the chapter moves through the research of the famous French scientist Paul Bert. The introduction of pressurised underwater working areas (Caissons) and the resulting discovery of Caisson's disease is detailed along with the experiences of workers involved in early Caisson construction projects. At about the same time, the first evidence of decompression sickness amongst divers was also documented.

The pioneering work of John Scott Haldane and his work for the British Admiralty in developing the first scientifically derived decompression tables sets the tone for future research on decompression theory. The contribution of the US Navy between the two world wars and in the early 1950s is described, as well as the significant contributions of Prof. Albert Bühlmann in Switzerland. Together, this research provides the basis of what we would consider traditional decompression theory.

In chapter two some of the key principles of decompression theory are explored. This combination of physical effects and their impact on our body provide an overview of exactly what happens to us when we breathe in a pressurized environment. Although dealing with concepts from physics and biology, this chapter is written in a descriptive style with no scientific jargon or complex equations.

Chapter three describes the various forms of decompression sickness, how they are caused and how they can be avoided. Various conditions, behaviours and environmental conditions that can increase the risk of decompression sickness are discussed. The medical effect of decompression sickness on the body, together with the treatment, both in a first aid and in recompression chambers, is discussed.

Saturation diving is discussed in chapter four. This type of diving is popular with commercial diving organisations but is not practical for the recreational diver. Saturation diving involves the divers staying on the sea bed until their bodies become saturated with the gas they are breathing, they can then work for indefinite periods – from days to weeks or even months – without incurring any further decompression penalties. This approach becomes cost effective for commercial divers undertaking long projects. Due to the interest in saturation diving amongst commercial and military organisations, a significant amount of research has been carried out in this area and in fact many aspects of decompression theory have arisen as a result of saturation diving research.

Chapter five discusses the use of Nitrox and its effect on decompression. Most recreational diving has traditional been carried out while breathing compressed air. Since the 1990s Nitrox, a combination of Nitrogen and Oxygen where the Oxygen content is higher than normal air, has become increasingly common. The use of Nitrox to reduce decompression obligations is discussed, as well as the use of an additional rich Nitrox mixture to speed up (or accelerate) decompression. Using the first of these techniques divers can spend up to twice as long on the bottom without having to go into decompression. With the second technique, divers can significantly reduce the amount of decompression they need to do for a given dive.

Modern approaches to decompression theory are summarised in chapter six. The emergence of inconsistencies in the traditional view of decompression which has led to the development of more recent theories are also discussed. More recent approaches, which can be described as deep stop or bubble model approaches, are covered in detail. The development of deep stops through both empirical trial and error as well as more scientific approaches is detailed. Empirical approaches such as Pyle stops are covered, along with the popular gradient factor approach. The work of researchers in the "tiny bubble" group, which has led to so called bubble models, is described as well as both the generic aspects of bubble models and some of the specifics of several of the more popular versions of bubble models.

For deeper diving, the use of Trimix – a mixture of Oxygen, Helium and Nitrogen – is becoming increasingly common. The introduction of Helium into the breathing mix provides significant advantages for deeper diving but introduces additional complications into decompression. Chapter seven gives a full discussion of all the factors involved in Trimix decompression.

A variety of other decompression models or approaches are discussed in chapter eight. Despite sponsoring the original research by JS Haldane, the British Royal Navy developed an alternative method of calculating decompression schedules. These tables were developed by the Royal Naval Physiological Laboratory and are known that RNPL tables. These tables adopt a quite different approach to decompression modeling to the traditional approach inspired by Haldane. The British Sub Aqua Club (BSAC) has also developed a set of tables based on an alternative model. The BSAC has never published the details of their model but by investigating the research of the scientist who developed them we can piece together some clues as to how they work. The US Navy has also looked at alternative models based on different assumptions as to how our body takes in and eliminates nitrogen. They have also put extensive effort into calculating decompression tables based on statistical or probability models.

For those who are interested in the details of the various decompression models discussed throughout the book, Chapter nine contains tables of the various key parameters as well as details of the mathematical models. All the mathematical details of the various models have been collected into a single chapter, providing a complete reference for those who would like to investigate the implementations of the various approaches. It also ensures that the rest of the chapters can remain relatively maths free which makes the main sections of the book more readable. For those who are not mathematically inclined, this chapter can be safely skipped!

In the main body of the text I have generally avoided giving specific references or including footnotes in order to avoid breaking up the flow of the narrative. The References and Further Reading section contains further reading on key areas of decompression theory as well as references to source material for each chapter.

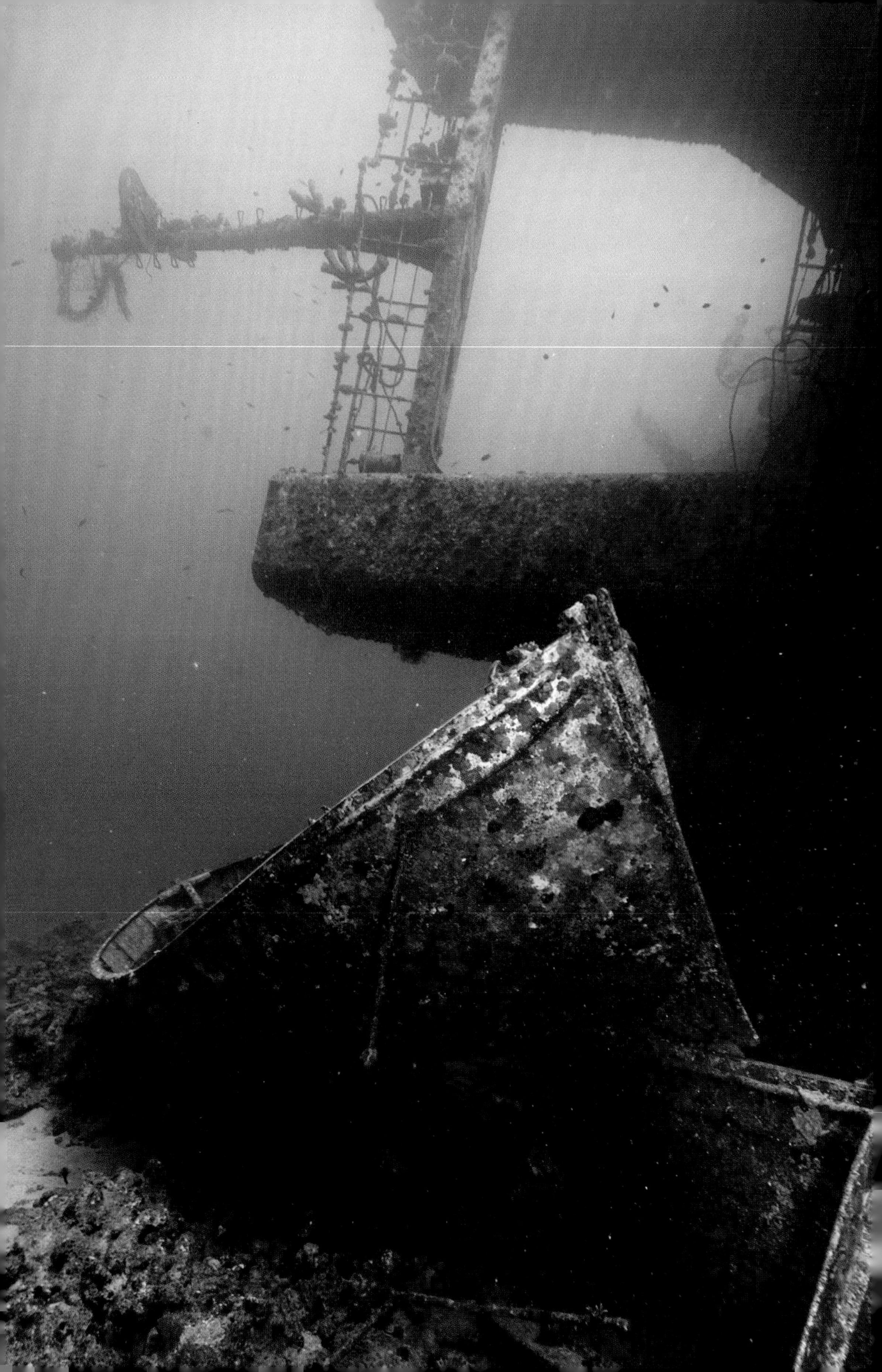

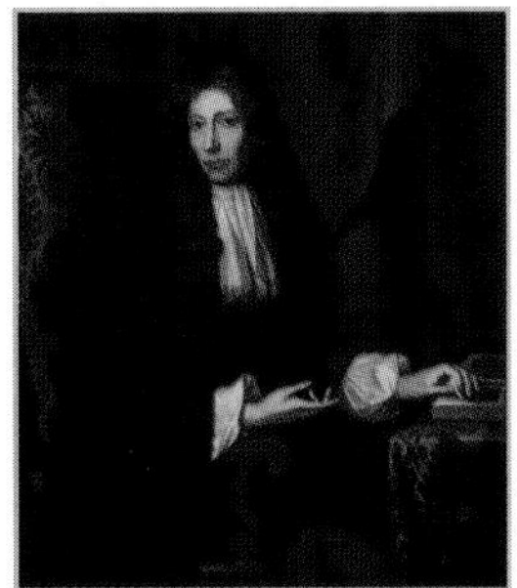

Robert Boyle was the first scientist to document an incident of decompression illness

1 Historical Perspective

Decompression theory has a long and involved history. Some of the greatest scientific minds have been involved in the story of decompression theory. Despite 350 years of study there are still many aspects of decompression theory which are still as unknown to us as they were to the earliest pioneers of deco theory. The story of decompression started in England in the seventeenth century and over the next 350 years the focus of our story jumped between England, the rest of Europe, as well as the United States and involved some of the most famous scientists of the ages. Great scientific minds like Robert Boyle, John Dalton and Paul Bert all played an important part in putting in place some of the foundations of modern decompression theory.

Robert Boyle (1627 - 1691)

The first of the great diving medicine innovators to describe decompression illness was Robert Boyle (1627-91), the Irish physicist and chemist who gave us Boyle's Law, so well know to diving students all over the world. In 1667, before 'diving' was even known, Boyle had discovered decompression illness.

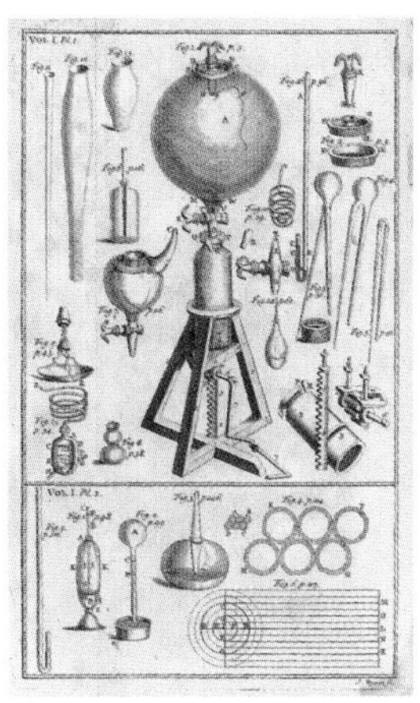

Boyle's vacuum globe

Boyle was the seventh son of Richard Boyle, 1st Earl of Cork and was born at Lismore Castle, Munster, Ireland. He studied at Eton and then travelled around Europe for 6 years before returning to his family's estates in Dorset. He moved to Oxford in 1654 where he carried out a range of experiments on vacuums, combustion and respiration.

Boyle was studying the behaviour of gases and built a small pressure chamber, based on Von Guericke's vacuum pump, to see how animals reacted to different pressures. He observed that a snake (a viper to be precise) became very distressed when the air was removed from the 'receiver' in which it resided. Boyle's experimental notes record 'I observed the viper furiously tortured in our exhausted receiver, which had manifestly a conspicuous bubble moving to and fro in the waterous humor of one of its eyes'. This was the first recorded observation of the bubble formation that leads to decompression illness. Boyle recorded his observations but had no idea as to why the bubble had been formed.

Rediscovery

Decompression illness was rediscovered in the early 19th century although at that time there was still no clear understanding of the cause of the disease. Workers involved in mining, tunnel construction or building work in pressurised underwater containers as well as the early hard hat divers began to notice a variety of symptoms when leaving the tunnel or construction chamber or when ascending after a hard hat dive.

In 1844 Royal Engineer Colonel William Pasley (later Major General Sir William Pasley) was allocated the task of clearing the wreck of *HMS Royal George* which had sunk in the Solent in 1787 and was proving a hazard to navigation for ships entering Portsmouth (United Kingdom), an important Naval harbour. Pasley decided to use the opportunity to test and evaluate hard hat diving equipment. Workers on the project regularly undertook long strenuous dives, frequently working up to seven hours a day at depths of 20m (65ft).

"Despite the success of the project, all of the divers involved reported a number of symptoms including aches and pains in various parts of the body. The cause of the symptoms was unknown and initially these symptoms were referred to as the "Mysterious Malady"."

During this same time diving bells were increasing in size. The industrial revolution produced high-capacity air pumps capable of sufficient pressure to keep water from entering these bells. Diving bells then evolved into dry underwater chambers allowing several men to work in a dry environment. In 1830 Lord Cochrane patented the use of compressed air to provide an air filled working environment underwater or in mines or tunnels which were below the level of the groundwater.

This innovation greatly simplified the task of constructing bridge footings and tunnels. These dry, pressurised work areas were known as plenum pneumatic or Caissons, French for "big box." This design was a major leap forward in engineering, as it allowed workers easy access from the surface and the pressure inside kept the work area dry. An air-lock was used to pass materials in and out or to change work shifts. The use of the Caisson grew rapidly as larger and more ambitious engineering works were undertaken. The men who worked in these big boxes became known as Caisson workers or just Caissons.

Caissons Disease

As the use of the Caisson grew a large number of workers began to complain of symptoms similar to those encountered by the hard hat divers. Caisson workers reported a number of symptoms including dizzy spells, shortness of breath and sharp acute pain in the joints or abdomen. After a period the symptoms would reduce, but the worker was sometimes left with symptoms which refused to disappear completely. It was also noted that those who suffered from the mysterious malady felt better when they returned to the pressured environment of the Caisson. As projects got bigger and working pressures increased, the attacks of the mysterious malady increased, not only in number of victims, but also in severity, so much so that fatalities started to occur frequently.

The term 'maladie du caisson' or Caisson's Disease was first used in 1841 by a French mining engineer named Triger who noticed that coal miners working under increased atmospheric pressure suffered from muscular cramping and pains after returning to the surface.

In 1851 Caissons were first used in the construction of a bridge when they were used by William Cubitt and John Wright in the construction of the Medway Bridge at Rochester in Kent, England.

In 1866, James Eads, was called on to bridge the Mississippi at St. Louis, Missouri. Instead of the usual truss bridge, he proposed to build three huge cantilever arches, 500 feet across. Eads was an unconventional choice for building the bridge; he had never built one before although, despite no formal education, he had a wide range of design and engineering experience. In his twenties he designed a diving bell and worked at salvaging cargo from sunken river boats. During the American Civil War, Eads built ironclad gunboats.

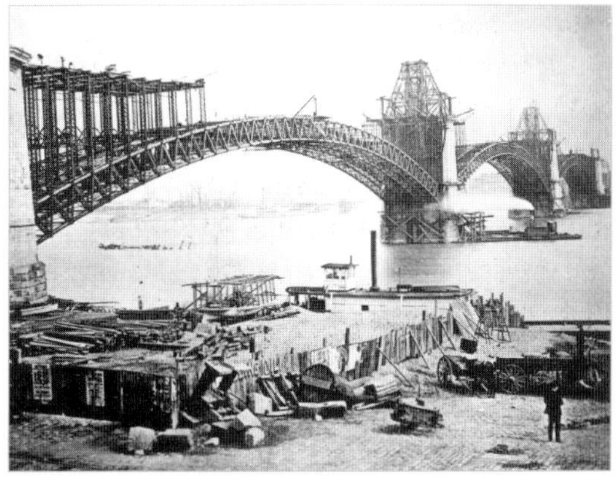

The Eads Bridge over the Mississippi River under construction in St. Louis, Missouri, in 1874 or earlier.

This project would stretch current engineering practice as it involved placing the piers right in the middle of the Mississippi river. Eads knew that the bottom of the Mississippi was made up of swirling mess of moving mud and silt. Furthermore he knew that the bedrock lay 30m (100 feet) below the mud and silt. Clearly the use of Caissons was the only answer, but they would need to be used on a scale that had not previously been imagined.

The Caissons were 82 feet long and 60 feet wide steel boxes, and open at the bottom. They were floated into position and then masonry piers were built on top of them, causing them to sink down to the riverbed. Air was pumped into the caisson under pressure in order to keep the water and mud out.

Workers descended a stairwell through the masonry to the caisson and entered it through an airlock. Inside, they dug out mud while the whole structure gradually settled downward toward bedrock. Workers above kept building up the masonry pier on top of the gradually sinking Caisson.

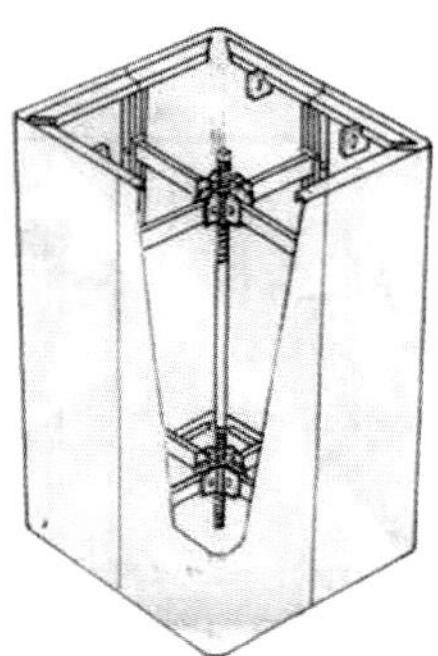

A Caisson

The approach seemed to be working well and it allowed workers to proceed with the project. However, when the pressure in the Caisson reached twice atmospheric pressure, workers felt pains in their joints as they returned to the surface. When they reached a depth where the pressure was three atmospheres the symptoms became worse and a number of workers were hospitalised. Some suffered total paralysis and in some cases the symptoms were so serious that the workers died of their injuries. Fifteen workers died, two other workers were permanently disabled, and 77 were severely afflicted..

It was noticed that visitors to the Caissons who only spent a short period of time under pressure and then returned to the surface never experienced any problems. Obviously, the less time you spent below, the less you suffered. It was also noticed that if you ascended slowly from the Caisson the symptoms were reduced. Eads gradually reduced the working shifts to only 45 minutes and in 1870 ordered that workers always carried out a slow return to the surface. These measures seemed to work. Doctors, however, were baffled and couldn't explain the etiology (physiological cause behind the disease).

Even in Webster's 1913 Dictionary the definition of Caisson's Disease shows a clear explanation of the symptoms but no clear understanding of the causes.

Definition: \Cais"son dis*ease"\ (Med.)
A disease frequently induced by remaining for some time in an atmosphere of high pressure, as in caissons, diving bells, etc. It is characterised by neuralgic pains and paralytic symptoms. It is variously explained, most probably as due to congestion of internal organs with subsequent stasis of the blood.

Caisson's disease continued to affect workers throughout the 1800s. During the construction of the Brooklyn Bridge between 1870 and 1883 three people died and 15% of those who suffered symptoms were left with some level of permanent paralysis. Unfortunately, due to personality conflicts between James Eads and Washington Roebling, who took over from his father John as Chief Engineer on the Brooklyn Bridge, Eads never passed on the knowledge that had been gained during construction of the St Louis Bridge. Washington Roebling was himself struck down with Caissons disease in 1872 and remained painfully paralysed for the rest of his life.

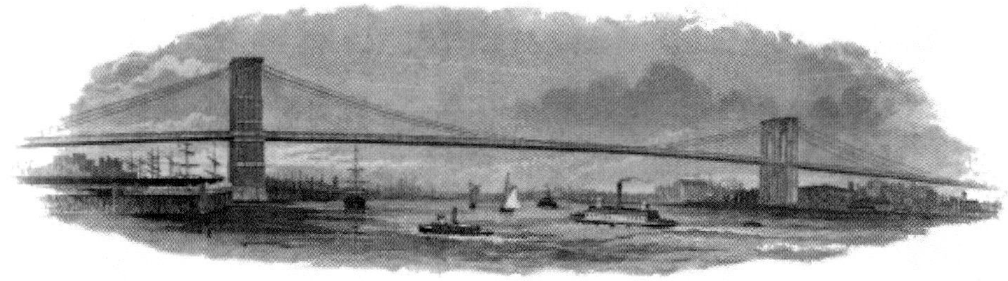

The Brooklyn Bridge

It was during the construction of the Brooklyn Bridge that the term "bends" was introduced for the first time. As the workers often had trouble standing straight their posture was similar to the "Grecian bend" adopted by fashionable women of the time and so they began to call the problem "the bends", a name which has stuck to this day.

Paul Bert (1833-1886)

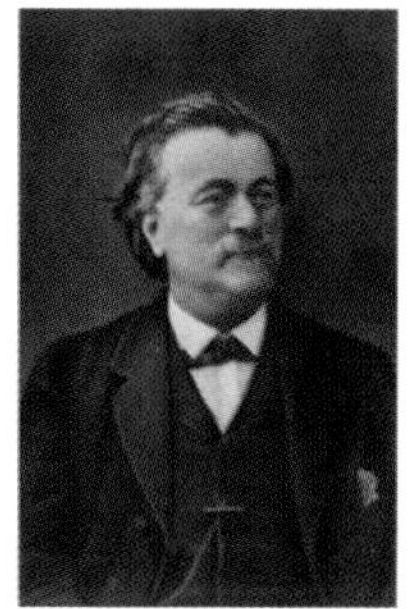

Paul Bert was born at Auxerre in 1833. He entered the Ecole Polytechnique at Paris with the intention of becoming an engineer; then changing his mind, he studied law; and finally, he took up physiology. After graduating at Paris as doctor of medicine in 1863, and doctor of science in 1866, he was appointed professor of physiology successively at Bordeaux and the Sorbonne. After the revolution of 1870 he began to take part in politics and four years later he was elected to the Assembly, where he sat on the extreme left. He was elected to the chamber of deputies and served as minister of education and worship. Early in 1886 he was sent to Indochina and appointed resident-general in Annam and Tonkin. Five months later in November 1886 Bert suddenly died of dysentery in Hanoi. He was 53 years old.

Bert is remembered more as a man of science than as a politician or administrator. His classical work, *La Pression Barometrique* (1878), laid the foundation of knowledge of the physiological effects of air-pressure, both above and below atmospheric pressure.

Bert became interested in the problems that low air pressure caused for mountain climbers and balloonists. This led him to study the problems that divers had with increased pressure as well. He reviewed the current reports of research in this area. He was struck in particular by the experiences that Dr. Alphonse Gal had while diving in Greece. Dr. Gal was the first doctor to actually dive in order to study how the body reacted underwater. Bert studied Gal's own diving experiences and his reports on divers who were injured or killed.

Bert's research and experiments led to his conclusion that pressure does not effect us physically, but rather chemically by changing the proportions of oxygen in the blood. Too little creates oxygen deprivation and too much creates oxygen poisoning. He showed that pure oxygen under high pressure can be deadly and to this day Central Nervous System (CNS) oxygen toxicity is known as the 'Paul Bert Effect'.

Perhaps his most important discovery was the effect of nitrogen under high pressure, which for the first time explained decompression. In investigating the causes of decompression illness Bert exposed 24 dogs to pressure of between seven and nine and three-quarter atmospheres (equivalent to a depth of 87.5msw or 290fsw) and decompressed them rapidly in one to four minutes. The result was that 21 died, while only one showed no symptoms. In one of his cases, in which the apparatus burst while at a pressure of nine and a half atmospheres, death was instantaneous and the body was enormously distended, with the right heart full of gas. However, he also found that dogs exposed, for moderate periods, to similar pressures suffered no ill effects provided that the pressure was relieved gradually, in between one and one and a three-quarter hours.

"Bert determined that the symptoms observed were due to the formation of gas bubbles in the blood and tissues. He also identified nitrogen as the gas which was producing the bubbles."

He went on to explain that it was the increase in partial pressure of Nitrogen which caused Nitrogen to become dissolved in the bodies tissues and then the subsequent reduction in pressure caused the nitrogen to come out of solution and form bubbles. As a result of this research Bert concluded that divers and caisson workers decompress slowly and at a constant rate *"for they must not only allow time for the nitrogen of the blood to escape but also to allow the nitrogen of the tissues time to pass into the blood".*

He also went on to suggest stopping divers halfway to the surface during decompression after a deep dive and as such was the first to suggest what are now known as deep stops.

Bert carried out a number of experiments into methods of treating the compressed air illness once the symptoms had appeared. His experiments showed that once bent - the symptoms could be relieved by returning into the compressed air environment of the Caisson or tunnel and then decompressing the patient slowly. This was clearly the start of recompression therapy which has been shown to be the most effective way of treating decompression illness. He also showed that breathing pure oxygen was highly effective in relieving the symptoms of decompression illness. In one of his experiments on animals he noted: *"The favorable action of oxygen was... evident; after several inhalations (of oxygen) the distressing symptoms disappeared."*

In a later entry, Bert attempted to explain why oxygen worked. *"I thought that if the subject were caused to breathe a gas containing no nitrogen — pure oxygen for example — the diffusion would take place much more rapidly and perhaps would even be rapid enough to cause all the gas (nitrogen) to disappear from the blood."*

This is indeed why oxygen is so useful in treating decompression illness. Bert was the first to propose the concept of oxygen recompression therapy, though the actual practice wasn't implemented until many years later.

John Scott Haldane (1860-1936)

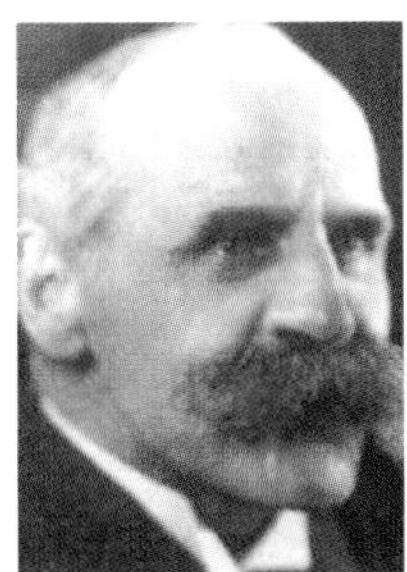

JS Haldane

Scottish physiologist John Scott Haldane is considered to be the father of modern decompression theory. Haldane was the first scientist to apply a scientific approach to predicting decompression and his methods form the basis of the majority of modern decompression theories. Haldane was born in Edinburgh into a notable family. Haldanes had been Lords of Gleneagles since the thirteenth century and his brother Richard, Lord Haldane of Cloan, was Secretary of War from 1905-1912, Lord Chancellor and was also the founder of the Territorial Army.

Haldane studied medicine at the University of Edinburgh and graduated in 1884. After graduation he moved to Queen's College, Dundee (which at the time was part of St Andrews University). Here he took on the relatively humble role of demonstrator before transferring to Oxford University. At Oxford he lectured on medicine and conducted medical research. In 1906, in collaboration with John Gillies Priestley (1880-1941), he discovered that the respiratory reflex is triggered by an excess of carbon dioxide in the blood rather than a lack of oxygen.

In his later years Haldane became an authority on the effects of pulmonary diseases on industrial workers and in 1912 was appointed Director of the Mining Research Laboratory in Doncaster. He was known to half the miners in Yorkshire as 'The Doctor' and was frequently seen underground taking samples of the air or measuring the thickness of the dust. Haldane's understanding of the dangers of carbon monoxide was used to increase safety in the mines. His findings led to the introduction of mice and canaries as early indicators of air quality. He also devised more effective mine rescue equipment.

Haldane and his wife Kathleen lived in the same house in Oxford for fifty years. The Haldane residence was an impressive house and would later become part of Wolfson College. In order to keep the household running the servants included a butler and housemaids, a nurse and a coachman who would later be replaced by a chauffer. Haldane often worked at home; he had a study in the attic as well as a comprehensive laboratory complete with a pressure chamber so that he could expose his test subjects to the effects of gases under pressure. Often Haldane would work through the night and then rise late next day in time for lunch. Haldane was notoriously eccentric and disorganized; according to his wife *'the carpet in his study was hidden under layers of papers, the desk piled high ... chairs laden with reports and notes and sheets of calculation'*. Sometimes, when entertaining, he would forget his guests and start to consider some physiological problem then wander off to his laboratory to continue his experiments.

Haldane also founded the *Journal of Hygiene* and it was in this publication that the first set of diving decompression tables were published. During his lifetime he also published *Organism and Environment* (1917), *Respiration* (1922) and *The Philosophy of a Biologist* (1936).

It is Haldane's work on decompression for which he is most widely remembered, especially amongst divers. In 1905 Haldane was approached by the Royal Navy's Deep Diving Committee to carry out research on a number of aspects of their diving operations. The most important aspect of this work was looking at ways to avoid the bends or "caissons disease" as it was then widely known.

It had long been observed that men working in pressurised bridge and tunnel construction areas, known as *caissons*, would sometimes complain of pain in their joints. As the depth at which they were working increased, and so the pressure inside the caisson increased, the severity of the symptoms worsened. Many suffered total paralysis and there were frequent deaths. Research and practical observation suggested that gasses, breathed under pressure by the workers, were diffusing into the body's tissues and when these gasses came out, in the form of bubbles in the body, the workers got caisson disease, or what we now call decompression illness (DCI).

The same symptoms were seen amongst divers who were breathing air under pressure. Divers were told to minimise this risk by ascending slowly to begin with, and then rising faster as they got nearer the surface. Thanks to Haldane's work, we know now that this was completely incorrect and potentially very dangerous.

Haldane began working with Dr Teddy Boycott from the Lister Institute in London. A team of Royal Navy divers including Lieutenant Guy Damant were also assigned to the research. Haldane began experimenting on goats as they were readily available subjects and are of a similar size to humans. He found that the body could tolerate a certain amount of excess gas with no apparent ill effects. Caisson workers pressurised at two atmospheres (10 m/33 fsw) experienced no problems, no matter how long they worked. Similarly goats saturated to 50 m (165fsw) did not develop DCS if decompressed to half ambient pressure.

Haldane wrote *"the formation of bubbles depends, evidently, on the existence of a state of supersaturation of the body fluids with nitrogen. Nevertheless there was abundant evidence that, when the excess of atmospheric pressure does not exceed about one-and-a-quarter atmospheres, there is complete immunity from symptoms due to the bubbles, however long the exposure to the compressed air may have been, and however rapid the decompression. Thus, bubbles of nitrogen are not liberated within the body unless the supersaturation corresponds to more than a decompression from a total pressure of two-and-a-quarter atmospheres to a total pressure of one atmosphere (i.e. that normally existing on the surface of the earth)."*
In order to explain these observations Haldane proposed four basic principles;

1. Gas absorption and elimination in a tissue occurs exponentially
2. Different tissues absorb and release gas at different rates
3. Decompression is achieved by decreasing ambient pressure
4. Gas tension in a tissue must not exceed approximately twice ambient pressure

"Haldane suggested that we consider the body as a group of tissues which absorbed and released gases at different rates."

This meant the tissues were all exposed simultaneously to the breathing gasses at ambient pressure, but each tissue reacted to the gas pressure in a different way. He then went on to suggest a mathematical model to describe how each of the tissues absorbs and releases gases and put limits on the amount of over-pressurisation that the tissues could tolerate.

Haldane introduced the concept of half times to model the uptake and release of nitrogen into the blood. The half time is the time required for a particular tissue to become half saturated with a gas. He suggested five tissue compartments with half times of 5, 10, 20, 40 and 75 minutes.

He also demonstrated that decompression was most dangerous nearest the surface. One of the key elements of Haldane's work, and one that is still as relevant today, is that he identified that it is the relative pressure differences that are important rather than just the absolute depth changes. As we are now well aware, a diver ascending from 60m would have to travel 35m before the absolute pressure on him was halved (7 bar to 3.5 bar), but only 15m to achieve the same result from 20m (3 bar to 1.5 bar). He wrote *"Hence it seemed to me probable that it would be just as safe to diminish the pressure rapidly from four atmospheres to two, or from six atmospheres to three, as from two atmospheres to one. If this were the case, a system of stage decompression would be possible and would enable the diver to get rid of the excess of nitrogen through the lungs far more rapidly than if he came up at an even rate. The duration of exposure to high pressure could also be shortened very considerably without shortening the period available for work on the bottom".*

Haldane also developed practical dive tables based on his research that included slower ascent rates as the diver approached the surface. The results of this research and Haldane's diving tables were published in 1908 in the *Journal of Hygiene.*

Following the report of the Admiralty's Deep Diving Committee it was decided to publish the committee's conclusions in the form of a blue book available to the public. The conclusions were universally accepted and it became the foundation of all diving operations, both in the UK and abroad.

In 1915 Haldane was asked to investigate the poison gas being used by the Germans in the trenches of France. During his research into these gases Haldane often ended up breathing samples of these gases while testing new designs of gas masks. Haldane's lungs were permanently damaged by this and would cause problems for the rest of his life. However the result of this work was that Haldane developed one of the first effective gas masks and as a result saved many thousands of lives. Haldane also invented several tests and measuring devices including a gas analysis apparatus that enabled physiologists to estimate the gases present in the blood from a small blood sample.

Haldane died of pneumonia in 1936 at the age of seventy-five. His lungs had never recovered from his experiments during the First World War. He had just returned from a trip to the Middle East where he had been investigating heat stroke amongst oil workers. He was cremated and his ashes scattered at the family graveyard at the mouth of Gleneagles.

US Navy

Prior to 1912, US Navy divers had rarely ventured below 18m/60 fsw. In that year, Chief Gunner George D. Stillson had proposed that the US Navy study the work of Haldane in order to allow US Navy divers to safely dive below 18m/60 fsw. Stillson set up a program to test Haldane's diving tables and methods of stage decompression. An additional goal of the program was to develop general improvements in Navy diving equipment and procedures. Throughout a three-year period, first diving in tanks ashore and then in open water in Long Island Sound from the *USS Walke*, the Navy divers went progressively deeper, eventually reaching 83m/274 fsw. Stillson also studied the affects of using pure oxygen during decompression. As a result of these studies the Navy published their own set of tables in 1915. The were known as the C&R tables as they were published by the Bureau of Construction and Repair.

The experience gained in Stillson's program was put to dramatic use six months later when the submarine *USS F-4* sank near Honolulu, Hawaii. Twenty-one men lost their lives in the accident and the Navy lost its first boat in 15 years of submarine operations. Navy divers salvaged the submarine and recovered the bodies of the crew. The salvage effort incorporated many new techniques, such as the use of lifting pontoons, but what was most remarkable was

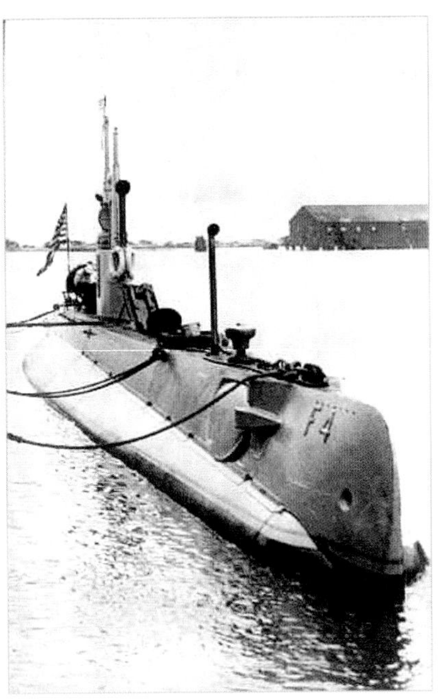

The USS F4

that three US Navy divers, Crilley, Loughman, and Nielson completed a major salvage effort working at the extreme depth of 92m/304 fsw, using air as a breathing mixture. These dives remain the record for the use of standard deep-sea diving dress.

Because of the depth and the necessary decompression, each diver could remain on the bottom for only ten minutes. Even for such a limited time, the men found it hard to concentrate on the job at hand. They were, of course, being affected by nitrogen narcosis.

In 1916 the US Navy established the Deep Sea Diving School based at the US Naval Torpedo Station in Newport, Rhode Island. It wasn't until 1924 that the results of Stilson's work in developing working practices and procedures were published as the first US Navy Diving Manual.

In 1930 Charles Shilling showed that existing tables didn't adequately cover decompression for longer deep dives. Five years later in 1935 J A Hawkins analysed Shilling's data and concluded that a surfacing ratio of 2:1 was too conservative for the faster tissues and not conservative enough for the slower tissues. Hawkins realised that rather than a single surfacing ratio for all the tissue compartments each compartment should have its own individual surfacing ratio.

In 1937 O D Yarbrough further developed Hawkins work. He observed that the 5 and 10 min compartments could tolerate such an over pressurisation ratio that they could effectively be ignored. However the ratio for the other compartments was reduced in order to make the tables more conservative. Revised tables were published without the 5 and 10 minute compartments, just with the 20, 40 and 75 minute compartments but each with their own over-pressurisation ratio. This was the first major development to the model since Haldane had developed the approach in 1907.

However there were still problems with Yarbrough's tables when applied to long, deep dives. In the late 1940s Otto E Van Der Aue was studying surface decompression. He was working at the US Navy Experimental Diving Unit conducting a large series of experimental dives in order to produce acceptable surface decompression schedules. The decompression schedules were the first in which a tissue half-time of 120 minutes was used in their calculation. All were completed in October 1945 with air. The first was to 10m/33ft for 24 hours with direct surfacing. No cases of DCS resulted in the four divers. The next two dives were to 10m/33ft for 36 hours with 4 divers in each exposure. Two of the divers developed bends. The last dive was to 36m/99ft for 12 hours followed by decompression to 10m/33ft for a stay of 24 hours. Both the divers using this schedule suffered DCS. The conclusion was that for decompression from longer dives long half-time tissues needed to be assigned lower ratios than short half-time tissues. In other words, the 2:1 ratio for decompression did not work.

As part of this series four dives were done which resulted in total saturation of all tissue compartments, Van Der Aue used the term 'Saturation Dive' to describe these dives and this is the first recorded use of this phrase.

In the early 1950s the US Navy decided to revise its tables in order to improve their safety. This was carried out my M Des Granges and Lt Cmdr J.V. Dwyer. They found that, as depth and time increases so must depth of decompression. They restored the 5 and 10 minute compartments and also added a much slower 120 minute compartment. This was to account for long deep dives which had proved to be the Achilles heel of a number of the previous tables. In 1956 the revised US Navy Standard Air Decompression Tables were published. A review of the tables in 1965 showed a DCS incidence of 0.69% as compared to 1.1% for the tables developed by Yarbrough in 1937.

Robert Workman

The approach to decompression modelling proposed by Haldane was used with minor modifications from 1908 through until the 1960s. These modifications were primarily changes to the number of compartments and half times used. As we have seen US Navy tables published in 1937 and based on research by O. D. Yarbrough used only 3 compartments as the two fastest compartments were dropped (5 and 10 mins). Later revisions in the 1950's restored the fast 5 and 10 minute compartments as well as adding a slower 120 minute compartment to give a total of six compartments.

It wasn't until the 1960s that any fundamental changes to the model were considered. Robert D. Workman of the U.S. Navy Experimental Diving Unit (NEDU) was a medical doctor with the rank of Captain in the Medical Corps. It had been observed that tables based on Haldane's work and subsequent refinements were still inadequate when it came to longer and deeper dives. Workman undertook a review of the basis of the model as well as subsequent research performed by the US Navy.

Workman revised Haldane's model to take into account the fact that each of the various tissue compartments can tolerate a different amount of over-pressurisation and that this level changes with depth. He introduced the term "M-value" to describe the amount of over-pressurisation each compartment could tolerate at any depth. Workman also added three further slow tissue compartments with 160, 200 and 240 minutes half times. M-Values still form a critical part of decompression theory and will be discussed in more detail in Chapter 2.

Rather than present his calculations as a completed table Workman presented his conclusions in the form of an equation which could be used to calculate the results for any depth. He also made the observation that "a linear projection of M-values is useful for computer programming as well" and so was one of the first people to identify the role that computers would come to play in the calculation of decompression tables.

Professor Albert Bühlmann (1923–1994)

Professor Albert A. Bühlmann, M.D., began research into decompression in 1959 at the Laboratory of Hyperbaric Physiology, part of the University Hospital in Zurich, Switzerland. Bühlmann continued his research for over thirty years and made a number of important contributions to decompression science.

Bühlmann specialized in the patho-physiology of the respiratory and circulatory systems. He took a particular interest in respiratory physiology under extreme atmospheric conditions, of the kind encountered at high altitudes or whilst diving. For the majority of his career his main interest was professional deep diving. In 1959 he supervised successful experimental dives to a depth of 120 metres in Lake Zurich using Trimix gas mixtures and changes of mixture during decompression. In the next two years Professor Bühlmann and Hannes Keller demonstrated the practical results of their research with simulated dives to 300 metres. In the following years Bühlmann worked with the US Navy who funded a series of experimental extended dives in the range of 150 to 300 metres. Bühlmann also worked with Shell Oil who were interested in the practical implications of his research as they could be applied to commercial dives involved with undersea oil fields.

Much of Bühlmann's research was intended to determine the longest half time compartments for Nitrogen and Helium. As a result of this work Bühlmann extended the number of half time compartments to 16. He also investigated the decompression implications of diving at altitude. A number of severe cases of DCS showed that high altitude diving was very dangerous when using standard 'sea level' decompression tables. Following a series of simulated high altitude dives decompression tables that could be used at a range of altitudes were published. Bühlmanns' method for decompression calculations was similar to the one that Workman had prescribed. This included M-values which expressed a linear relationship between ambient pressure and the maximum inert gas pressure in the tissue compartments. The major difference between the two approaches was that Workman's M-values were based on depth pressure (i.e. diving from sea level) and Bühlmann's M-values were based on absolute pressure (i.e. for diving at altitude).

In 1983 he published the results of his years of research in the first edition (in German) of a successful book entitled *"Decompression - Decompression Sickness"*. An English translation of the book was published in 1984. This book was the first nearly complete reference on making decompression calculations that was widely-available to the diving public. As a result, the "Bühlmann algorithm" became the basis for most of the world's in-water decompression computers and do-it-yourself desktop computer programmes.

Three more editions of the book were published in German in 1990, 1993, and 1995 with the revised title *"Tauchmedizin"* or *"Diving Medicine."* An English translation of the 4th Edition of the book (1995) has still not been published.

Bühlmann's model was also used to generate tables which became the standard diving tables for a number of sport diving associations. Max Hahn used Bühlmann's model to develop tables which were adopted by the Swiss Underwater Sport Association and the Association of German Sports Divers. In the UK Bob Cole developed a set of tables for the Sub-Aqua Association. In 1987, working in conjunction with Bühlmann, he developed the SAA Bühlmann System which is made up of the tables themselves together with a set of rules and procedures for using them safely.

Prof. Bühlmann died suddenly of heart failure in 1994 at the age of 70. Although he was not himself a diver he made a great impact on the science of decompression. He constantly tried to create tables which resulted in the lowest possible risk while avoiding unnecessarily long decompression. His work gained worldwide recognition and in 1993 he received an award from the Divers Alert Network (DAN) for his life's work in the service of decompression science.

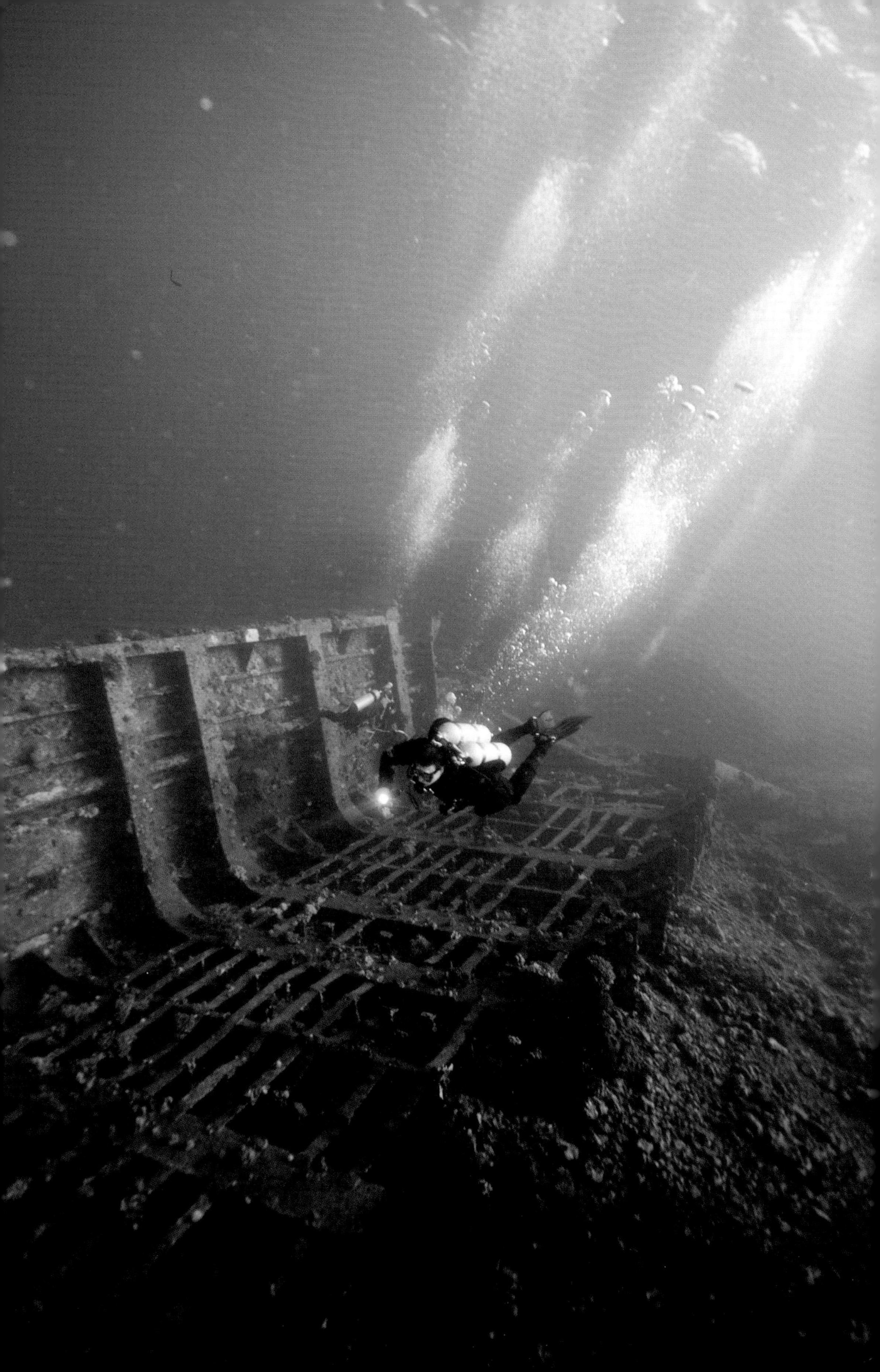

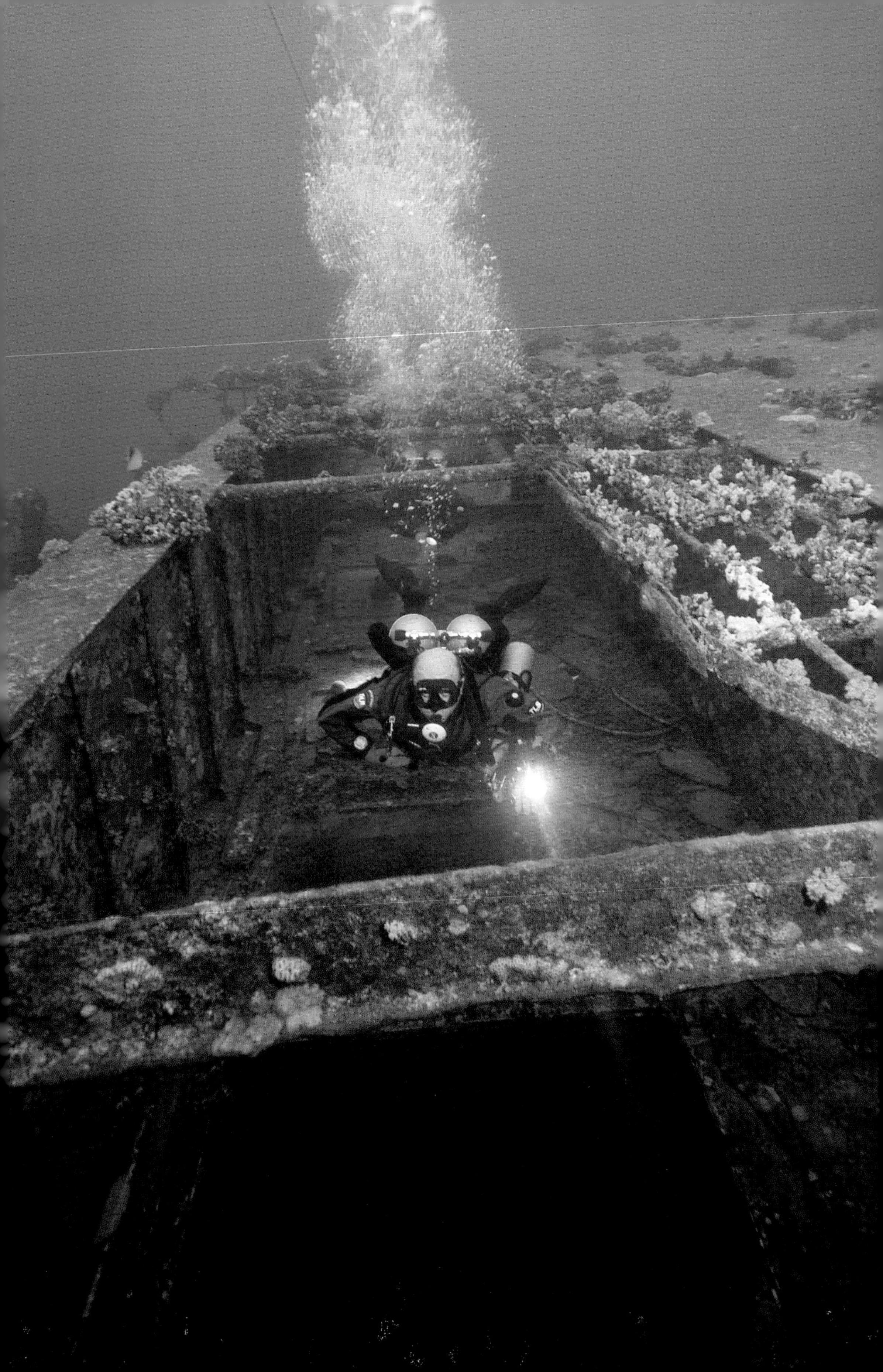

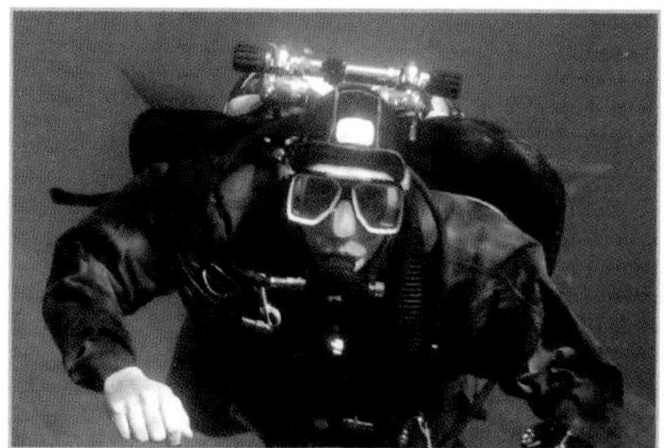

The deeper we dive and the longer we stay down, the more nitrogen is absorbed into our body

2 Decompression Principles

Overview

When we are at the surface, breathing normal air, the nitrogen dissolved in our body is in equilibrium with the nitrogen in the air. Even the bodies of those people who have never dived will contain dissolved nitrogen in equilibrium with the nitrogen in the air.

When we dive, the weight of the water around us increases the ambient pressure acting on us and we must breathe compressed air, or some other compressed breathing gas, in order to counteract the pressure of the water and allow our lungs to expand. As this breathing gas is compressed or pressurised then we are breathing a gas at a higher pressure than we would be breathing at the surface. This higher pressure means that there is more nitrogen than in the air we breathe at the surface. This increased pressure of nitrogen in the gas we are breathing results in more nitrogen being absorbed by the tissues of the body.

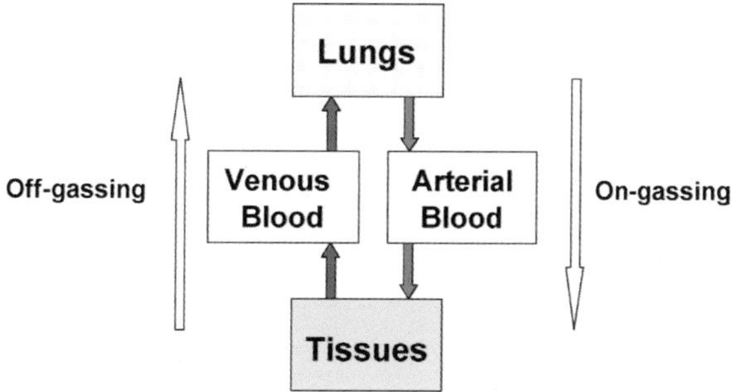

Overview of the flow of nitrogen during a dive

The deeper we dive and the longer we stay down, the more nitrogen is absorbed into our body until after some time our bodies are once again in equilibrium with the gas we are breathing. It will take many hours, even days for our tissues to reach this equilibrium or to become saturated. Once we reach this level then we will not take on any more nitrogen at that depth. However if

Left: A diver using a twinset and decompression cylinder

we were to descend to a greater depth and the pressure were once again to increase then we would again start to take on nitrogen until we were once again saturated.

As we ascend at the end of the dive the situation is reversed. In ascending we are reducing the ambient pressure around us and as a result the pressure of the gas we are breathing. We are now in a situation where the nitrogen in our tissues is potentially at a higher pressure than the gas we are breathing. At this point the nitrogen starts to come out of our tissues into the lungs and is breathed out with each breath.

If we have too much nitrogen in our body then the nitrogen cannot come out fast enough and bubbles may form in the body. This is the cause of decompression illness or the bends. If we have stayed down too long or ventured too deep then we may have to pause during the ascent to allow the nitrogen to escape. This is the reason why we have to perform decompression stops.

The Air we Breathe

The human body is well adapted to breathing air at one atmosphere (ATA) or one bar of pressure. For thousands of years the atmospheric pressure at the Earth's surface has been effectively constant and so through years of evolution we have come to consider this pressure to be the norm. Despite concerns over pollution and greenhouse gases the composition of air is remarkably consistent around the world. The air that we breathe contains:

Gas	% by Volume	% by Weight	Parts per Million	Chemical Symbol
Nitrogen	78.08	75.47	780840	N_2
Oxygen	20.95	23.20	209460	0_2
Argon	0.93	1.28	9340	Ar
Carbon Dioxide	0.03	0.046	300	CO_2
Neon	0.0018	0.0012	18.21	Ne
Helium	0.0005	0.00007	5.24	He
Krypton	0.0001	0.0003	1.14	Kr
Hydrogen	0.00005	Negligible	0.50	H_2
Xenon	8.7 x 10-6	0.00004	0.087	Xe

Composition of Normal Air

For most physiological or medical situations we are primarily interested in the oxygen content of the air we breathe. It is the oxygen that the body uses to burn fuel and to create energy. Nitrogen and the other trace gases are chemically and biologically inert at atmospheric pressure which means that on the surface they have no chemical or biological affect on us. Combined with the fact that there are such small traces of Argon, xenon and the other trace gases it is customary to group all of the inert gases together and to assume that air is made up of 21% Oxygen and 79% Nitrogen.

This air is taken into the lungs and mixes with the gas already in the lungs which includes carbon dioxide generated by the respiration within the body's cells as well as some water vapour. This means that the gases within the lungs have a slightly different make up to the atmosphere in general.

Gas	% in Atmosphere	% in Lungs
Oxygen	20.95	14
Water Vapour	0	6
Nitrogen	79	75
Carbon Dioxide	0.03	5

Table 2: *Composition of air in the atmosphere and air in the lungs*

This can be seen more clearly in a diagram of the percentage composition of air in the atmosphere and air in the lungs.

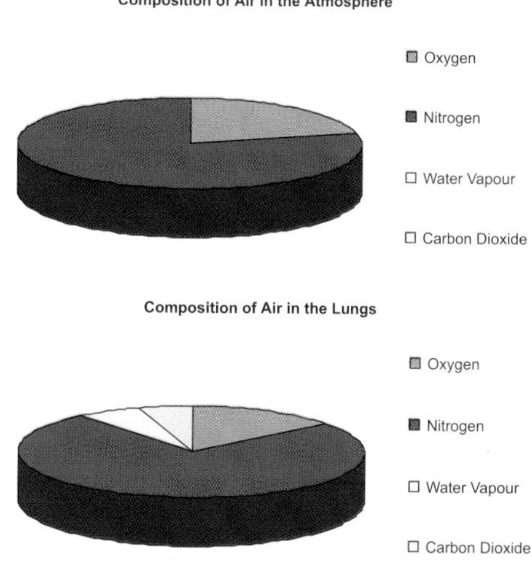

Oxygen passes from the lungs, through the walls of the lungs and into the blood vessels surrounding the lungs. From here the oxygen is carried to all parts of the body by the blood in the arteries where it is used by the cells to create energy. Carbon Dioxide is also produced in this process as a waste product and is carried back to the lungs by the veins. As well as Oxygen the blood also absorbs some of the nitrogen from the lungs and this is also carried around the body. As Nitrogen is inert it is not used up by the body and is carried back to the lungs. This means that on the surface the amount of Nitrogen in the body is constant. Some may flow from the lungs into the blood stream and some may flow from the blood stream into the tissues but an equal amount flows back out of the tissues into the blood and from the blood into the lungs. On average the total amount of nitrogen stays the same.

The Effects of Pressure

If we stay at the same pressure then this situation remains constant. For the majority of people, as they are non-divers and non-mountaineers, this is the end of the story. However, as divers, when we descend we increase the pressure surrounding us. Ambient pressure on the surface is 1 bar but if we descend to 10m then the 10m of water above us adds a further 1 bar of pressure and the ambient pressure increases to 2 bar. In other words that first 10m of water adds the same pressure as the entire weight of the atmosphere above us. For every further 10m we descend a further 1 bar is added to the ambient pressure.

Depth (m)	Pressure (Bar)
0	1
10	2
20	3
30	4
40	5
50	6
60	7
70	8
80	9
90	10
100	11

Pressure in Bar at Depth

In order to continue breathing at depth it is essential that the gas we breathe is at the same pressure as ambient pressure. If the gas we were breathing were still at 1 bar pressure then we would be unable to inflate our lungs. Scuba equipment supplies us with gas that is at ambient pressure which means that at 10m the gas we are breathing is at 2 bar and at 50m the gas we are breathing is being supplied to us at 6 bar. Scuba regulators are designed to achieve this automatically and so a diver just needs to breath in and the regulator will automatically provide gas at ambient pressure.

As the diver descends the gas he is breathing increases in pressure. As a result the pressure of each constituent part of that gas is also at a higher pressure. This is known as the partial pressure. So we can see that as the diver descends the partial pressure of Nitrogen being breathed will increase. If there is more Nitrogen present in the lungs then more Nitrogen will flow through into the blood and be carried to the tissues where the tissues will absorb more Nitrogen. As the Nitrogen is inert and so is not used up by the tissues it is held in solution within the tissues.

As the diver ascends at the end of his dive the pressure is reduced and the pressure of the breathing gas is also reduced. This now means that there is a higher concentration of nitrogen in the body's tissues than in the breathing gas. Nitrogen now flows from the tissues into the blood and then into the lungs where it is then breathed out. If the pressure is reduced too quickly or if there is too much nitrogen in the tissues then instead of coming out of the tissues into the blood and into the lungs the nitrogen can form bubbles within the body. This is what happens when a diver suffers from decompression illness or the bends. It is essential therefore that the amount of nitrogen is allowed to escape from the body in a controlled manner in order to avoid suffering from decompression illness.

Lets look at each of the stages in more detail:

Dalton's Law

John Dalton (1766-1844) was an English chemist born at Eaglesfield near Cockermouth on the edge of the Lake District. He was the son of a Quaker weaver and a very bright student; so much so that he was put in charge of the local Quaker school at the age of 12. At this age Dalton was reading Newton's Principia in the original Latin. He also studied meteorology and kept a meteorological journal recording more then 200,000 observations over his lifetime. In 1793 he was appointed teacher of mathematics and science at New College Manchester where he stayed for the remaining 50 years of his life. In 1794 he first described colour blindness, which was known for many years as Daltonism, as both he and his brother suffered. Despite his wide ranging scientific interests his main areas of research were on mixed gases, the forces of steam, the elasticity of vapours, the expansion of gases by heat and the absorption of gases in water and other liquids.

Dalton was unquestionably one of the greatest of pioneering chemists, but as a person he was known to stick to his Quaker upbringing. He is described as having simple habits, grave manners and being reserved but kindly. Despite gaining significant fame and recognition as a result of his many contributions to science; including membership of the Royal Society, numerous medals and a generous government pension, he continued teaching elementary arithmetic to boys in a small school in a Manchester backstreet. When he died in 1844, forty thousand people viewed the coffin and the funeral procession stretched for two miles.

As far as decompression is concerned Dalton's major contribution was in the area of partial pressure and the framing of what came to be know as Dalton's Law of Partial Pressures.

Dalton's law states that: the total pressure exerted by a mixture of gases is the sum of the pressures that would be exerted by each gas if each occupied the total volume.

The partial pressure of any constituent gas in a breathing mixture can easily be calculated by multiplying the fraction of that particular gas by the total pressure. So if a diver is breathing air at 20m the fraction of Nitrogen in the gas would be 0.79 and the total pressure would be 3 bar. This means that the partial pressure of nitrogen is equal to the fraction of nitrogen multiplied by the total pressure or:

$$ppN_2 = FN_2 \text{ x } P(total)$$
$$ppN_2 = 0.79 \text{ x } 3$$
$$ppN_2 = 2.37 \text{ bar}$$

So the partial pressure of Nitrogen when breathing air at 20m is 2.37 bar. We can see from the diagram below that the percentages of each gas stays the same, there is still 79% Nitrogen

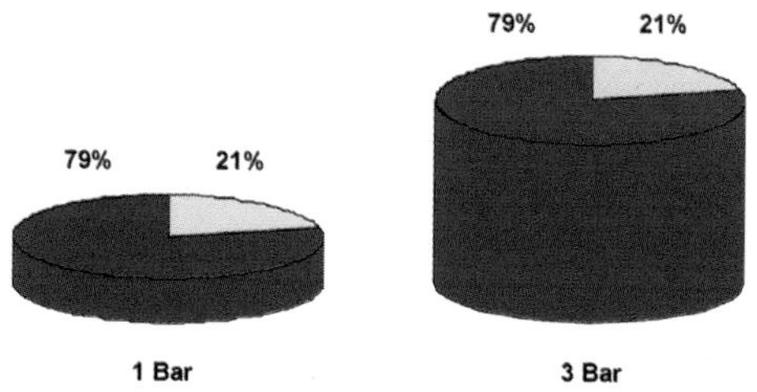

Partial pressure of gasses at different ambient pressures

in air no matter what the pressure of that air. However the partial pressure of that Nitrogen is higher as the total pressure increases.

The partial pressure of the oxygen in the mixture can be calculated the same way;

$$ppO_2 = FO_2 \text{ x } P(total)$$
$$ppN_2 = 0.21 \text{ x } 3$$
$$ppN_2 = 0.63 \text{ bar}$$

If we add up the partial pressure of Nitrogen (2.37) and the partial pressure of oxygen (0.63) then we get the total pressure (3.0). Which is exactly what Dalton's law predicts when it states that the total pressure exerted by a mixture of gases is the sum of the pressure that would be exerted by each gas if it occupied the total volume.

Depth (m)	Pressure (Bar)	ppO_2 (Bar)	PPN_2 (Bar)
0	1	0.21	0.79
10	2	0.42	1.58
20	3	0.63	2.37
30	4	0.84	3.16
40	5	1.05	3.95
50	6	1.26	4.74

Partial pressure of Oxygen and Nitrogen at various depth

The table above shows the partial pressures of Nitrogen and Oxygen at a range of depths when breathing air.

The Lungs

When we take a breath (inhalation) the external intercostal muscles of the ribcage contract and the internal intercostals relax. This has the effect of pulling the ribcage up and outwards. The diaphragm is also pulled down and away from the lungs. This causes a reduction in pressure in the lungs which causes air to be drawn into the lungs. When we breath out (exhalation) the opposite occurs: the external intercostal muscles relax and

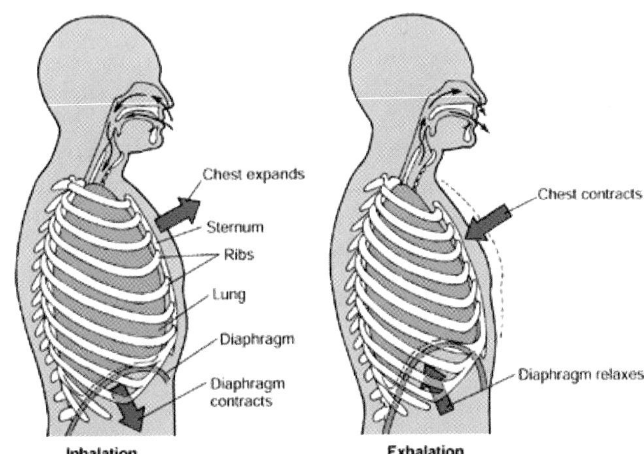

The Mechanics of Inhalation and Exhalation

the internal intercostals contract causing the ribcage as a whole to contract. The diaphragm also relaxes. The result of this is that the air is squeezed from the lungs and we release the breath we took.

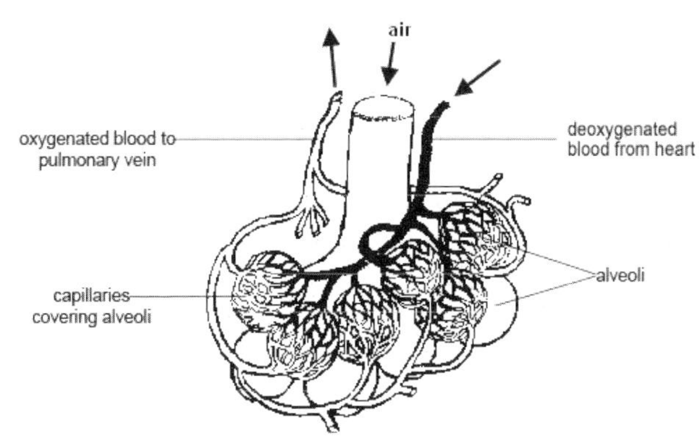

Diagram 9.1 - Alveoli with blood supply

The Function of the Alveoli

The gas we are breathing comes in through the nasal cavity, or, in the case of diving through the mouth. It then passes down the trachea, which subdivides into the two bronchi, one of which enters each of the lungs. Inside the lungs the bronchi split into secondary bronchi and keep on separating into smaller and smaller branches called bronchioles which form a tree like network. The splitting has the effect of increasing the surface area available for gas exchange. At the end of these fine tubules are millions of small groups of sacks called alveoli. Each lining of the alveoli forms the gaseous exchange surface. There are over 600 million alveoli present in the human lung, with a total surface area of 100 m^2, about the same area as a singles tennis court. The wall of the alveolus is only 0.1μm thick, which is just 1/1000th the thickness of a human hair.

The outside of every alveolus is a dense network of capillaries, all of which have come from the pulmonary artery. The walls of the alveoli are composed of a single layer of flattened cells called epithelial calls, as are the walls of the capillaries, so gases need to diffuse through just two thin cells. By reducing the distance the gas has to travel this increases the speed of gas exchange. Water diffuses from the alveoli cells into the alveoli so that they are constantly moist. The water also contains a surfactant which, just like a soap bubble, reduces its surface tension and stops the alveoli collapsing. Oxygen dissolves in this water before diffusing through the cells into the blood, where it is taken up by haemoglobin in the red blood cells. The blood from the pulmonary artery flows through the capillaries surrounding the alveoli taking about 1 second to pass through the lung capillaries. In this time the blood becomes nearly 100% saturated with oxygen and loses its excess CO_2.

The alveoli also contain phagocyte cells which are immune system cells which will kill any bacteria that have not been trapped by the mucus.

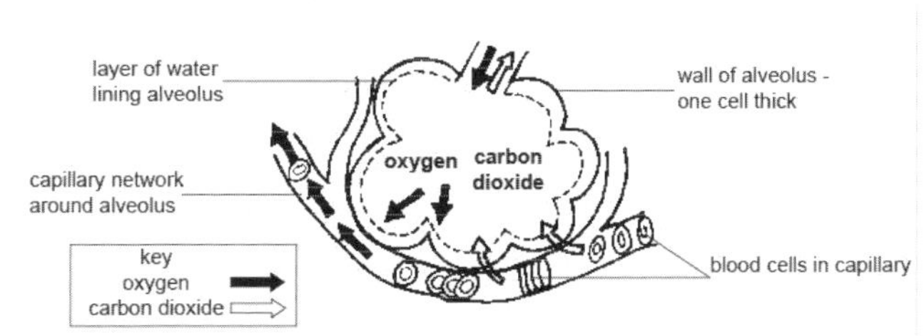

Figure 11: *Details of the alveoli.*

The trachea and some of the lung space such as the bronchioles are dead space and do not exchange gases. Only the air in the alveoli can exchange O_2 and CO_2 with the blood.

In the alveoli the partial pressure of oxygen is less than that of the surrounding air because alveolar gas is diluted with carbon dioxide and water vapour already present in the lungs. Inspired air has a partial pressure of Oxygen (ppO_2) of 159 mm Hg at sea level whereas the Alveolar ppO_2 is 100 mm Hg at sea level. The lung capillary blood is nearly in equilibrium with alveolar oxygen with ppO_2 of 95 mm Hg. In the tissues oxygen level is lower because it is being used up by the metabolism. Typical tissue ppO_2 is 30 mm Hg.

Gas	Inspired	Alveolar	Arterial	Venous	Tissues
Nitrogen	596	573	573	570	573
Water Vapour	5	47	47	47	47
Carbon Dioxide	0	40	40	46	50
Oxygen	159	100	95	40	30
Total	760	760	755	703	700

Gas pressures at various stages of the respiratory and circulatory systems

For carbon dioxide the gradients are reversed. CO_2 is high in the tissues ($ppCO_2$ = 50 mm Hg) where it is produced as a by-product and is much lower in the air (> 1 mm Hg or 0.03%) where it is breathed out.

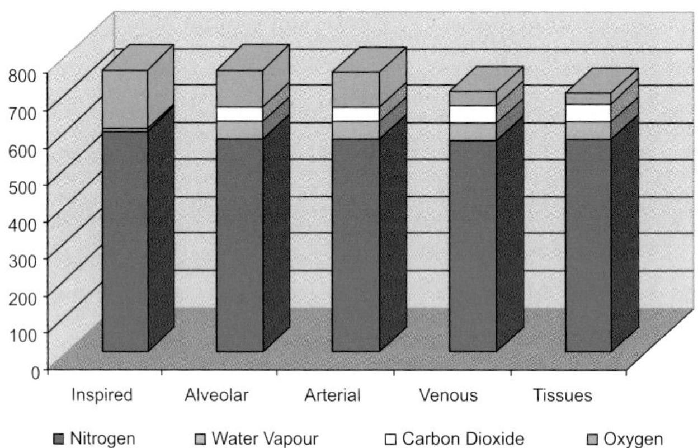

Gas Pressures

Henry's Law

The amount of gas that travels through the walls of the lungs is determined by Henry's law which states

"At a constant temperature the amount of given gas dissolved in a given type & volume of liquid is directly proportional to the partial pressure of that gas in equilibrium with that liquid."

" In other words if the partial pressure of the gas in contact with a liquid is increased then the amount of gas that will dissolve in the liquid is also increased.

This law was first proposed in 1800 by the chemist J. William Henry (1774-1836) as an empirical law well before the development of modern ideas of chemical equilibrium.

A simple rationale for Henry's law is that if the partial pressure of a gas is twice as high, then on average twice as many molecules will hit the liquid surface in a given time interval, and on the average twice as many will be captured and go into solution.

The number of molecules in a given volume depends on the partial pressure of the gas. Therefore the partial pressure controls the number of gas molecule collisions with the surface of the solution. If the partial pressure is doubled the number of collisions with the surface will double. The increased number of collisions produces more dissolved gas.

The illustration below shows that if the pressure is doubled then the concentration of dissolved gas will also double.

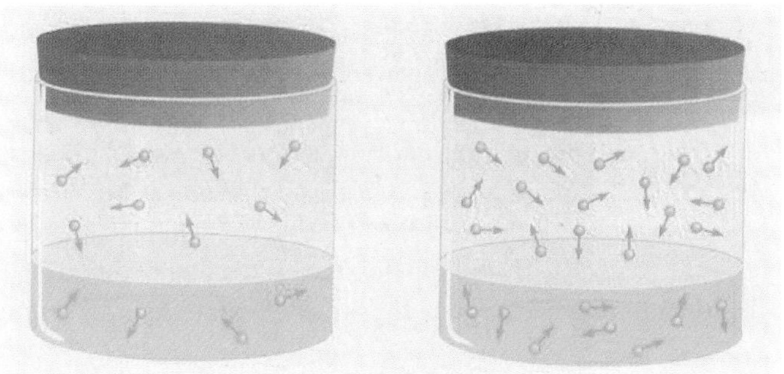

Henry's law

For a gas mixture, Henry's law helps to predict the amount of each gas which will go into solution, but different gases have different solubilities and this also affects the rate. The constant of proportionality in Henry's law must take this into account. For example, in the gas exchange processes in respiration, the solubility of carbon dioxide is about 22 times that of oxygen when they are in contact with the plasma of the human body.

The Henry's law constant "k" is different for every gas, temperature and solvent. The units on "k" depend on the units used for concentration and pressure.

Diffusion

Diffusion is the process whereby a gas or liquid will move from an area of higher concentration to an area of lower concentration. This can be seen if you drop an ink drop into a glass of water. The ink will diffuse out from its initial position and over time will spread itself evenly throughout the glass of water until all parts of the glass are equally diffused with ink.

Diffusion occurs by random movement of the molecules. If there is a concentration of a substance in one area then random movement will mean that it is more likely that molecules will move away from the area of concentration as it is more likely that any movement will result in a movement from a high concentration area (where they are plentiful) to a low concentration area than vice versa. Once the substance is equally distributed then random movements of the molecules will continue but on average the random movements will keep the substance equally distributed.

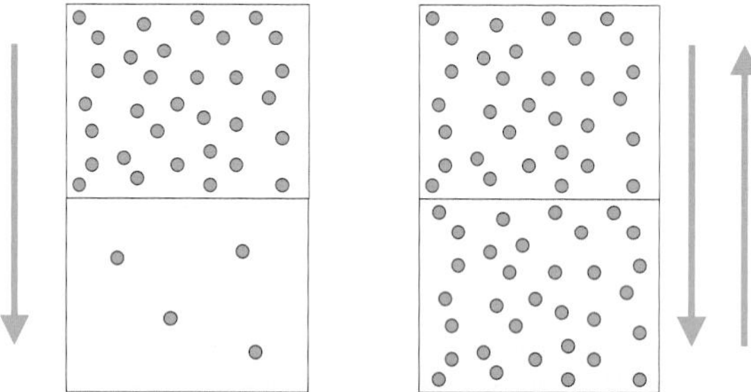

Diffusion from high concentration area to low concentration area

In the body gasses dissolve into the liquid lining the walls of the alveoli, as predicted by Henry's law. They then diffuse through the walls of the alveoli into the blood and then diffuse from the blood into the tissues.

On the surface the body is saturated with nitrogen and so there is very little diffusion of Nitrogen as the concentrations in the lungs, blood and tissues are all equal. It is only the metabolic gases Oxygen and Carbon Dioxide that have varying concentrations. As deoxygenated blood returns to the lungs, the partial pressure of oxygen in the alveoli is higher than in the blood and so oxygen diffuses from the alveoli into the blood. The oxygenated blood is then carried around the body and the oxygen diffuses into the tissues. Carbon Dioxide diffuses out of the tissues into the blood and is carried back to the lungs where it diffuses through the wall of the alveoli.

Diffusion occurs when there is an imbalance or gradient in the concentration between two areas. The rate at which a substance can diffuse is given by Fick's law which states that in terms of gas diffusion from the lungs into the capillaries the movement of gas transferred across the alveolar-capillary barrier is related to the solubility of the gas, the diffusion area, the length of the diffusion pathway from the alveoli to the blood, and the driving pressure. These factors are all included in the simplified version of Ficks law shown below. The solubility is often referred to as the Bunsen solubility quotient.

$$\textbf{Rate of Diffusion} = \textbf{Solubility} \times \frac{\textbf{surface area} \times \textbf{concentration gradient}}{\textbf{Distance}}$$

The human lungs have a very high surface area relative to the size of the lungs (600 million alveoli with an area of $100m^2$) and the walls of the alveoli are very thin, just 1 cell thick, so the distance to be diffused is very short. The steep concentration gradient across the respiratory surface is maintained in two ways: by blood flow on one side which is constantly removing blood which has had a chance to exchange gas with the lungs and replacing it with blood from the body's tissues and by air flow on the other side which replaces the air in the lungs with air from the atmosphere. This means oxygen can always diffuse down its concentration gradient from the air to the blood, while at the same time carbon dioxide can diffuse down its concentration gradient from the blood to the air.

When we dive then we increase the partial pressure of the gasses we breathe. This means that we are now breathing a higher partial pressure of Nitrogen than is in the blood or tissues. This differential in the partial pressure of nitrogen in the lungs and the partial pressure of nitrogen in the blood causes the nitrogen to diffuse from the lungs to the blood and then into the tissues.

Although diffusion is a result of a partial pressure gradient, gases are not pushed into the tissues by the force of the pressure. When we pump air into a cylinder, the pressure is used to push air into the cylinder. However, diffusion works in a different way. It is the movement of individual gas atoms or molecules due to random atomic or molecular movement that cause the gas transfer. This means that diffusion of an individual gas into or out of a tissue is dependent only on the partial pressure gradient of that particular gas, and not on other gases present in the tissue. In other words the diffusion of one gas is unaffected by the partial pressure gradient of a second gas.
This can be seen if we consider the interchange of Oxygen and Carbon Dioxide. Oxygen diffuses from the lungs into the blood whilst at the same time Carbon Dioxide is diffusing in the opposite direction from the blood to the lungs. The diffusion of Oxygen one way is not affected by the diffusion of Carbon Dioxide the other way. In the same way when we get diffusion of an inert gas such as Nitrogen the diffusion of this gas is unaffected by and does not affect the diffusion of any other gas.

Gas Transport

Oxygen is transported around the body, from the lungs to the tissues by the blood. Oxygen is carried in the blood by two distinct methods: Bio-chemically bound to haemoglobin, and physically dissolved in plasma, which is the liquid part of blood.

Once oxygen has crossed through the lining of the alveoli and into the capillaries surrounding the alveoli, it joins with haemoglobin to form oxyhaemoglobin. Haemoglobin is a complex protein molecule which lives within the red blood cells and its primary purpose is to carry oxygen in the blood so it binds chemically with oxygen to form a strong bond.

At sea level with a pressure of 1 ATA and an Oxygen partial pressure of 0.21 Bar haemoglobin is already 97% saturated with Oxygen. At this saturation level the blood has an oxygen content of about 19.8 ml of oxygen per dl blood. Oxygen dissolved in the plasma of the blood does not play a big part in Oxygen transport at this pressure, only 1.5% of the Oxygen being carried at sea level is dissolved in the plasma. This means that at atmospheric pressure haemoglobin is the main mechanism for the transfer of oxygen in the blood.

As the haemoglobin is already 97% saturated with Oxygen it only takes a slight increase in the partial pressure of Oxygen for the haemoglobin to become completely saturated. Once this happens it cannot bind with any more Oxygen. If we further increase the partial pressure additional Oxygen can only be carried dissolved in the plasma. As the partial pressure of Oxygen is increased past this saturation point the amount of Oxygen carried by the blood is determined by Henry's law. This means that the amount of Oxygen dissolved in the blood increases linearly as the partial pressure increases.

This is shown in Figure 15. The partial pressure of oxygen in the alveoli is shown along the bottom axis. As the partial pressure increases the amount of oxygen bound by the haemoglobin, represented by the pink line, increases rapidly. The oxygen dissolved in solution, represented by the yellow line, is negligible. The total oxygen content of the blood is the combination of the oxygen carried by the haemoglobin and the dissolved oxygen and is represented by the blue line. Due to the very low levels of dissolved oxygen the total oxygen content of the blood is effectively the same as the oxygen content of the haemoglobin.

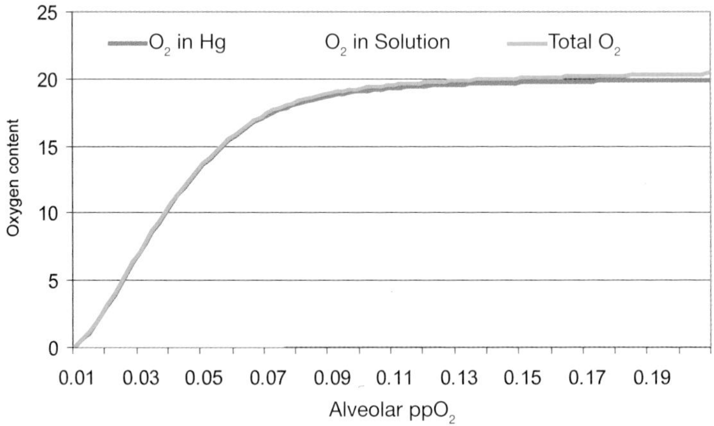

Figure 15: *Oxygen in the blood at increasing partial pressure*

As the haemoglobin reaches saturation, the amount of oxygen that can be carried reaches its limit. Any additional oxygen must now be carried in solution. This is the reason why the amount of oxygen in solution starts to increase towards the right hand side of the graph. We can also see that the total oxygen content starts to increase above the haemoglobin content.

Nitrogen as we know is chemically inert and so no reactions take place. All Nitrogen transport is due to the fact that it dissolves in the blood. The same is true of Helium or indeed any other inert gas that we breathe.

Perfusion

Blood rich in oxyhaemoglobin is carried from the lungs by the arteries. These spread out and carry the oxygen rich blood to the various areas of the body. As they spread out they branch out into smaller and smaller vessels until, when they reach the tissues to be supplied, they have become tiny vessels known as capillaries. The capillaries are only one red blood cell wide and supply blood to the areas that require oxygen. At the tissues the blood gives up its oxygen to the cells and removes carbon dioxide from the cells. Nitrogen is also carried in solution in the blood and if the gas tension of the nitrogen in the blood is higher than the tension of the nitrogen in the tissues then Nitrogen will diffuse from the blood into the tissues. On the other hand, if the Nitrogen tension in the tissues is higher than the Nitrogen tension in the blood, then the Nitrogen will diffuse from the tissues into the blood.

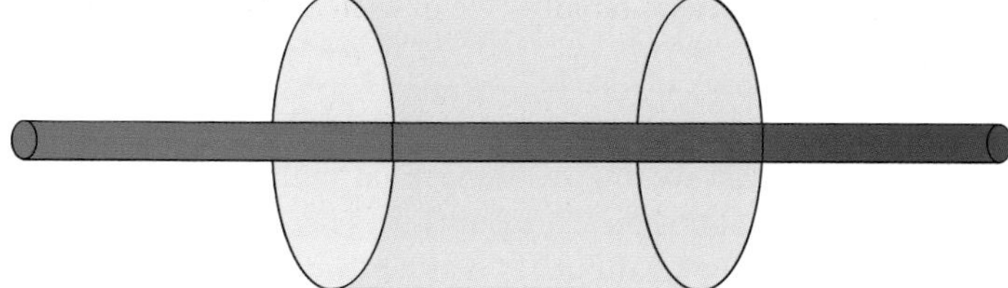

Diffusion from blood vessel into surrounding tissue

Different areas of the body are supplied or perfused by different amounts of blood. Some areas such as the muscles, brain and heart have very high levels of blood flow. Other areas such as fatty tissues and bones have a low blood flow.

Clearly tissues with good blood flow will receive a regular flow of fresh blood from the lungs. This allows for a rapid exchange of gases via diffusion. If the blood tension is higher than the tissue tension then when blood with a high nitrogen gas tension is brought to the tissues the nitrogen will diffuse into the tissues. The blood is quickly replaced by further nitrogen rich blood which can also diffuse into the tissues. As such nitrogen uptake is rapid when blood flow is high. In the opposite case, where the tissue tension is higher than the blood tension, the nitrogen in the tissues diffuses into the blood and the high blood flow removes the nitrogen and quickly carries it back to the lungs. The nitrogen rich blood is quickly replaced by blood following it which can also remove additional nitrogen from the blood and carry it back to the lungs.

Tissues which are poorly supplied with blood will be limited in the amount of gases that can be exchanged by the amount of blood that arrives at the tissue to supply additional gas or remove surplus gas.

By means of an analogy consider a distribution depot which receives deliveries by truck, unloads the truck and then loads it up with another load for the return journey. The depot may be able to load and unload a truck in a matter of minutes, but if a truck only arrives every six hours then it is the arrival of the trucks (perfusion) rather than the rate of loading/unloading (diffusion) that will govern the overall rate of loading. Another depot may receive trucks every 5 minutes and here it is the rate of loading/unloading (diffusion) which will be key to the overall rate as the depot is well supplied with trucks (perfusion).

Haldane's 1908 paper made the assumption that the rate of uptake and release of gas by the body was limited by the rate of blood flow to the various tissues. The implication being that the rate of diffusion from the capillaries to the rest of the tissue was of secondary importance. This is known as a perfusion limited model and for almost 60 years this assumption was held to be true. However, as we shall see in later chapters, subsequent models were based on the assumption that it was the rate of diffusion that was the limiting factor and these are predictably known as diffusion limited models. Hybrid models which take into account both diffusion and perfusion have also been proposed.

Saturation

When we breathe air here on the surface we are breathing air with 21% Oxygen and 78% Nitrogen. The other 1% is made up of Carbon Dioxide, Carbon Monoxide, Argon and other trace gases. The 78% Nitrogen and the 1% of other trace gases are inert and so are not used up by the body. For the purposes of the following discussion we will ignore the makeup of the 1% trace gases and consider air to include 79% Nitrogen. At a normal atmospheric pressure of 1 bar this means that we are breathing a gas with a 0.79 bar partial pressure of Nitrogen. After spending time at this pressure our tissues become saturated with Nitrogen at the same partial pressure. Although Nitrogen is constantly diffusing in and out of our tissues it stays in balance with the ambient partial pressure of 0.79 bar.

Pressure	ppN_2 Lungs	ppN_2 Blood	ppN_2 Tissues
1	0.79	0.79	0.79

When we dive we rapidly increase the ambient pressure surrounding us. The pressure differences in diving are much greater than ascending to altitude whether climbing a mountain, driving over a mountain pass or flying in an aeroplane. At the surface we are at 1 bar of pressure. If we were to travel all the way to space the pressure would drop from 1 bar to 0 bar, a difference of only 1 bar. When we dive the ambient pressure changes by this amount for every 10m we descend.

As the depth increases our regulator provides us with gas at ambient pressure. This means that we are now breathing gas at an increased pressure and the partial pressure of Nitrogen within that gas has also increased. At 10m the ambient pressure is 2 bar and so the partial pressure of Nitrogen is 1.58 bar. This is higher than the partial pressure in the tissues and so the tissues start to absorb or "on-gas" more Nitrogen. Nitrogen will quickly diffuse into the blood in the capillaries surrounding the lungs and the ppN_2 in the blood will increase to 1.58. This blood is then carried to the rest of the body where the other tissues also start to on-gas Nitrogen. Eventually the tissues will have on-gassed enough Nitrogen that the partial pressure in the tissues is also 1.58 bar and so the tissues will be in equilibrium with the gas being breathed. This is known as saturation.

Pressure	ppN_2 Lungs	ppN_2 Blood	ppN_2 Tissues
1	0.79	0.79	0.79
2	1.58	0.79	0.79
2	1.58	→ 1.58	0.79
2	1.58	1.58	→ 1.58

Saturation is only relevant for the particular depth that we are at. As we saw above we are saturated on the surface, but started to on-gas once we descended to 10m until we were saturated at 10m. Once this occurs we could descend to 20m where the ambient pressure is 3 bar and the partial pressure of nitrogen in our breathing gas would be 2.37 bar. Once again our body would start to on-gas until the tissues were eventually at a partial pressure of 2.37 bar and we were once again saturated.

Pressure	ppN_2 Lungs	ppN_2 Blood	ppN_2 Tissues
2	1.58	1.58	1.58
3	2.37	1.58	1.58
3	2.37	→ 2.37	1.58
3	2.37	2.37	→ 2.37

The difference between the pressures of inert gases is known as the inert gas gradient. If the gradient is such that the inert gas pressure in the lungs is higher than the pressure in the blood and tissues then we will be on-gassing. If the inert gas gradient is such that the pressure in the tissues is higher than that in the lungs then we will be off-gassing.

Tissue compartments

Due to the fact that various parts of the bodies are perfused to a greater or lesser degree they will receive varying amounts of dissolved gasses from the blood. In addition different tissues will absorb and release gasses at differing rates due to tissue composition.

This means that some areas of the body will increase their levels of dissolved inert gasses faster then others. The human body is an incredibly complex mechanism and calculating the amount of dissolved inert gas in each part of the body would be a very complex problem. Haldane proposed a solution to this problem; he suggested that similar areas of the body which absorb inert gas at the same rate should be considered together. Haldane grouped all parts of the body into one of five categories.

Haldane used the term "tissue" to describe each of the categories but this has often lead to confusion amongst divers as none of these categories maps directly onto a single tissue in the body. Even within a distinct body part such as a muscle there are a number of constituent tissues, muscle fibres, tendons, ligaments, etc. All of these may have different perfusion levels and may absorb and release inert gas at different rates. For this reason we should not think of what Haldane called tissues as having a one-to-one correspondence with any single tissue in the body. Instead the term compartment has become commonly accepted.

Different models have adopted varying numbers of compartments. As we have seen Haldane's original paper assumed five compartments with half times of 5, 10, 20, 40 and 75 minutes. US Navy tables published in 1937 and based on research by O. D. Yarbrough used only three compartments as the two fastest compartments were dropped (5 and 10 mins). Later revisions in the 1950's restored the fast 5 and 10 minute compartments as well as adding a slower 120 minute compartment for a total of six compartments. In further revisions Robert Workmann expanded the number of compartments to nine by adding slower still compartments at 160, 200 and 240 minutes.

Bühlmann also varied the number of compartments he used in different versions of his model. The 1983 and 1990 Editions of his book used 16 compartments while the 1994 Edition used 8 compartments.

Half times

The key factor for each of the tissue compartments is the half time for that compartment. Half times are a common concept in science. The most famous use of half times is in relation to nuclear materials where the half time is the time it takes a radioactive substance to decay to half of the original number of atoms. This is exactly the same concept applied to the uptake of Nitrogen by a tissue compartment. The half time of a compartment is the time it takes for the compartment to become half saturated, or if we are ascending to become half desaturated.

So if we consider a compartment with a half time of 5 minutes this means that compartment will become 50% saturated within 5 minutes. It will then take a further 5 minutes for the compartment to move from the current state to half way to saturation, i.e. 75%. The table below shows the progression of the tissue saturation at 5 minute intervals.

5 min	50%
10 min	75%
15 min	87.5%
20 min	93.75%
25 min	96.88%
30 min	98.44%

Tissue saturation after a series of half time periods

We can see from this that the largest movement takes place during the first half time, each subsequent half time period then sees a smaller and smaller change. If we draw a graph of gas uptake over time we can see a smooth line that initially shoots up but then gets ever shallower as it reached 100%.

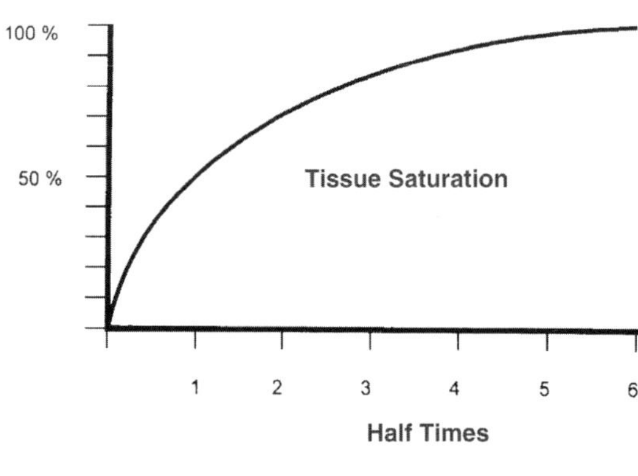

Half time graph

Mathematically the tissue will never reach 100% saturation as it only moved half of the way from where it is towards 100% at each stage so it takes smaller and smaller steps towards it's goal but always has the other half of the last step to cover. However, for practical purposes, after 6 periods we can consider the tissue saturated as it is at 98.44% saturation and after 24 hours we would consider the tissue to be completely saturated.

Each compartment will saturate at a different rate. As we have seen after five minutes the 5 min tissue is 50% saturated but the 10 min tissue will take ten minutes to become 50% saturated and so on. This means that each of the tissues will have a different level of saturation with the fast tissues absorbing gas and moving towards saturation faster than the slow tissues. However, as the diver ascends and the pressure is reduced the fast tissues will also release inert gas faster as the half time also refers to the time it takes to release 50% of the absorbed gasses. This means that fast tissues will also release gases faster then slow tissues.

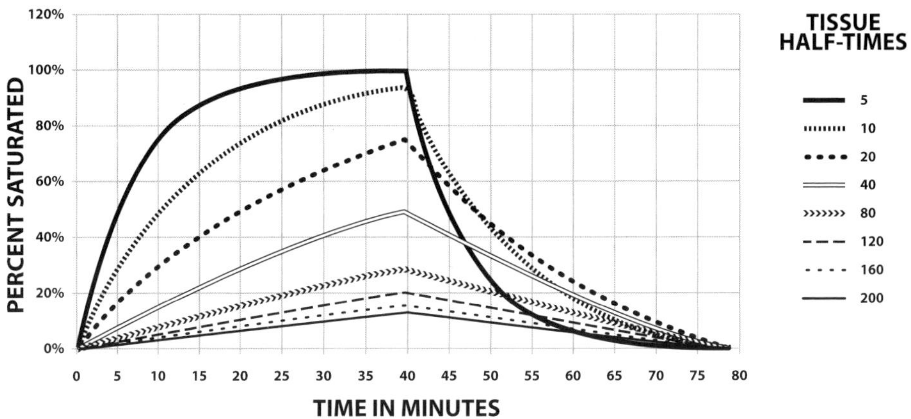

Figure 18: *Nitrogen Saturation and Desaturation curves*

From Figure 18 we can see the behaviour of a number of compartments when considered together. As we have seen above the 5 min compartment is 50% saturated after 5 minutes, at 10 minutes it is 75 % saturated and so on until 30 minutes or 6 half-time periods it is effectively saturated (98.44%). The 10 min compartment is 50% saturated after 10 minutes. After 40 minutes the compartment is not yet saturated as this has only been 4 half time periods. It would require 6 half-time periods (60 minutes) for this compartment to become effectively saturated. The 40 min compartment is at 50% saturation at 40 minutes but all of the slower compartments; 80, 120, 160 and 200 min, are less then 50% saturated.

At 40 minutes the pressure is released and the compartments start to desaturate. The 5 min compartment was the most saturated but as it desaturates equally fast the level of saturation quickly drops to below that of the 10 min compartment and soon drops below the other compartments until at time 60 minutes, 20 minutes after the pressure was released, the 5 min compartment is less saturated than all of the other compartments. The 10 min compartment also drops quickly so that at 48 mins it drops below that of the 20 min compartment.

Supersaturation

At the end of most dives it is likely that some of the tissues, at least the fastest tissues, will be saturated with inert gases. With longer dives more of the tissues will be saturated. This means that the tissue tension in these tissues is the same as the partial pressure of the inert gas in the mixture being breathed at depth. As the tissues are saturated they cannot physically hold more gas. As the diver ascends the ambient pressure is reduced and so is the pressure of the inspired gas. The internal tissue tension is now higher than the partial pressure of the inspired gas and may even be higher than ambient pressure. This is known as "Supersaturation".

A certain amount of supersaturation is allowed. In fact it is desirable, as the supersaturation or pressure gradient is required in order to allow the Nitrogen to escape from the tissues.

The middle and slower tissues may not be saturated at the end of the dive but as the diver ascends, and the ambient pressure is reduced, there will come a point where the ambient pressure drops below the tissue tension. This means that although the tissue was not saturated at depth it will become supersaturated during the ascent. Once each tissue becomes supersaturated it will begin off gassing.

Depth	Ambient Pressure	Inspired Nitrogen Pressure	Tissue 1 Nitrogen Tension	Tissue 2 Nitrogen Tension
30	4	3.16	3.16	2.50
20	3	2.37	3.10	2.42
10	2	1.58	2.50	2.30

Table 7: *Inspired pressure and tissue tension*

In Table 7 above you can see the Ambient pressure, inspired nitrogen pressure and the tissue nitrogen tension for tissues 1 and 2. At 30m the Inspired Nitrogen pressure is 3.16 bar. Tissue 1 is already saturated and so the tissue nitrogen tension is also 3.16 bar. Tissue 2 is not yet saturated and it's tissue nitrogen tension is only 2.5 bar, it is still on gassing and would continue to on gas until it too reached 3.16 bar. If we now ascend to 20m the ambient pressure drops to 3 bar and the inspired nitrogen pressure drops to 2.37 bar. We can now see that tissue 1 is supersaturated as its tissue nitrogen pressure is higher than the inspired nitrogen pressure and is also higher than the ambient pressure. As a result Tissue 1 starts to off gas. Tissue 2's nitrogen tension is now higher than the inspired nitrogen pressure and so it too starts to off gas although the nitrogen tissue tension is not yet higher than ambient pressure. If we then continue the ascent to 10m ambient pressure drops to 2 bar and the inspired nitrogen pressure is now 1.58 bar. Tissue 1 is still higher then the inspired and ambient pressure. Tissue 2 is now also higher then both the inspired nitrogen pressure and the ambient pressure and so it too is supersaturated even though it was not saturated at depth.

When a tissue compartment becomes supersaturated it will start to off-gas. The rate of off-gassing will be related to the amount of supersaturation. The half time concept described earlier says that a particular tissue will go 50% of the way from its current level to saturation in its half time period. So if it is supersaturated it will go 50% of the way from its current level of supersaturation to saturation in the half time period. It doesn't matter what the absolute difference is between the current level of supersaturation and saturation it will still go half way. So if the level of supersaturation is low then it only has to go 50% of a short distance but if the level of supersaturation is high then it will go 50% of a larger difference.

So for example, if we have a situation where the 5 minute tissue has a tissue tension of 4 bar and we reduce the inspired inert gas pressure to 3 bar then the tissue is supersaturated by 1 bar. Our half time period is 5 minutes and so in 5 minutes the tissue tension would have moved half way from the initial tissue tension to the inspired pressure, in other words the tissue tension would have dropped from 4 bar to 3.5 bar. This is shown in the top example in Figure 19. In another 5 minutes it will again drop from 3.5 bar to 3.25 bar.

However if we reduce the inspired inert gas pressure by a greater amount, say to 2 bar instead of 3 bar then we are making a bigger difference between the tissue tension and the inspired gas tension. The tissue will still only travel 50% of this distance but now it is 50% of a bigger difference. This is shown in the bottom example in Figure 19. In this case in the first 5 minutes it will drop from 4 bar to 3 bar and then in the second 5 minutes from 3 bar to 2.5 bar. It is clear that a larger difference between the tissue tension and inspired gas pressure will result in faster off-gassing.

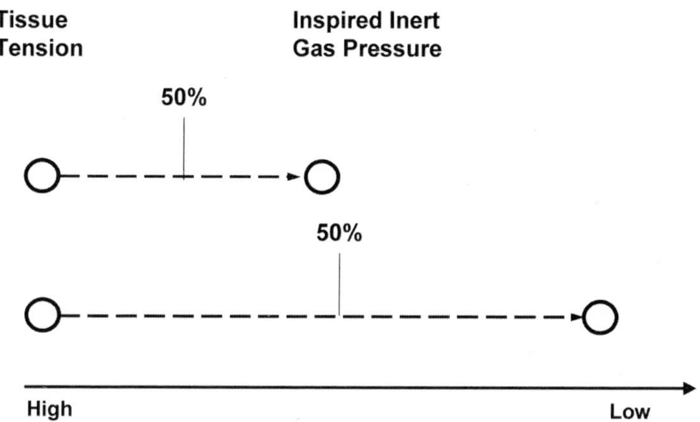

Figure 19 *Greater inspired gas gradient leads to faster off-gassing*

The difference between the tissue inert gas tension and the inspired inert gas pressure is often called the inert gas gradient and the examples above show that a larger inert gas gradient will lead to faster off-gassing. Unless we can change the gas we are breathing the only way to reduce the inspired inert gas pressure and so create a larger inert gas gradient is to reduce the ambient pressure which (by Dalton's Law) will also reduce the inspired inert gas pressure. Reducing the ambient pressure can only be achieved by reducing our depth in the water column. This means that moving as shallow as possible increases our inert gas gradient and increases the rate of off-gassing.

Critical supersaturation

As we have said a certain amount of supersaturation is desirable in order to allow off-gassing and the greater the amount of supersaturation (in other words the larger the inert gas gradient) the faster we will off-gas. However, there is a limit to the difference between the tissue tension and the ambient pressure that can be tolerated. This limit is known as critical supersaturation. Once the inert gas pressure in a tissue reaches critical supersaturation it will start to form bubbles.

This is analogous to releasing the pressure in a bottle of fizzy drink. As the top is slowly released and the pressure difference is kept small (supersaturation) the carbon dioxide in solution is released. However if the top is opened too much and the pressure difference is too great (critical supersaturation) then the drink becomes overly fizzy and bubbles out of the top.

Controlling ratio - M-Values

We know that we need some supersaturation in order to allow off-gassing, but too much supersaturation and we reach critical supersaturation where bubbles start to form, leading to decompression illness. So how do we know how much supersaturation is too much? How can we ensure that we are off-gassing efficiently but not allowing bubbles to form?

The critical consideration is the ratio between the inert gas tissue tension and the ambient pressure. There is a maximum value, or M-Value, that we can allow this ratio to reach. If we exceed this Maximum value then we have reached critical supersaturation. Other terms that have been used for M-Values and that you might see in some of the references are “limits for tolerated overpressure,” “critical tensions,” “supersaturation ratios” and “supersaturation limits.”

In Haldane’s original work he assumed a supersaturation ration of 2:1. This was based on the observation that a diver could ascend from 10m (2 bar) to the surface (1 bar) without experiencing any signs of decompression illness. Equally an ascent from 50m (6 bar) to 20m (3 bar) seemed to produce no ill effects and so he proposed a constant supersaturation ratio of 2:1.

The term "M-value" was coined by Robert D. Workman in the mid-1960's when he was carrying out decompression research for the U.S. Navy Experimental Diving Unit (NEDU). It had been observed that tables based on Haldane’s work and subsequent refinements were inadequate when it came to longer and deeper dives. Workman undertook a review of the basis of the model as well as subsequent research performed by the US Navy.

Workman recognised that Haldane's original ratio of 2:1 was really a ratio of 1.58:1 if you considered only the partial pressure of Nitrogen as the inert gas in air. Workman also found that the "tissue ratios" for tolerated overpressure varied between the different half-time compartments and by depth. The data showed that the faster half-time compartments could tolerate a greater overpressure ratio than the slower compartments, and that for all compartments the tolerated ratios become higher with increasing depth. Then, instead of using ratios, Workman described the maximum tolerated partial pressure of nitrogen and helium for each compartment at each depth as the "M-value".

Rather than list his M-Values as a table Workman expressed them as an equation that could be used do draw a line showing the M-Value for any depth for each of the tissue compartments. This approach has been adopted by subsequent decompression researchers as at it allows the concept of a linear relationship between depth pressure [or ambient pressure] and the tolerated inert gas pressure in each "tissue" compartment.

The concepts introduced in the previous section, saturation, supersaturation, critical supersaturation, M-Values, etc can be illustrated using a diagram as shown in Figure 20. The axis along the bottom shows the ambient pressure, which increases with depth. As we go further along the axis to the right the depth, and as a result the ambient pressure, increases. Further to the left the depth and hence the ambient pressure decreases. The vertical dotted line near the zero point shows the surface pressure at sea level. This is not at the zero point because the surface pressure at the surface is still 1 Bar. The axis on the left hand side shows the inert gas pressure in the tissue compartment under consideration.* As we go higher up this axis this represents a higher inert gas pressure in the tissue which can also be described as a higher tissue tension. Each tissue compartment will be at a separate point on the graph but in the discussions that follow we will only consider a single tissue compartment at a time.

Point A on the diagram represents a situation where the ambient pressure is higher then the tissue tension. This corresponds to a point near the start of the dive where the diver has descended to depth but the tissues have not had time to absorb much inert gas. This means that the tissues are under-saturated and will be on-gassing as represented by the arrow at point A which shows that the tissue tension will be increasing. If we stay at depth long enough then the tissues will become saturated and the tissue tension will be equal to inspired inert gas pressure at ambient pressure. Point B on the diagram represents the point where the tissue tension and inspired inert gas pressure at ambient pressure are equal, that is the tissue is saturated. The grey line, labelled Ambient Pressure Line, shows the point for any depth where the inspired inert gas equals the tissue tension. Once saturated, the tissues will not take on any more inert gas so if the diver stays at this depth the tissue tension will stay at point B indefinitely.

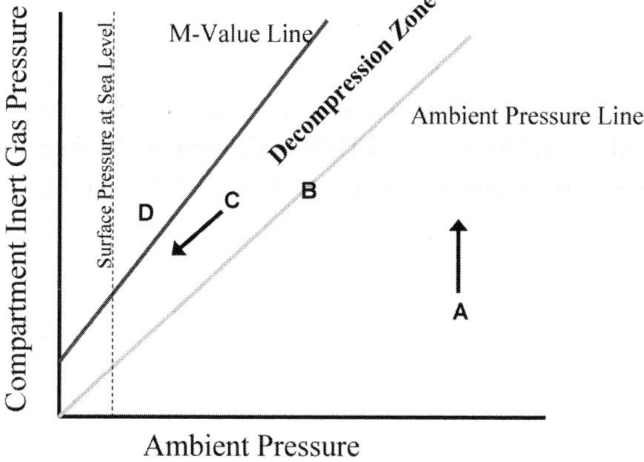

Figure 20 *The Decompression Zone*

* In other words the pressure of the nitrogen dissolved in that particular tissue.

As the diver ascends the ambient pressure surrounding him will drop quickly. This causes the tissues tension to be higher then the ambient pressure, i.e. the tissue is supersaturated. This is represented by point C on the diagram. We are now in what is known as the decompression zone as the reduction in ambient pressure and subsequent supersaturation allows the inert gas to come out of the tissues into the blood and return to the lungs. The arrow on point C indicates the direction the point will move. The reduction of ambient pressure causes the point to move to the left but off-gassing from the tissue means a decrease in tissue tension which also results in the point moving downwards. These two movements together mean that point C will move diagonally down and to the left.

The dark line on the graph is the M-Value line and for any depth represents the maximum tissue tension which can be tolerated without bubbles being formed. If the reduction in ambient pressure is rapid enough so that the tissue does not have enough time to off-gas sufficiently then the tissue can cross the M-Value line and can end up at point D. We can see that in order to prevent this we must reduce the ambient pressure at a gradual enough rate so that the tissue tension also drops enough to ensure we stay within the decompression zone and do not break the M-value line.

The number of compartments in the model, the half time of each compartment and the M-value of each compartment will together serve to determine the characteristics of the model. A higher M-Value allows a greater level of supersaturation which results in longer no-stop times and a more ‘aggressive’ set of tables. On the other hand lower M-values allow less supersaturation and a more conservative set of tables. Table developers have used test dives on animals as well as volunteer divers to determine a suitable set of M-values. Compartments, half times and M-values for a range of tables are reproduced in Chapter 9 for reference.

Professor Albert A. Bühlmann published a number of sets of M-values which have become well-known in diving circles. He published the ZH-L12 set in the 1983 edition of his book, the ZH-L16 set(s) in the 1990 Edition and finally the ZH-L8ADT set in the 1994 Edition. The "ZH" in these designations stands for "Zurich" (where the laboratory was located), the "L" stands for "limits," and the "12", "16" or “8” represents the number of pairs of coefficients (M-values) for the array of half-time compartments for helium and nitrogen. The ADT in the latest set stands for Adaptive.

The ZH-L12 set has twelve pairs of coefficients for sixteen half-time compartments and these M-values were determined empirically (i.e. with actual decompression trials). The ZH-L16A set has sixteen pairs of coefficients for sixteen half-time compartments and these M-values were mathematically-derived from the half-times based on the tolerated surplus volumes and solubilities of the inert gases. The ZHL16 set of M-values for nitrogen is further divided into subsets A, B and C. The reason for the various subsets is that the mathematically-derived set A was found to be overly aggressive in the middle compartments when used for real world dives. The modified set B is slightly more conservative and is suggested for use in table calculations. Set C is slightly more conservative again is suggested for use with personal dive computers which calculate decompression schedules in real-time.

Unlike the first two models, which used 16 compartments, the newer model ZH-L8ADT uses only 8 compartments. It also includes the effects of temperature and work or breathing rate during the dive as well as taking into account microbubble formation. Unfortunately the ZH-L8ADT model is described only very superficially in the latest edition of Bühlmann's book and doesn't include many details of the parameters of the model. The model was adopted by Uwatec and is the basis for their range of dive computers, as such it has been extensively dived by recreational divers around the world.

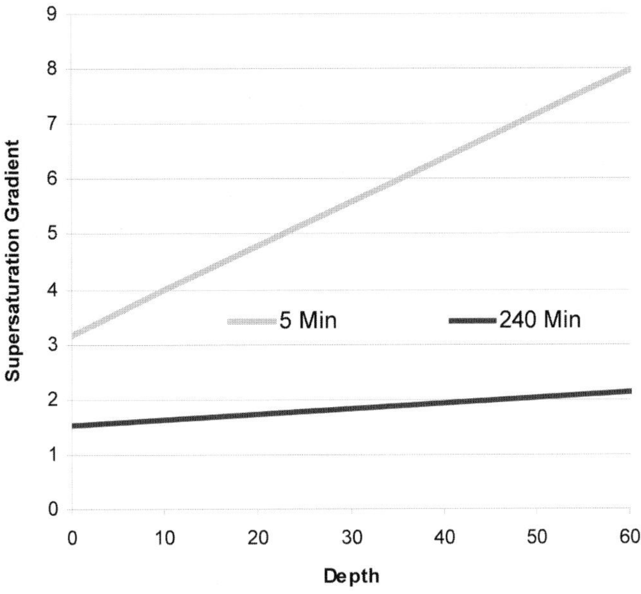

Figure 21 *M-values at varying depths for fast and slow compartments*

The graph in Figure 21 shows the range of supersaturation limits (M-Values) for two compartments from the ZHL16C set of M-Values. From this it is easy to see that the fastest compartment, represented by the grey line, has a greater change in the M-Value as the depth changes. The M-value at 60m is almost twice as high as at 10m. The graph also shows that the slower compartment, represented by the dark line has a lower M-Value at any depth than the faster compartment and furthermore that the amount of allowed supersaturation does not increase anywhere near as much at deeper depths when compared to the faster compartments.

Ascent rates

Each decompression model or set of decompression tables specifies a maximum ascent rate. The RNPL and BSAC-88 tables specify an ascent rate of 15m/min while the Bühlmann model specifies a 10m/min ascent rate, The PADI Recreational Dive Planner (RDP) gives an 18m/minute rate. The ascent rate is an important part of the model. If the actual rate of ascent is faster than the recommended rate then a dive, which would otherwise have been uneventful, can cause DCI.

There is clearly a considerable variation in the ascent rate for various tables and indeed there is a great debate as to what is the correct ascent rate. It is interesting to look at the development of ascent rates and the reasons why we are left with the ascent rates in use today.

In 1878, French physiologist Paul Bert suggested a rate of 1m/3ft per minute. In 1907 John Scott Haldane recommended ascent rates between 1.5m/5ft and 9m/30ft per minute. Between 1920 and 1957, rates of 7.5m/25ft per minute were commonly used. In 1958, during the production of the U.S. Navy Diving Manual, the rate of ascent to be specified in the manual was reviewed. US Navy Scuba divers wanted a faster rate of ascent and argued for an ascent rate of 30m/100ft per minute or even faster. The hardhat divers, on the other hand, considered this impractical for the heavily suited divers who were used to coming up a line at 3m/10ft per minute. As a compromise a rate of 18 m/60ft per minute was agreed. Conveniently this resulted in rate of 1 foot per second.

So from 1957 until 1993 the U.S. Navy tables have consistently advocated an ascent rate of 18m/60ft per minute, based on a historical comprimise. Many recreational diving tables, and even some early personal dive computers, adopted the same ascent rate. In recent years there has been a push to reduce ascent rates and typical rates have been slowed to 10m/30ft per minute combined with a recommended safety stop for three to five minutes at 3-6m (10-20 feet).

Slow ascents allow the faster tissues, some of which may be saturated, to offgas safely. The ascent rate is analogous to the speed at which the top on a bottle of fizzy drink is opened. A slow, gradual opening will allow the gas to escape without excessive bubbling whereas a rapid opening will cause many more bubbles. A bottle of fizzy drink is one of the most common visual aids for any lecture on decompression but it is also one of the oldest analogies to have been applied to the field of decompression. In fact the first reference to using a bottle of fizzy drink as an analogy for decompression was in 1860 when Professor Leroy do Mericourt, writing in the Ann d'Hygiene Publique et de Medicine Legale, 1860 2e SerieXXXI stated that

"the greater the depth, and the longer the stay at the bottom, the more will the blood be charged with an excess of gas in solution. The diver is really, from a physical point of view, like a bottle charged with carbonic acid".

As the diver ascends the ambient pressure drops, this has two effects. It creates a pressure differential between the dissolved gas within the tissues and the ambient pressure but also a tension differential or gradient between the dissolved gas in the tissue and in the blood and lungs. This second gradient means that tissue becomes supersaturated and so Nitrogen starts to diffuse out of that tissue. However, if the differential between the dissolved gas within the tissue and the ambient pressure is allowed to exceed the M-Value, it will result in bubble formation.

This means that the rate of change in ambient pressure, i.e. the ascent rate, must be kept under control so that the faster tissues are allowed to offgas a sufficient amount before the pressure differential between the tissue tension and ambient pressure exceeds the M-Value.

From this we can see that a rapid ascent may result in the situation where not enough inert gas has been allowed to offgas from the tissues and the M-Value limit is breached. This is shown in the diagram overleaf, where the almost horizontal angle of line A indicates a rapid ascent. As we can see, this rapid ascent has not allowed the tissue tension to drop, whereas the ambient pressure has dropped rapidly and the tissue compartment will quickly exceed the M-Value.

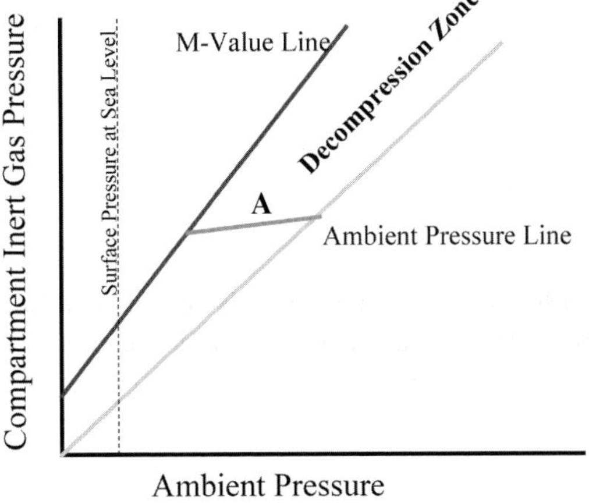

Figure 22 *Impact of a rapid ascent*

We can contrast this with the following example, where a slower ascent rate (represented by line B) has allowed the tissues to offgas sufficiently. The tissue tension has dropped as the ambient pressure is reduced and the ascent can continue all the way to the surface without breaching the M-Value.

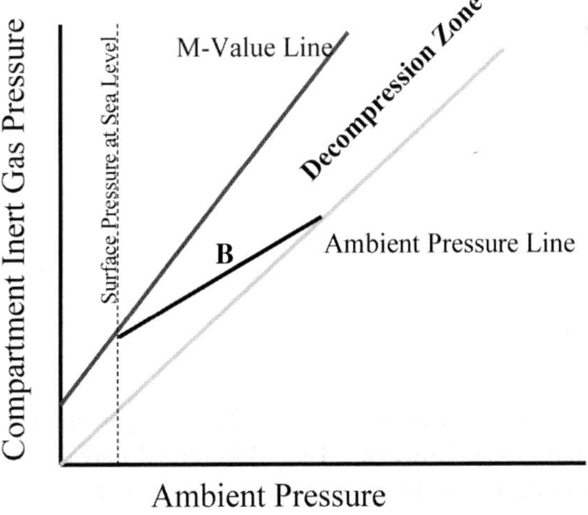

Figure 23 *Impact of a slower ascent rate*

The trend in recent years has been for ascent rates to be slowed considerably and significantly slower ascents are much more common than just a few years ago. In general this is a significant factor in decreasing the risk of decompression illness.

If a slower ascent is judged to be safer then is there such a thing as an ascent rate that is too slow? Recent research by Divers Alert Network (DAN) investigated the effects of varying ascent rate and deep safety stops on the number of silent bubbles formed during ascents.

They carried out a number of dives which were identical except for the ascent. Linear ascent rates of 18, 10 and 3 metres per minute were investigated. A linear ascent rate just means that the same ascent rate was used throughout the whole ascent. The research showed that 10m/min was the most effective ascent rate but it also showed that 3m/min was the last effective.

These results are interesting as many divers now ascend much slower then the recommended ascent rates. For recreational depths of 30m or less then this is not a major problem; as we have seen above a slower ascent rate gives the tissues more time to off-gas and reduces the likelihood of exceeding the M-Value of highly saturated tissues. However for deeper dives a very slow ascent from depth can introduce additional problems. A slow ascent taking 10 minutes to ascend from 10m to the surface is a good thing but a slow ascent taking 10 minutes to ascend from 50m to 40m is not such a good thing. The reason for this is that a slow ascent from depth will allow additional time for compartments which are not yet fully saturated to absorb more inert gas. At a normal ascent rate these tissues might not have absorbed enough gas to subsequently reach critical supersaturation. However with the slower ascent rate and greater on-take of inert gas they may now have absorbed enough gas to exceed their M-Value during a later part of the ascent. This can result in a no-stop dive becoming a decompression stop dive or for decompression stop dives can result in longer stops or additional stops at deeper depths.

This situation is shown in Figure 24 where line A shows the decompression profile for the dive when the correct ascent rate is followed. If the initial ascent from depth is excessively slow, resulting in effectively a greater bottom time, the subsequent decompression profile may involve a deeper initial stop followed by a longer overall decompression.

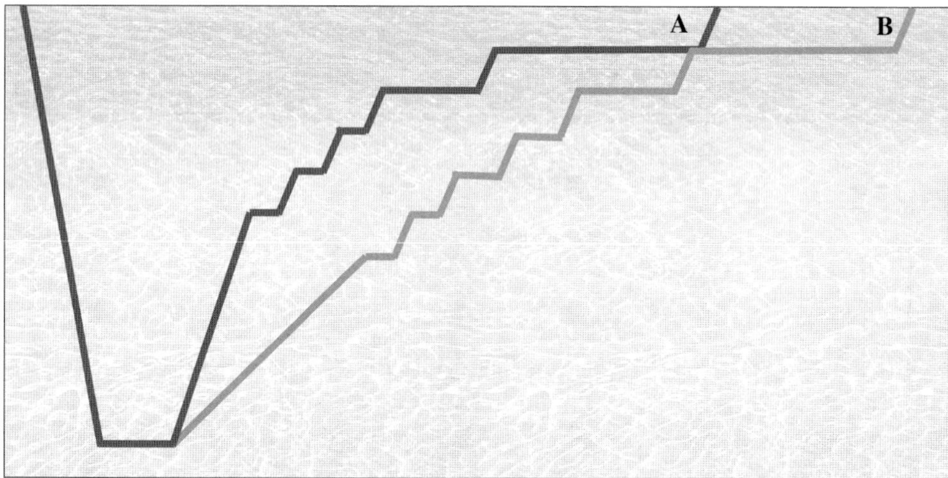

Figure 24 *Excessively slow ascent from depth can change the decompression profile*

As we saw earlier a rapid ascent is also to be avoided. This means that we should not ascend too fast or too slow but should aim to ascend at the correct rate. An ascent rate of 10m/minute for the initial part of the ascent followed by an ascent rate of 3m/minute for the shallower part of the ascent has become popular.

For divers planning dives using pre-printed decompression tables it is essential that you match the ascent rate specified in the table. A table will give you the ascent profile shown as line A in Figure 24 based on the specified ascent rate. A slower ascent rate, as shown by line B, will invalidate the decompression profile specified by the table. For divers using PC based decompression planning software it is usually possible to specify the ascent rate and even to vary the ascent rate at different depth ranges to allow a much slower ascent rate for the shallower portions of the ascent. However it is still essential that you follow the ascent rate specified when cutting the plan. For wrist mounted decompression computer users your decompression computer will take into account your ascent rate when calculating your decompression obligation and so in the example above your decompression computer will switch from profile A to the profile B as a result of your ascent rate.

No-Stop dives

A no-stop-dive, also known erroneously as a no-decompression dive, is a dive in which no-decompression stops are required. It is defined as a dive in which the diver can ascend directly to the surface at the recommended ascent rate without any of the tissue compartments exceeding their M-Values and hence without needing to do a decompression stop.

The term no-decompression dive is a misleading name. As we have seen every dive involves a degree of on-gassing and every ascent involved a degree of off-gassing and so decompression of some sort is required on every dive. The tissues may decompress enough on the ascent so that no additional stops are required but that does not mean they are not decompressing.

In addition, as we have seen above, a rapid ascent, even on a no-stop dive, can still result in exceeding the M-Value for one or more tissue compartments. This is shown in Figure 25. The graph on the right shows an ascent from depth where at the normal ascent rate we do not exceed the M-Value. In other words this is a no-stop dive. However the graph on the left shows what happens with a rapid ascent. The ascent rate does not give enough time for the tissues to offgass and so the M-Value is exceeded, despite it being a no-stop dive.

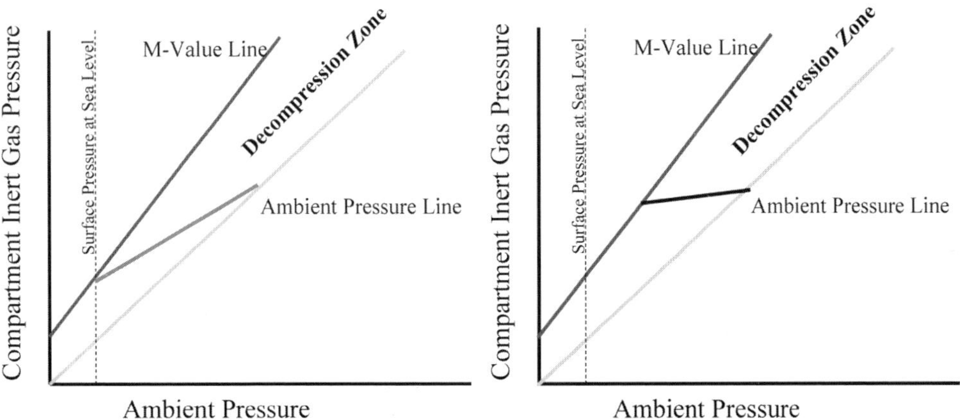

Figure 25 *Impact of a rapid ascent on a no-stop dive*

Bubble Formation

Despite over a hundred years of research into decompression theory even something as apparently basic as the exact mechanism of bubble formation is still not known. What we do know is that there are two principal ways in which bubbles can form: de novo formation (from nothing) and formation from pre-existing gas nuclei or gas seeds. We also know that despite everything we just learnt about M-values, bubble formation is not solely dependant on the reduction in pressure. If we compressed a glass of pure water to 200 bar, equivalent to a depth of approximately 2000 metres, and then left it there until it was completely saturated with Nitrogen then we could decompress it immediately back to 1 bar and no bubbles would be formed via the de novo mechanism. This is because the water has a very high tensile strength, which means that it is very difficult to force the water molecules apart in order for the dissolved gas to form bubbles.

If there are any impurities or disturbances in the water then these will act to will disturb the tensile strength and allow bubbles to form. Our bodies are not made of pure water and the cells and blood are constantly in movement. Blood flowing through the body creates a turbulent flow just like a stream tumbling over the rock stream bed. These impurities and turbulence within the body create numerous opportunities for bubbles to develop and are know as gas seeds or gas micronuclei.

Gas nuclei also form in other tissues throughout the body as the relative movement of the various tissues generates negative pressure which creates localised supersaturation. This supersaturation is mechanical in nature rather than gaseous and is known as tribonucleation. Tribonucleaton is responsible for introducing gas nuclei in almost every joint of the body, including the spine. These silent bubbles are always present and are seen in people who have never been diving.

The creation and destruction of gas nuclei appear to be balanced so that there is always a similar amount of nuclei present within the body. Various factors can increase or decrease the overall number of gas nuclei. Exercise, particularly pre-dive weightlifting, can encourage the creation of nuclei. Increased ambient pressure promotes the destruction of nuclei which reduces bubble formation and the subsequent risk of DCS.

Bubble formation is rare in tissues such as the liver, kidneys or brain as it is postulated that they do not have moving structures necessary for gas nuclei formation.

Silent Bubbles

The traditional Haldane model and subsequent refinements such as the Bühlmann model are based on the assumption that bubbles are only formed if the M-Value is exceeded. However in the late 1960's Merrill Spencer showed using Doppler ultrasound that in fact bubbles are commonly found in divers who have been diving well within the limits of normal tables. This contradicts the traditional Haldane approach but it shouldn't have been a great surprise. The body just doesn't work in absolutes and to suggest that on one side of an arbitrary line no bubbles are formed but as soon as that line is crossed bubbles will start to form should have set alarm bells ringing for anyone with a passing knowledge of physiology.

These bubbles are known as Silent bubbles or Asymptomatic bubbles as they do not cause any of the traditional signs and symptoms of decompression illness. They do not cause any major problems and the lungs act as an effective filter to trap and disperse them. The bubbles get trapped in the fine capillaries of the lungs where the Nitrogen diffuses back out through the lining of the lungs.

These 'silent bubbles' do not cause any of the traditional symptoms of DCS but can cause excessive tiredness. However an excess of silent bubbles can cause a reduction in the ability of the lungs to perform effective gas exchange. The lungs will trap the bubbles but an excess of silent bubbles will result in more bubbles being trapped in the capillaries of the lungs and reducing the surface area in contact with the lungs. This will reduce the opportunities for the blood to give up the dissolved Nitrogen. In addition an excess of silent bubbles can cause problems for repetitive dives.

This just shows us that decompression is not an absolute science and that an M-Value can be thought of as a solid black line through a large grey area. Divers have exceeded an M-Value and ended up with no bubbles and no signs or symptoms of decompression illness, whilst other divers have stayed within the M-Value and ended up with silent bubbles or even symptomatic bubbles.

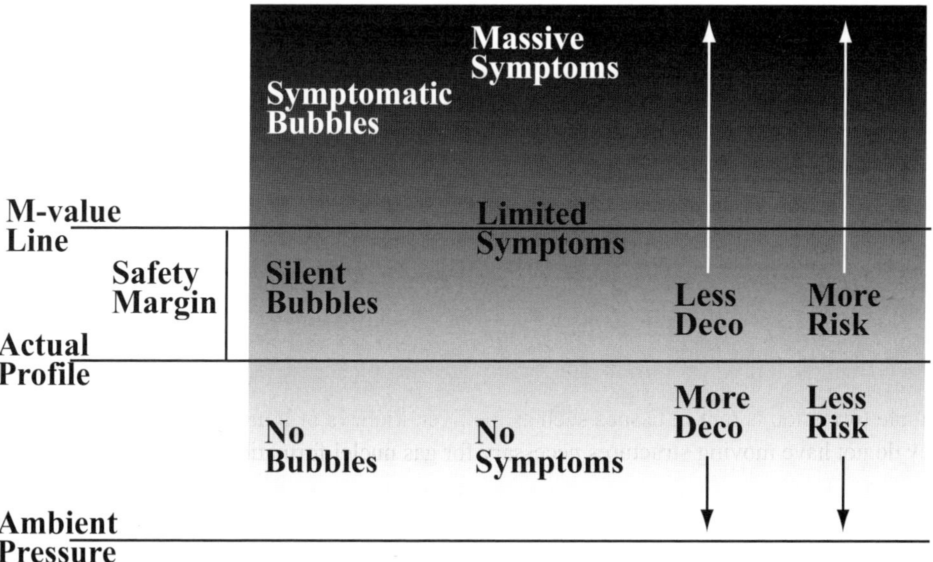

M-Values, a solid black line through a very grey area

The discovery of silent bubbles is actually a significant blow to the traditional theory of decompression. The traditional view is that if we stay within our supersaturation levels then bubbles will not be formed and we won't get decompression illness. In other words it is the formation of the bubbles that cause decompression illness. If we can routinely get bubbles forming and yet we have no signs or symptoms of decompression illness then what is it that causes decompression illness? This is a key question and we will be returning to it later but for now we will stick with the traditional view of decompression theory.

Safety stops

A safety stop is a non-mandatory stop that is performed on a no-stop dive as an additional safety factor. The idea of a safety stop is to allow the body a few extra minutes before ascending to the surface. A safety stop is usually carried out between 6m and 3m as it is in the shallower depths that the greatest pressure change occurs. Various agencies recommend safety stops of 1 minute at 3m, 1 minute at 6 or 3 min at 5m. Many modern dive computers also display an optional safety stop, often a 3 minute stop. This safety stop is optional and no penalty is incurred if it is ignored. However as we shall see there are good reasons why they should be followed.

As the dives in question are considered to be no-stop dive then traditionally the safety stop has been considered as good practice but not essential. However, recent research using Doppler bubble detection to measure the amount of bubbling experienced on no-stop dives shows the benefits of these 'optional' safety stops.

In a series of experiments researchers in the US conducted a set of dives to test the effectiveness of safety stops in reducing the formation of silent bubbles. A number of divers performed a dive to 30m for a bottom time of 25mins. This dive was a no-stop dive according to the tables in use. After the dive the first set of divers ascended to the surface at the correct ascent rate but did not perform a safety stop. The divers were then tested using a Doppler ultrasound detector on surfacing and at intervals of 15 minutes. The results from the first set of divers are shown in Figure 27 as the blue area. This shows a high level of bubbling on ascent, followed by an increase in silent bubbles after 15 minutes which drop off slowly so that there are still a significant number of bubbles in the system, even after 2 hours. Despite the number of bubbles detected no signs or symptoms of decompression illness were detected in any of these divers.

The second set of divers performed an ascent at the same rate but performed a 2 minute safety stop at 3m. The results of Doppler testing this second set of divers is shown in the graph as the purple area. This shows a significant reduction in the number of bubbles detected with just a 2 minute safety stop. Again no signs or symptoms of decompression illness were detected in this group.

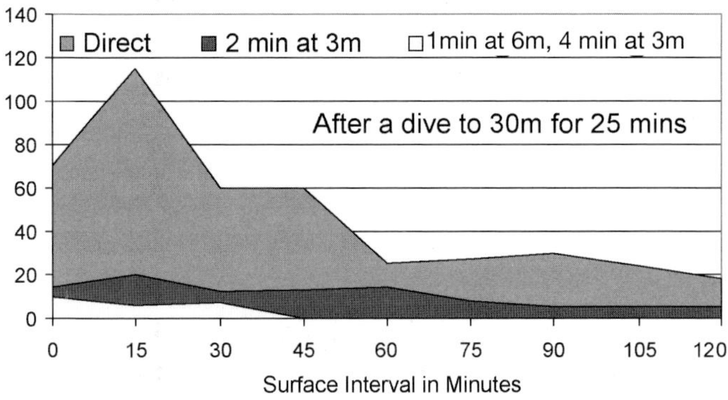

Impact of safety stops on no-stop dives. Source AAS

The third set of divers used the same ascent rate but carried out a 1 minute safety stop at 6m and a 4 minute safety stop at 3m. We can see from the white area on the graph that the number of silent bubbles is reduced even further. So much so that immediately after the ascent there are less bubbles then were present in the first group after a surface interval of 2 hours and after 45 minutes the number of bubbles for the third group had reduced to zero.

The implications of this experiment and the benefits of performing a safety stop are clear. For divers undertaking repetitive dives the implications are even more important. If the first set of diver were to carry out a repetitive dive after a surface interval of 90 minutes they would still have a large number of silent bubbles present in their system. The group that performed a safety stop at 6m and 3m would however have no silent bubbles left after a surface interval of only 45 minutes.

It is interesting to note that at various points after ascent the number of bubbles detected seems to go up rather then decreasing. For the first two groups the reading after 15 minutes was higher than the reading taken immediately after surfacing. For the third group there is a slight increase from 15 minutes to 30 minutes. This shows that bubble formation and growth is not immediate and can occur some time after the pressure reduction has been completed."

A similar experiment was carried out for a no stop dive to 36 metre for 12 minutes. In the first case an ascent was carried out using an ascent rate 18m/minute and with no Safety-Stops. In the second case a three minute safety stop was carried out at 4.5m.

Tissue Half-Time	% Change Tissue Tension	% Change Bubble Radius
5	-21	-68
10	-11	-39
20	-6	-24
40	-2	-18
80	1	-2
120	2	1

SOURCE: AAS

The tissue tension and the average bubble radius in each of the compartments was calculated for each of the ascents. The table overleaf shows the percentage change in gas tension and bubble tension between the direct ascent and the ascent with a three minute safety stop at 4.5m. From this we can see that the percentage change in the tissue tension and bubble radius is quite significant in the faster tissues. This is due to the fact that these tissues would have had a relatively higher saturation level and during the ascent would probably have become supersaturated. The mid range tissues show a smaller change as they would have had a comparatively lower level of saturation and would probably not have become supersaturated. Interestingly the slower tissues show a slightly higher tissue tension and bubble radius. This is due to the fact that these tissues had reached such a low level of saturation that there was no supersaturation and in fact it is likely that they would have continued to on-gas even during the safety stop.

Decompression stops

A dive is defined as a no-stop dive if the diver can ascend directly to the surface at the recommended ascent rate without any of the tissue compartments exceeding their M-Values.

If any one of the tissue compartments would exceed it's M-Value during the ascent then a direct ascent to the surface is impossible and a decompression stop is required. In this case the diver has an ascent ceiling which, if they ascend above this limit, they will exceed the M-Value. The stop allows the tissue to off-gas to the extent that the ascent can continue, either to the surface or to the next decompression stop.

The ascent ceiling is traditionally rounded down to the next multiple of 3m/10ft. For example if a diver has stayed well beyond his no-stop time then he may have an ascent ceiling of 8m/17ft. This means that if he ascends to a shallower depth than 8m/17ft he will exceed the M-Value for at least one tissue. The ascent ceiling is rounded up to the next multiple of 3m/10ft and so 9m/30ft is considered the divers first decompression stop. The diver must then remain at 9m/30ft until their ascent ceiling is above 6m/20ft, at which point he can then ascend to 6m/20ft. This continues until the diver reaches the surface.

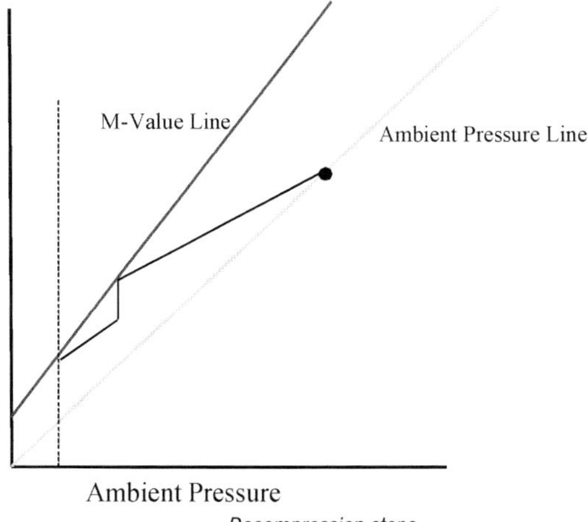

Figure 28: *Decompression stops*

This is shown in Figure 28 where as the diver ascends the ambient pressure drops. The compartment inert gas pressure is above the ambient pressure line, indicating that it is supersaturated and although the inert gas pressure drops as the tissue off-gasses it eventually reaches a level of supersaturation where it is about to cross the M-Value line into the area of critical supersaturation. The depth at which this occurs is known as the ascent ceiling. At this point a decompression stop is inserted into the decompression schedule.

On a decompression stop the diver maintains a constant depth which means that the reduction in ambient pressure is halted. The tissues continue to off-gas and this can be seen as the supersaturation level drops. Eventually it will drop to a point where the supersaturation is low enough to allow an ascent to the next decompression stop depth or the surface without exceeding the M-Value limit. Figure 28 is actually a simplification as it only shows a single tissue compartment. With multiple compartments there will be a supersaturation level and an M-Value line for each compartment. For a Bühlmann model with 16 compartments the decompression calculation will therefore need to check that the supersaturation level is not exceeded in any of the 16 compartments. As soon as any of the compartments is about to reach its M-Value level a decompression stop is inserted which will hold the diver at that depth until they can ascend to the next decompression stop without breaking the M-Value in either that or any of the other 15 compartments.

M-Values are not constant amongst all compartments. Faster tissues are allowed to be supersaturated to a higher degree than slower tissues. In addition the allowable supersaturation, even for a single compartment, will vary with depth. As depth increases, the allowable supersaturation increases, and correspondingly, at shallower depth the allowable supersaturation decreases.

This is shown in Figure 29 where the grey line represents the allowed supersaturation gradient at various depths for the 5 minute tissue compartment. At 60m a supersaturation gradient of 8 can be tolerated but at 10m a gradient of only 4 can be tolerated. For the 240 minute tissue compartment much lower supersaturation levels are allowed. At 60m a supersaturation level of just over 2 is allowed. At 10m this is reduced to approximately 1.6.

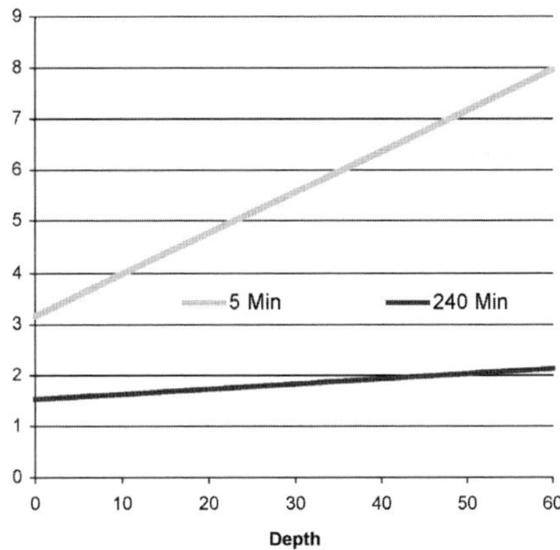

Figure 29: *M-values vary between different compartments and also vary with depth*

The difference in allowable supersaturation limits between different tissue compartment and the reduction in allowable levels at shallower depths give rise to the shape of a decompression profile. Fast tissues are allowed a higher level of supersaturation, and at depth each tissue is allowed a higher level of supersaturation. This means that high levels of supersaturation may be seen in the fast tissues during the ascent but due to the high level of supersaturation allowed the M-Value is not exceeded and no stop is required until we reach the shallower depths where the level of allowable supersaturation is reduced and where the slower tissues are likely to be the controlling tissues. The lower supersaturation limits coupled with the slower off-gassing of the slower tissues means that the shallow stops are likely to be long. This leads to the distinctive shape of a Neo-Haldanean model with a long initial ascent pulling the diver close to the surface followed by a short number of shallow but long decompression stops.

If we combine the concepts of multiple tissue compartments, critical supersaturation and M-values then we can see how this all fits together to produce a total decompression schedule. In Figure 30 we can see the situation that arises during an ascent and the effects on the various tissue compartments. For this example we will simplify things by only having three tissue compartments; a very fast tissue compartment (1), a medium tissue compartment (2) and a very slow tissue compartment (3). At the end of the bottom time we are in the situation represented by point A at the far right of the bottom axis. The fast tissue compartment 1 has on-gassed a significant amount of nitrogen and is saturated at ambient pressure. The medium tissue compartment 2 has on-gassed some nitrogen and so the tissue loading is higher than at the start of the dive but is not yet saturated. The slow tissue compartment 3 has on-gassed very little nitrogen and so its loading is only slightly above the starting point.

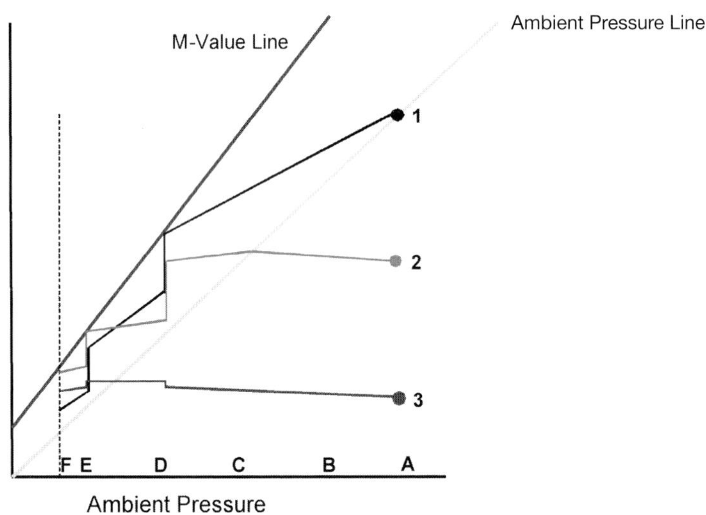

Figure 30: *Decompression with multiple tissue compartments*

As the ascent begins we reduce the depth and as a consequence the ambient pressure is also reduced. This is represented by point B on the bottom axis. The ambient pressure is now lower than the compartment inert gas pressure in tissue 1. This is represented by the line of tissue 1 which is now above the ambient pressure line. In other words tissue 1 is now supersaturated and so it starts to off-gas. As a result the compartment inert gas pressure starts to drop. Tissue compartment 2 on the other hand was not saturated and even when we reduce the ambient pressure to point B it is still above the compartment pressure and so this compartment continues to on-gas during the initial part of the ascent. This is shown by the fact that the line of tissue 2 is sloping upwards as we travel from point A to point B. It is only when we reach point C that the ambient pressure is reduced sufficiently that it is now lower than the tissue tension in tissue 2. If we now consider tissue compartment 3 we can see that the inert gas pressure was much below ambient pressure at point A and continues to be below ambient pressure a points B and C. As a result this tissue continues to on-gas but at a very slow rate as represented by the slight upward trend of the line from points A to C.

As the ascent continues and the ambient pressure drops we reach point D where, if we continued to ascend, the line of tissue 1 would cross the M-value line. For this reason a decompression stop is inserted. At point D tissue 2 is also supersaturated but tissue 3 is still undersaturated. During the decompression stop tissue 1 off-gasses, as does tissue 2, but as it is a fast tissue it will off-gas more than tissue 2. Tissue 3, on the other hand, is still undersaturated and so continues to on-gas as the other two tissues off-gas.

As the ascent continues we can see that, at point E, the situation changes. The reduction in ambient pressure means that tissue compartment 3 has finally become supersaturated. We can also see that as tissue 1 is a fast tissue and is off-gassing faster than tissue 2 it has overtaken tissue 2 and now has a lower level of supersaturation. As a result, at point E, it is the line of tissue 2 which is the controlling compartment and which forces the decompression stop. This stop lasts until we can ascend to the surface without tissue 2, which is still the controlling tissue, exceeding its M-Value.

Point F is where we reach the surface and here we can see that tissue 2 is still the controlling compartment as it has the highest level of supersaturation. Tissue compartment 1 has off-gassed so much that, despite being the only tissue to be saturated at the start of the ascent, it now has a lower level of supersaturated than the very slow tissue 3.

Despite the complexity of Figure 30 it is still a simplification as it only shows three tissue compartment and single M-value line is used for all of the compartments. As we have seen above real decompression models use eight, sixteen or in some cases even more tissue compartments. In addition we know that each tissue has its own M-value line.

Figure 31 shows the output from a PC based decompression planning programme. This program uses the Bühlmann ZHL16 model and so has sixteen separate compartments, each with its own M-value. This produces a more complicated diagram but the principle is exactly the same as shown in the example above.

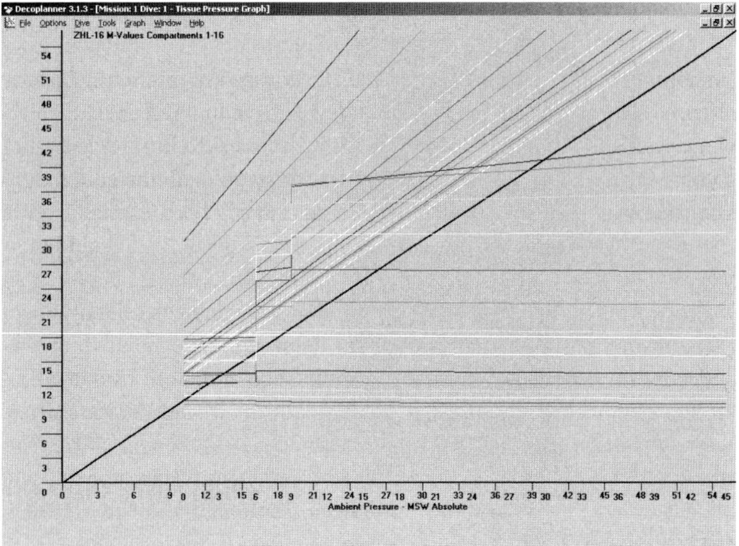

Figure 31: *Tissue loadings and M-values*

The process described above, where the diver halts at a specific depth until he is able to ascend to the next decompression stop depth, results in a 'stepped' profile. For divers following pre generated decompression tables this is an easy way to control their decompression. However a stepped decompression profile is not strictly necessary because as soon as the diver arrives at the decompression stop his ascent ceiling will gradually creep upwards as he further off-gasses until it reaches the next decompression stop depth. This makes intuitive sense, the body doesn't work on such an artificial, stepped basis. As a result, instead of halting for a set period at a given depth and then ascending up to the next depth it is possible to slowly ascend from the first decompression stop at a slow rate that always puts the diver below his ascent ceiling. If he makes his ascent slow enough then by the time he reaches his next stop depth the ascent ceiling will have already moved up to the subsequent stop depth and he can carry on the slow ascent. This process is known as 'following the ascent ceiling' or 'flying the curve'. As shown in Figure 32 this produces a much smother decompression profile.

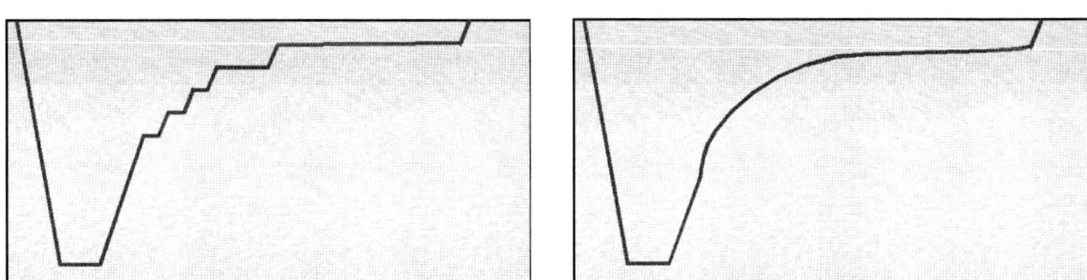

Figure 32: *Stepped decompression stops versus a smooth gradual ascent*

This can also be represented as in Figure 33 where we gradually decrease the ambient pressure in order to stay within our supersaturation limit. This figure gives a feel for what is happening but again it is a simplification as the controlling compartment will vary throughout the ascent.

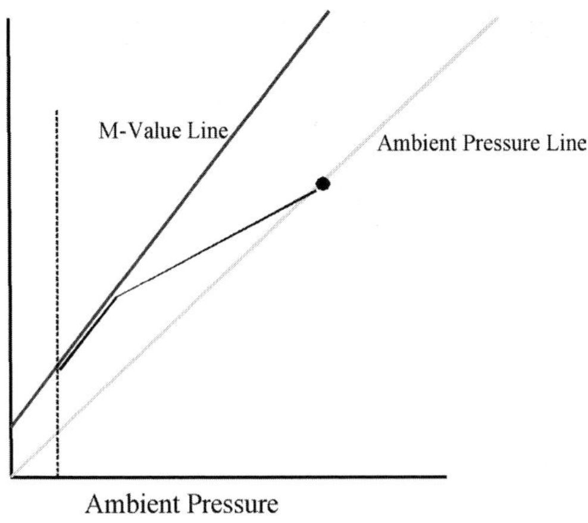

Figure 33: *Flying the curve*

Oxygen Window

One of the confusing aspects of decompression theory is that some terms are used in different ways by different people. The oxygen window is just such a term. There are several uses of this term; each use is closely related to the others but is subtly different. This can cause problems in any discussion of the oxygen window as people end up talking at cross purposes. In this section we will look at the basic and most widely used use of the term. This usage of the term is applicable to normal physiology at the surface as well as decompression and mixed gas diving whereas the other usages only become relevant when using multiple gases and so will be considered later in the mixed gas decompression sections.

At its most simple level the oxygen window is created when oxygen in the arterial blood is consumed by tissues and only partially replaced by carbon dioxide in the venous blood. This results in a pressure drop of approximately 8-13% in the venous system as opposed to the arterial system. This pressure drop provides a cushion or window which reduces the overall gas pressure in the venous system and reduces the chances of bubble formation.
The idea that blood and tissues may be under saturated when compared to the surrounding air and alveolar air was first discovered in 1910 when August Krogh showed that the gas pressure of arterial blood was less than the gas pressure of air in the alveoli. The idea has also been referred to as inherent unsaturation or partial pressure vacancy. It was Albert Behnke in 1951 who first coined the term 'The Oxygen Window' and it is this term which has become the most commonly used. Other terms that have been used are 'partial pressure vacancy' and 'inherent unsaturation'.

To see how the Oxygen window works we have to revisit the mechanisms of gas transport. When we breathe in and gas diffuses through the alveoli and into the blood, the component gasses of our breathing mixture are transported by the blood in two different ways. The metabolically inactive (inert) gases such as Helium and Nitrogen are transported in solution in the blood and Henry's Law tells us that the amount of gas present in blood is directly related to the gas partial pressure. However the story is quite different for Oxygen and Carbon Dioxide which are metabolic gases and the body has developed highly specialized transport systems to move these gases to and from the cells. Haemoglobin is a specialised protein present in red blood cells (RBCs) that chemically binds to Oxygen. At normal atmospheric pressure most Oxygen is transported around the body bound to haemoglobin in the blood; approximately 97% is carried in this way with only 3% of Oxygen is carried in solution in the plasma of the blood. Once chemically bound to haemoglobin the Oxygen no longer exerts any partial pressure and so the partial pressure in the blood is effectively provided by the 3% that is in solution.

As arterial blood travels through the capillaries and perfuses the tissues it reaches areas of low Oxygen concentration and high Carbon Dioxide (CO_2) concentration. The low partial pressure of Oxygen in the tissues causes the Oxygen dissolved in the blood to diffuse into the surrounding tissues. This then causes the Oxygen bound to the haemoglobin to be released into the blood where it too can diffuse from the blood into the tissues. At the same time Carbon Dioxide diffuses in the opposite direction, from the tissues into the blood. If the pressure of O_2 absorbed from the blood were replaced by an equal pressure of CO_2 from the tissues, then there would be no change in total partial pressure from the arterial to the venous blood. However, as blood flows through the tissue, the increase in the pressure of CO_2 is much less than the decrease in the pressure of O_2. This is due to two reasons: First not all of the Oxygen consumed is converted to Carbon Dioxide. Under normal conditions, only 80% of O_2 is converted to CO_2. The second reason is that Carbon Dioxide is 20 times more soluble in blood than Oxygen. Gases that are more soluble produce a lower partial pressure when a given volume of gas is absorbed into a liquid. In other words, if the same volume of O_2 and CO_2 were to be absorbed into the blood the CO_2 would have a lower partial pressure than the same volume of O_2.

The result of this is that the tissues and venous blood have a lower overall pressure then the arterial blood or the alveolar air. On the surface the pressure of the Air we breathe and of the air in our lungs is 760 mm Hg. Arterial blood has a slightly lower pressure of 752 mm Hg but the tissues and venous blood has a pressure of 706 mm Hg. A drop of 46 mm Hg from the arterial to the venous system. It is this drop in pressure that causes the Oxygen window.

This is shown in Figure 34 where we can see that the overall pressure in the tissues and the venous system is less than in the arterial system and also less than the ambient pressure represented by the inspired gas.

So what advantage does the Oxygen window give us? Well one thing it doesn't do is that it doesn't help us to off-gas any quicker. The rate of off-gassing is dependant only on the individual inert gas gradient, in other words gases off-gas at the same rate no mater what the other gases are doing. So the fact that the Oxygen partial pressure is lower on the venous side has absolutely no impact on the rate that Nitrogen (or any other inert gas) off-gasses. Where the Oxygen window does give us an advantage is in controlling bubble formation. Remember that we said bubbles formed when the supersaturation level – the ratio between tissue gas pressure and ambient pressure exceeded the M-Value. Bubble formation is different to off-gassing in that we must consider all of the gas pressures together when calculating the supersaturation ratio. If the sum of all of the gas pressures exceeds the M-Value then bubbles will start to form.

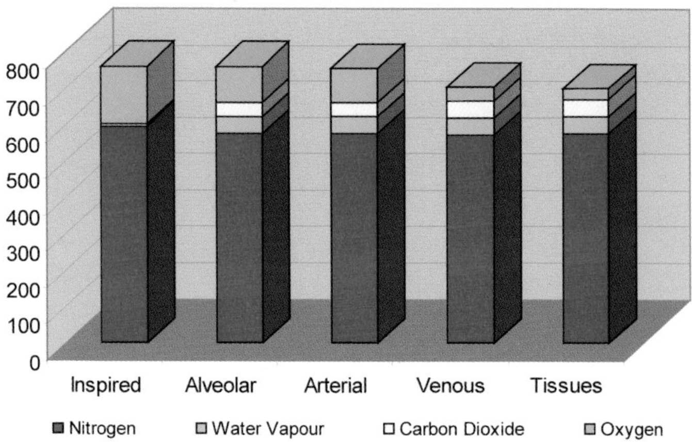

Figure 34: *Oxygen window*

So each gas acts independently of the other gases for the purposes of off-gassing but they act together when it comes to forming bubbles. This means that the reduction in overall pressure from the uptake of Oxygen reduces the total gas pressure which in turn reduces the supersaturation ratio and means that bubble formation is less likely. The oxygen window can be illustrated using the simple analogy of a pan of potatoes being boiled on a cooker. As the water heats up and starts bubbling there is a risk of the water bubbling over. The potato itself is not boiling and does not contribute to the boiling over. However, if one of the potatoes is removed then there is less overall volume in the pan and the water will not boil over as quickly.

We will return to the Oxygen Window in Chapter 5 where two other definitions of this term will be discussed.

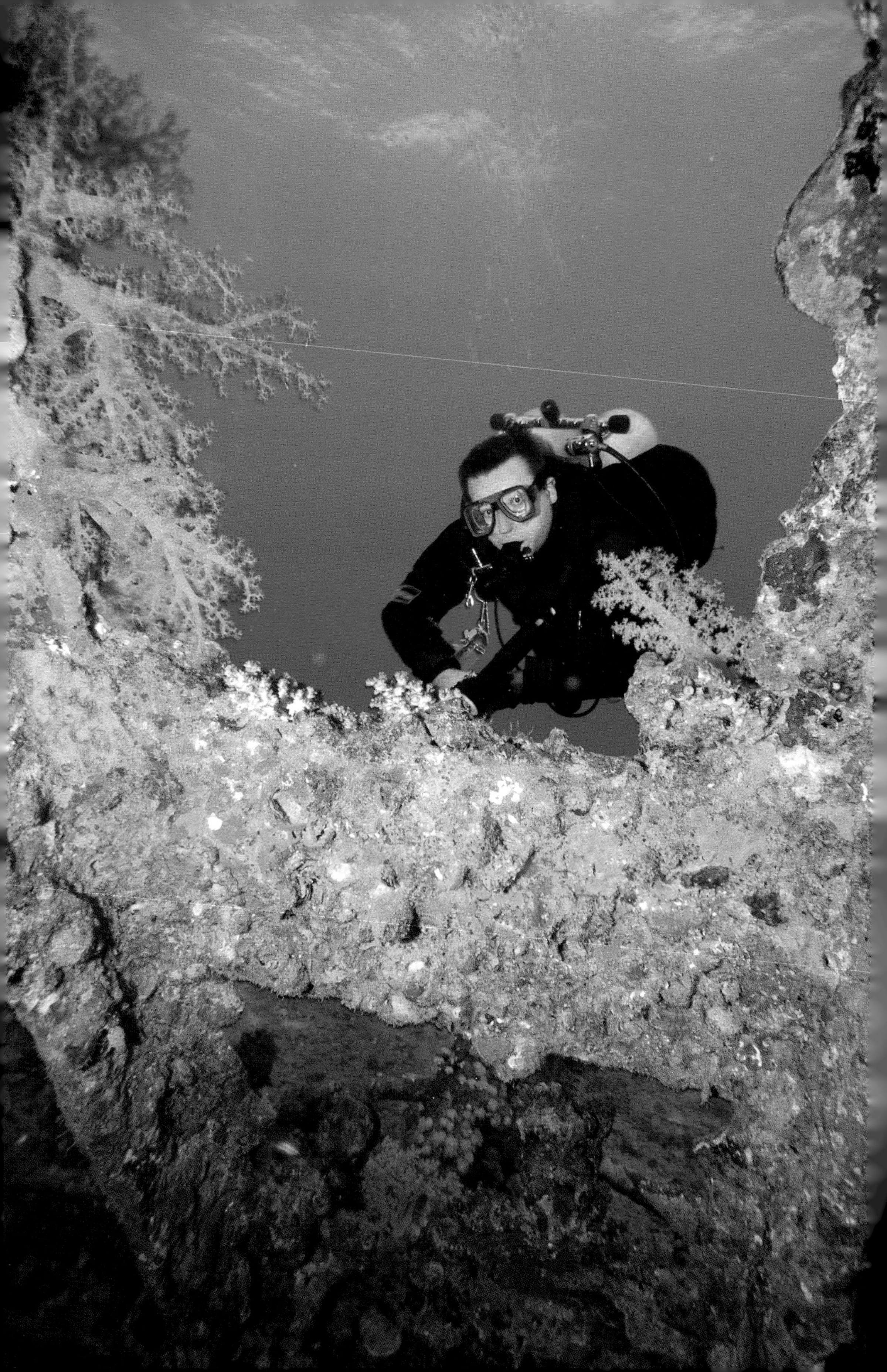

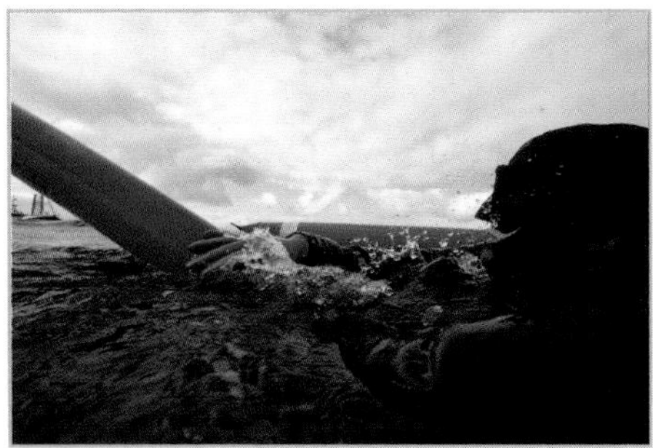

3 Decompression Illness

There are many aspects of decompression that are not fully understood. Unfortunately the symptoms of decompression illness are all too well understood as research into decompression has often been on a trial and error basis. This, combined with the fact that there is always a risk of decompression illness on even the most conservative dive, has lead to a constant stream of caisson workers, hard hat divers and scuba divers who have suffered the effects of decompression illness. In this chapter we will look at some of the different types of decompression illness, some of the predisposing factors that can increase the risk of DCI as well as some of the techniques that have been developed to treat the condition.

Burst Lung

As the diver ascends pressure drops and any gas volume in the body will expand, as predicted by Boyle's law. Expanding gas can result in excess pressure in the lungs which can cause damage to the lungs and is known as Pulmonary Barotrama. This term and it's associated meaning can be broken down into Pulmonary (of the lungs) Baro (pressure related) Trauma (damage). This is most likely to occur during a rapid ascent or an ascent where the diver holds their breath. Our bodies had no evolutionary need to develop any mechanism to detect a dangerous level of over-pressurisation within the lungs and so there are no nerves or any other sensory input which tells us when our lungs are overly full. As a result it is relatively easy to inflict a burst lung on ourselves if we hold our breath during an ascent.

Anything which interferes with the normal air passage through the lungs may lead to lung overpressurisation in certain areas of the lungs. Smoking, lung infection, congestion, constriction from respiratory illness, previous lung injuries may all lead to the situation where gas becomes trapped in a pocket in the lungs and as the diver ascends this pocket expands causing lung damage.

Left: A diver carries out a no-stop dive on the Carnatic

Burst lung is sometimes also referred to in medical references as Pulmonary Over Pressure Syndrome (POPS) or Pulmonary Over Inflation Syndrome (POIS). There are a number of different categories of burst lung, each of which is described below.

Arterial Gas Embolism (AGE)

Arterial Gas Embolism is caused by excess gas pressure in the lungs which means that the lungs expand to their maximum amount and can expand no further. Any further over-pressurisation causes the alveolar membrane to stretch and rupture which forces gas bubbles or emboli directly into the blood stream. Once in the blood stream they may be carried by the arteries throughout the circulatory system directly to the tissues. The gas bubbles will continue to grow as the pressure drops and several smaller bubbles may unite to form a larger bubble. When the bubbles encounter a blood vessel which is too small to let them pass they will block the blood vessel and form an embolus or blockage where they can cause direct damage to the surrounding tissue as well as prevent the flow of blood to tissues down stream of the obstruction. AGE can be caused by relatively small over-pressurisation of the lungs and the damage to the lungs can otherwise be undetectable.

AGE can, in some cases, cause cardiac arrest. Various theories have been suggested as to the cause of cardiac arrest. The earliest theories were that bubbles causes a vapour lock in much the same way that air bubbles can cause a blockage in your central heating system. However experiments that introduced vapour locks into the ventricular chamber of a dog showed that this does not produce cardiac arrest. This means that we still don't know how AGE can cause cardiac arrest in humans or dogs for that matter.

AGE is potentially more dangerous than DCS as the arterial circulation is designed to quickly and efficiently carry oxygen and nutrients to key body tissues but unfortunately, in the case of an arterial gas embolism, it also carries the gas embolism directly to the key body tissues and in particular the brain. This is known as a Cerebral Arterial Gas Embolism (CAGE). CAGE can result in severe neurological symptoms as parts of the brain are damaged by the embolism and starved of oxygen by the blockage in the capillaries bringing oxygen to the brain.

The onset of AGE is very much shorter than DCS. Unlike DCS it can even present itself while the diver is still surfacing.

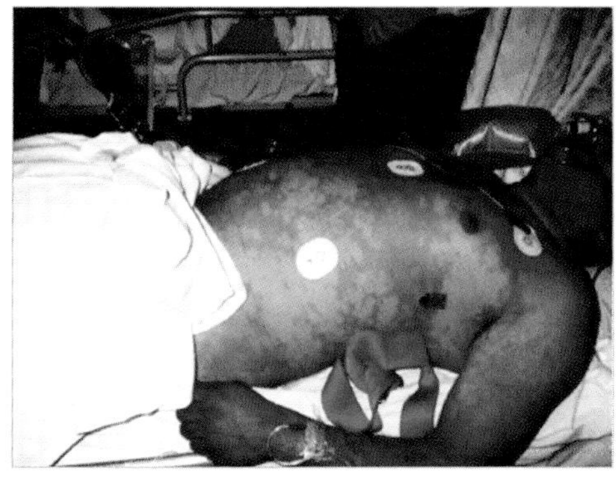

Figure 35: *Skin Marbling*

Interstitial Emphysema

As the level of over-pressurisation in the lungs increases this can result in tears in the alveoli which will allow gas to escape into the lung cavity. Bubbles of air will become trapped within the tissues of the lung. There the build up of gas can apply pressure on airways, blood vessels, the heart and the lung sacs.

Divers suffering from Interstitial Emphysema are likely to show a shortness of breath, they may have difficulty swallowing and there may be a swollen appearance at the base of the neck. Interstitial Emphysema will almost certainly be accompanied by Arterial Gas Embolism and so severe neurological symptoms may also be present.

Pneumothorax

Pneumo is Greek for Air and the Thorax is your chest cavity. The space between the lining of the lungs and the chest wall is called the pleural space and is normally airtight. Pneumothorax is caused when excess gas pressure in the lungs causes the lining of the lung to rupture as well as the alveoli. This allows gas to escape from the lungs into the pleural space. The gas build-up and subsequent increase in volume from expansion of the gas results in pressure on the lungs and can cause a collapsed lung, this drastically reduces the surface area of the lung available for gas exchange and severely impairs the divers ability to breathe properly. The pressure can also affect the heart and major blood vessels and so affect the circulation and even cause the heart to stop.

Divers suffering from Pneumothorax are likely to show a shortness of breath, they may be coughing blood and may report pain on breathing. The chest area may also appear swollen or distorted and the reduced lung function may result in signs of cyanosis. Pneumothorax will almost certainly be accompanied by Arterial Gas Embolism and again severe neurological symptoms may also be present.

Decompression Sickness

Decompression Sickness (DCS) is caused when inert gas (usually Nitrogen or Helium) dissolved in the tissues comes out of solution and forms bubbles. The immediate signs and symptoms of DCS are caused by the physical pressure of the bubbles pressing on tissues and nerves. Longer term damage is caused by the bubbles restricting the flow of blood to tissues downstream of the bubble and causing tissue damage through oxygen starvation.

Decompression Classification

Historically Decompression Sickness (DCS) was classified into a number of categories or types.

Type I

Type I decompression sickness was historically described as a minor or pain only bend. Typical symptoms are localized pain in the joints and irritation or itching of the skin.

Pain – An aching pain in the joints is the classic and most common occurrence of decompression sickness, it is observed in 75% of all decompression sickness casualties. Usually it is the larger joints, shoulders or elbows that are affected. The pain is usually described as a deep, aching pain and is usually steady, though it will sometimes throb. The location of the pain may be difficult to specify. Despite the frequent occurrence of this type of DCS very little is known about the location or cause of the pain. The formation of bubbles within the joints themselves is almost certainly not the cause of the pain and current theories suggest that bubble formation in ligaments and tendon sheaths are the cause, although this is unproven.

Pain may occur by itself or with other forms of DCS. The pain of type I decompression sickness can be distinguished from the pain of sprains or other injuries by its prompt reduction on recompression. In fact limb bends are so responsive to recompression treatment that casualties occasionally report that the pain is relieved even before the chamber has reached the final treatment depth.

Itching (Pruritis) — In this mild form, no signs are visible, and the itching is temporary, mild, comes and goes and is more marked around the ears, wrists and hands. If itching is the only symptom, then it will usually resolve itself on its own or with 100% oxygen and the diver not need to be recompressed. However, there have been reports from the UK Sports Diving Medical Committee (UKSDMC) of a possible association between skin bends and patent foramen ovale (PFO) and there are now recommendations that divers with regular occurrences of this condition be checked for PFO.

Cutis marmorata (skin marbling) — See Figure 35, page 62. Although still a skin bend this should not be considered a minor bend as it is usually a sign of impending worsening of DCS. This condition may be preceded by a burning sensation and itching over the shoulders and torso. Patchy, reddish-purple mottled areas can occur, especially around the shoulders and trunk. These are extremely itchy and are due to a local vascular reaction from bubbles in the tissues below the skin.

This has a more serious connotation and is thought of as an initial sympton of decompression sickness and is often associated with other more serious types of DCS, such as chokes. Any diver showing these symptoms should be treated with recompression.

Localized pitting edema – Blockage of the dermal and subcuticular lymphatics with bubbles usually results in edema and a peculiar pitting of the skin called peau d'orange (French, meaning skin of the orange, or, orange-peeling). This is pigskin appearance more often seen over the trunk of the body and again is evidence of a more serious form of DCS.

Type I DCS often resolves by itself; however, most physicians recommend observation for at least 24 hours to ensure symptoms do not progress. For this reason, all cases of suspected DCS must be evaluated. It must be stressed to these patients that they should seek immediate care. Even though the condition may be self-correcting, proper diagnosis and treatment are essential to prevent permanent damage or reoccurrence.

Type II

Cardiovascular/Pulmonary – Bubbles forming in the capillaries and moving into the venous system will be carried back to the heart and then onwards via the pulmonary artery to the lungs. Large volumes of bubbles may interfere with the efficient operation of the heart as they will form a 'froth' that can accumulate in the chambers of the heart.

Once pumped through the pulmonary artery to the lungs the bubbles are then trapped within the capillaries surrounding the alveoli. Small numbers of bubbles can be caught in the capillaries and allowed to diffuse back into the lungs. This can be achieved without affecting the overall efficiency of the lungs. However with a large number of bubbles being trapped in the lungs eventually the volume of bubbles will start to have a negative effect on the efficiency of the lungs. The casualty will then start to suffer discomfort on breathing and a shortness of breath. A dry, persistent cough is also likely to be observed. Pulmonary DCS is often known as the *chokes*. The chokes are not particularly common amongst recreational divers although there is an increased risk for dives at high altitude.

Neurological – Inert gas bubbles forming or being transported to any part of the nervous system can have effects far beyond the localized site of the bubble. If bubbles form in the spinal column or nerves then sensations in the effects may be seen in the limbs or other areas controlled by those nerves. Pressure on a nerve can cause pain in the associated area which is quite a different case from the 'pain only' bend described above.

Pressure on a nerve can also cause numbness, tingling or even paralysis of the affected areas as the bubble interferes with the normal signals being sent from the brain to the remote location or from the location back to the brain. If instructions from the brain to move a limb are blocked from reaching the limb then paralysis will be the observed result. Conversely if a bubble is blocking signals being sent from the limb to the brain then numbness of the limb will be experienced. If the bubble is causing spurious messages to be sent to the brain then pain, tingling, heat or other sensations may be perceived in the affected limb.

Bubbles directly affecting the brain and spinal cord can cause symptoms in any of the other areas of the body, for example loss of bladder or bowel control, visual disturbances, hearing impairment, as well as a loss of balance and coordination. Lower back pain or a pain which encircles the abdomen is often a symptom of a spinal decompression problem.

Cerebral bends can also affect some of the higher cognitive areas such as memory, reasoning and speech. Casualties who are suffering from a cerebral bend may appear confused or disoriented, they may have trouble remembering simple information or answering simple questions. They may discount what are obvious symptoms of decompression sickness and as such it is important that others assess their condition to determine the likelihood of DCS.

Type III

Type III DCS was a term originally used by Bove and Neumann to describe a combination of DCS and AGE. It is now more common to use the term DCI to cover the combination of DCS and AGE and the term Type III has been used to describe DCS incidents relating to the inner ear or vestibular organs. It should be noted however that the classification Type III and indeed Type IV DCS was never as widely adopted as Type I and Type II.

Vestibular or Inner Ear DCS is much less common than Type I or Type II DCS. In fact, for sports divers it is irrelevant and even for technical divers at depth of less than 100m it is not common. However with deeper dives it has become more common. Type III DCS has been closely associated with Isobaric Counter Diffusion (ICD) (See Chapter 7 for more details on ICD)

In 2003, in response to a number of specific incidents and a growing focus on this area, Doolette and Mitchell, published a paper which provided a biophysical basis for inner ear DCS. Gas pressures in the inner ear were modelled and showed that for deep and/or long dives followed by a relatively rapid ascent significant supersaturation could occur during the early stages of decompression, prior to any gas switch. This supersaturation alone was enough to potentially result in bubble formation.

Doolette and Mitchell described the inner ear as three compartments: a well perfused, (i.e. well supplied with blood) vascular compartment that contains many of the critical functional structures of the inner ear; and the endolymph and perilymph compartments which are two poorly perfused "water" filled chambers separated from the perfused vascular compartment by a membrane.

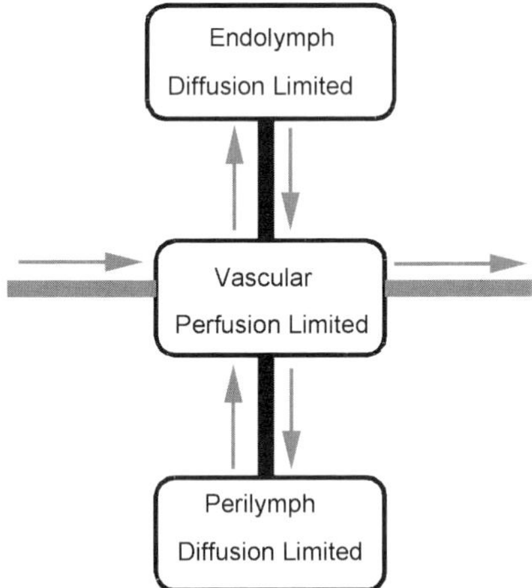

Figure 36: *Gas flows in the inner ear*

All gas enters and leaves the inner ear (all 3 compartments) via the blood flow into the well perfused vascular compartment. Under increased ambient pressure the watery endolymph and perilymph compartments on gas helium quickly as it diffuses from the vascular compartment. During decompression, helium will be trying to leave all the compartments as the ambient pressure falls. To do this, the helium in the endolymph and perilymph compartments diffuses into the vascular compartment to be carried away in the blood. The constantly decreasing ambient pressure resulting in the diver's ascent means that the rate of off gassing is lagging behind the fall in ambient pressure so all compartments are supersaturated with helium. At a gas switch, the diver then changes from breathing a high helium mix to a high nitrogen mix. The blood quickly carries this nitrogen to the perfused vascular compartment of the inner ear. Here the rapid diffusion of helium from the endolymph and perilymph compartments into the perfused vascular compartment exceeds the transfer of nitrogen in the opposite direction and the washout of helium from the vascular compartment by the blood flow away from the tissue. For a short period, this process will further raise the inert gas tensions in the already supersaturated vascular compartment. This increase in inert gas tension can be enough to result in bubble formation in the vascular compartment. As mentioned earlier, the vascular compartment contains many of the critical functional structures of the inner ear and bubbles forming in this area will result in the symptoms of inner ear or vestibular DCS.

Type IV

Type IV DCS has occasionally been used to describe the condition usually referred to as Dysbaric Osteonecrosis. Dysbaric can be translated as 'bad pressure' osteo means 'bone' and necrosis means 'cell death'. Therefore Dysbaric Osteo Necrosis (DON) is simply bone cell death as a result of pressure changes." This condition is also known as aseptic bone necrosis. This is a long term condition which is assumed to be caused by the blockage of blood vessels in the bones by bubbles caused during decompression. Swelling of fat cells in enclosed areas of the bone has also been suggested as the cause of DON. There are a number of other causes of bone necrosis but exposure to hyperbaric conditions is the usual reason when it occurs in someone who dives or has dived in the past.

In 1888, Twynam suggested that the areas of dead bone often seen in caisson workers were caused by their exposure to pressure. In 1913, Bassoe suggested that DON was somehow related to decompression sickness as he noticed that the caisson workers who had been bent the most also had the most incidence of DON.

In 1931 *HMS Poseidon*, a Royal Navy submarine, had an accident and five men were trapped at 38 meters (120 ft) for two to three hours before they escaped to the surface. All five developed DCS soon after surfacing. Twelve years later, when three of the five had x-rays taken, all three had DON, one with partial collapse of both femoral heads. None of the five were divers or had other known pressure exposures. Therefore we know that DON can develop from a single exposure to pressure.

Symptoms of DON can occur many years or even decades after exposure to pressure. It results in the weakening of the mechanical strength of the bone. It starts as a symptomless lesion detectable only by x-ray. It typically occurs in the longer bones such as the Humerus, Femur or Tibia although it has been detected in other bones. If these dead areas of bone are next to a joint this can result in severe joint damage and this may make joint replacement necessary. When a dead area affects the shaft of a bone it causes no symptoms, but there is still cause for concern because bone necrosis can change to a form of bone cancer.

The risk of dysbaric osteonecrosis appears to increases with depths of dives, their duration and the number of exposures. Amateur sports divers were considered to be at low risk because their dives were usually short and shallow. This means that until recently it was thought that DON was an occupational illness occurring in only professional divers and caisson workers. However in the last few years the members of the UK Sports Diving Medical Council (UKSDMC) have become aware of cases occurring in amateur divers. As amateur divers go deeper, for longer and use gas mixtures containing helium it is possible that more cases of dysbaric osteonecrosis may come to light.

Different studies have shown highly variable incidences. In caisson workers the average is around 19%. Up to 60% of caisson workers with more than 15 years experience have DON and those caisson workers who have a history of DCS are more likely to have DON. In addition, caisson workers who work at higher pressures are more likely to suffer DON.

In divers, the incidence of DON is even more confusing. The following table lists the findings of several studies into the incidence of DON in a range of diving communities. These show that the risk of DON is highest in divers who have the least training and by implication the least adequate decompression. From other studies we know that these same groups also have a very high incidence of DCS and that it is often inadequately treated.

Date	Exposure	Number	% DON
1974	Japanese Shellfishermen	301	50.5
1974	Gulf Coast Commercial Divers	330	27.0
1976	Royal Navy Divers	350	4.0
1976	US Navy Divers	611	2.5
1978	Hawaiian Fishermen	20	65.0
1981	North Sea Commercial Divers	4422	4.4
1983	Japanese Shellfishermen	747	25.0
1986	Australian Abalone Divers	108	56.4

Table 8: *Incidence of DON in divers in several retrospective studies. From Edmonds, Lowry and Pennefather, "Diving and Subaquatic Medicine", 3rd edition.*

Reclassification of DCS and AGE

For sports diving it was typical to simply talk about Type I and Type II decompression sickness as these were the most common types and Type III and Type IV were not normally considered as relevant.

However this classification was found to be problematic as it focused on the diagnosis of the type of DCS rather than on treatment. For example, skin manifestations (mottling) could be considered as mild manifestation of Type I DCS and as such a minor hit. However skin mottling has been associated with a Patent Foramen Ovale (PFO). This means that the 'minor' skin symptoms could be a precursor to more serious damage to the central nervous system (brain and spinal cord).

In addition the distinction between DCS and AGE was found to be counterproductive as the signs, symptoms and first aid for both are identical.

It doesn't matter if the signs are symptoms are the result of a nitrogen bubble formed due to improper decompression or an air bubble caused by arterial gas embolism. In both cases oxygen and recompression are required immediately.

The term Type III was suggested by Bove and Neumann to cover the combination of DCS and AGE but this was not widely adopted.

As a result a 1991 working party of the UHMS (Undersea Hyperbaric Medical Society) proposed the alternative terminology of Decompression Illness (DCI) to encompass all types of DCS and AGE. This terminology has now been adopted and the older term DCS is now less commonly used.

The classification of DCI is now based on the evolution of the symptoms, that is how the symptoms progress; the manifestations of the symptoms and any additional information. Figure 37 shows some of the various terms that are used by hyperbaric professionals to describe the evolution, manifestation and additional information relating to a case of DCI.

Alternative Classification of Decompression Illnesses

Evolution
- Progressive
- Static
- Spontaneously improving
- Relapsing

Manifestations
- Pain: musculoskeletal, girdle
- Neurological
- Audiovestibular
- Cardiopulmonary
- Cutaneous
- Lymphatic
- Constitutional

Additional information
- Presence of barotrauma
- Inert gas burden
- Response to treatment
- Investigations

Figure 37: *Alternative classification of DCI*

Signs and Symptoms

As we have seen in previous sections there are many signs and symptoms for decompression illness. The following is an alphabetical list of some but by no means all possible signs and symptoms.

Back pain
Blood in stools
Blotchy skin
Chest pain
Confusion
Convulsions
Coughing
Death
Diarrhoea
Difficulty urinating
Dizziness
Extreme fatigue
Headaches
Hearing loss
Itching
Lack of co-ordination
Loss of balance
Loss of bladder/bowel control
Nausea
Numbness
Pain/discomfort in or near joints
Paralysis
Pins and needles
Rash
Ringing in ears
Shortness of breath
Swelling
Stomach cramp
Torso pain
Unconsciousness
Visual disturbances
Vomiting blood
Weakness

Table 9: *Signs and symptoms of decompression illness*

Due to the wide range of potential symptoms any symptom observed after diving should be considered as a potential indication of DCI.

Symptoms of the Bends by Frequency

Some symptoms of DCI are much more common than others. Joint pain in the elbows, shoulder and other larger joints being by far the most commonly observed symptom of DCI. Studies by the US Navy reveal the following distribution of symptoms.

89%	Local Joint Pain
30%	Leg symptoms
70%	Arm symptoms
5.3%	Dizziness
2.3%	Paralysis
1.6%	Shortness of breath
1.3%	Extreme Fatigue
0.5%	Collapse/unconsciousness

USN DIVING MANUAL

Time of Onset of Symptoms

For divers using air or Nitrox the development of symptoms while the diver is still in the water is uncommon. Symptoms usually develop a short time after a dive. In a large sampling of cases the time of onset after surfacing was:

50%	Within 30 minutes
85 %	Within 1 hour
95%	Within 3 hours
1%	More then 6 hours

USN DIVING MANUAL

The delay in the onset of symptoms is due to the fact that bubbles do not form immediately even when the supersaturation level is very high. In addition the symptoms will become more noticeable in time as the body's reaction to bubbles causes additional symptoms in addition to those caused purely by the physical effect of the bubble formation.

Delays of more than 6 hours are usually associated with the diver not recognizing or not acknowledging the symptoms rather than a true delay in the onset of symptoms.

The timeframe for the onset of AGE is much shorter and symptoms may well be observed while the diver is still in the water.

For diver using helium the timeframe for the onset of symptoms is also much shorter with symptoms of Helium bends being reported during the ascent or on a decompression stop.

The distribution of symptoms of DCS also varies by the sample population. This is believed to be due to the fact that different exposure profiles will result in different forms of DCS and so will present different symptoms. Studies have shown that Caisson workers predominantly develop limb bends, as do aviators. When recreational divers develop limb bends they are more commonly in the upper limbs whereas Caisson workers tend to develop limb bends in the lower limbs. Cardiopulmonary DCS (Chokes) is rarely seen in divers but was a common risk for aviators until the causes and preventative use of Oxygen pre-breathing was discovered. Recreational divers, especially when undertaking repetitive dives, will have a higher incidence of spinal DCS whereas aviators and saturation divers do not seem to develop this type of DCS and Caisson workers only rarely develop it.

	Saturation	Caisson	Recreational
Pain only	82	85	41
Neurological	5.5	1	19
Vertigo	3	5	8
Difficulty Breathing	0.4	2	2.5

Table 10: *Distribution of DCS occurrence by sectors*

Predisposing Factors

There are certain factors that can increase the risk of DCS. Awareness of these predisposing factors can help to reduce this risk.

Dehydration

Dehydration is widely believed to be one of the more common factors affecting DCS hits. However there is very little clinical evidence to prove this link. Roughly half of our body weight is water with 75% of muscle tissue and 25% of fat tissue being made up of water. It is the primary transport and reactive medium of the body and is fundamentally important for a wide range of functions within the body.

Luckily dehydration is one factor that is under our control and is relatively easy to eliminate. Proper hydration is essential when diving. This doesn't just mean a cup of tea or coffee the morning before the dive or a swig of water when preparing for a dive but should begin at least 24 hours before the dive. It takes some time for the body to absorb the liquid it needs when you are dehydrated and simply drinking a large volume of water the morning of the dive is likely to result in you just passing most of it straight through.

One of the easiest ways to check on your hydration levels is to check the colour of your urine. Clear or very pale yellow generally means that you are well hydrated; darker yellow means that you are dehydrated and should be drinking more water. Many people are permanently dehydrated and the general recommendation is to drink at least 8-10 glasses of water a day. Ordinary water is the best way to rehydrate for the majority of people. Sports drinks are not necessary for most people and soft drinks and fruit juices, whilst they will help, will not be as effective in rehydrating you as pure water.

Dehydration can be caused by a number of factors. Flying, sweating, excess consumption of diuretics such as tea, coffee or alcohol, as well as diarrhoea or nausea can all cause dehydration. When these are combined, for example when you arrive off the plane at the start of your holiday in a hot climate and spend the first evening in the bar then it is likely that you will be heavily dehydrated for the first dive of your trip.

Diving itself can cause dehydration. If you are wearing a thick undersuit under a drysuit and kitting up in the sun then you are likely to sweat heavily. The air from your cylinders is very dry and you are continually moistening the air you breathe with moisture from the mouth and throat. Breathing dry air alone will double the rate of loss of moisture from the body. In addition, on dry land the force of gravity means that much of our available blood is pooled in our legs. When we enter the water and the force of gravity is reduced this blood redistributes itself around the rest of the body. Our body's reaction to this is to try and reduce the volume of blood in circulation by removing some of the water and transferring it to the bladder. This is one of the reasons why you often get that urge to go just after you have entered the water. The cold has the same effect as it causes peripheral vasoconstriction which drives fluid back into the core increasing the blood pressure and further stimulating the removal of water from the circulation and into the bladder.

Despite the widespread belief and anecdotal evidence of dehydration causing DCS it is not really known why, or how, dehydration contributes to the risk of DCS. One common theory is that it's because we need a good level of fluid in the circulatory system in order to off-gas the increased levels of inert gas in the body. If we are dehydrated then gas transport in the blood will be less efficient due to the reduction in plasma.

As bubbles grow and combine to form larger bubbles, they affect the surrounding tissue, making it more permeable to liquid. (See later in this chapter for more details). This results in a loss of fluid from the circulation and an increased level of dehydration. This means that dehydration is thought to be a cause of DCS but is also a result of DCS. This is why hydration is one of the key aspects of first aid treatment for DCS. It is also the reason why we should continue to drink water after the dive.

Dive profiles

Dive tables assume that a dive consists of a square profile which includes descent; some time spent on the bottom followed by an ascent which may include an optional safety stop or mandatory decompression stops.

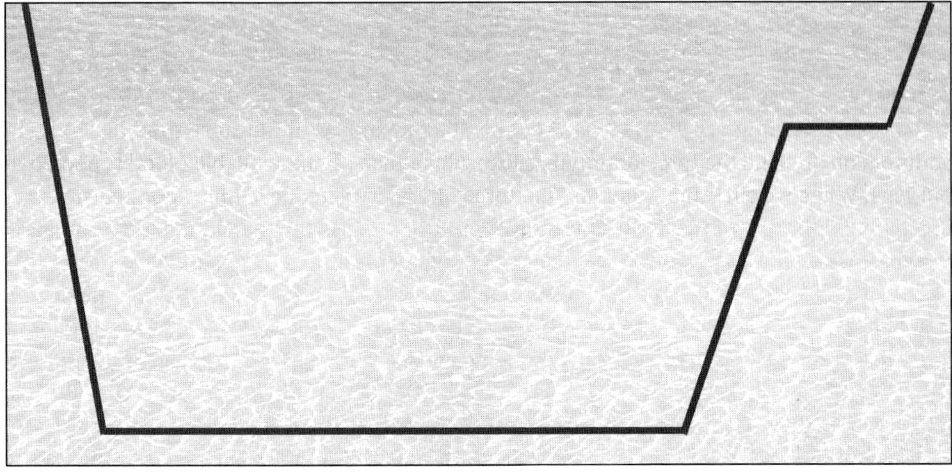

Figure 38*:* *Square profile*

Profiles with ascents to the surface (yo-yo profiles) or profiles where there is frequent changes in the depth (saw-tooth profiles) may increase the risk of decompression illness.

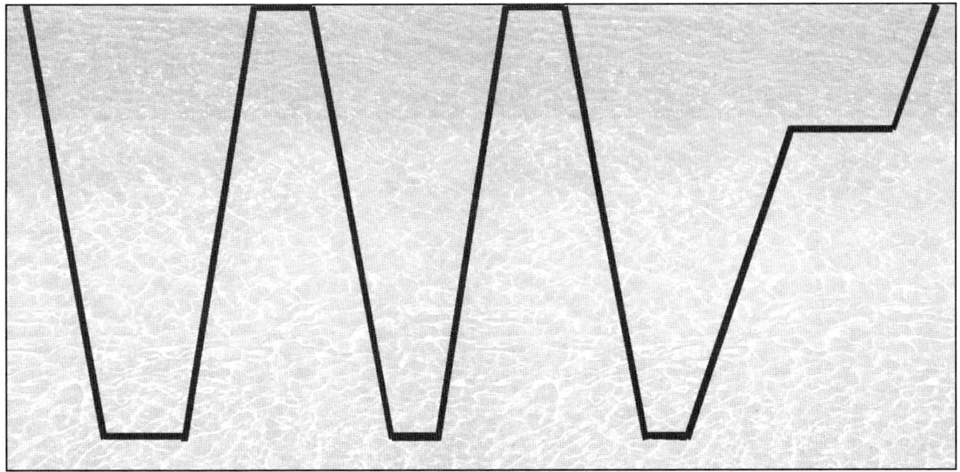

Figure 39: *Yo-Yo profile*

Figure 38 shows a traditional 'square' dive profile. After the descent all of the bottom time is spent at the maximum depth. This is the dive profile assumed by a diver using tables. Even if part of the dive is spent at shallower depths the whole bottom time is taken at the maximum depth. Figure 39 on the other hand shows a yo-yo profile where the diver has ascended to the surface and then re-descended twice during the dive. If we compare the two dives then the square profile dive involved much more time at depth whereas during the yo-yo profile dive the diver spent much less time at the maximum depth. We know that Nitrogen loading is related to the partial pressure of the inert gas being breathed and the time spent at that partial pressure. For the yo-yo profile dive we spent much less time at the maximum depth and so much less time breathing at the maximum partial pressure so we would assume that at the end of the dive we would have a lower inert gas loading. Why then would the yo-yo profile dive be considered more of a risk than the square profile dive?

The answer to this question lies not in the time spent at depth or the time spent breathing a particular partial pressure. The answer lies in the ascents during the dive. During these ascents the ambient pressure surrounding the diver is reduced and some of the tissues may move from being under-saturated to being supersaturated. When this happens there is a chance that silent bubbles are formed. When the diver descends for the second time these bubbles will remain in the body and can cause problems during the subsequent ascents by acting as a catalyst for further bubble formation. The existing bubbles will also slow down the efficiency of off gassing during subsequent ascents and this may cause more bubbles to form than would have otherwise have occurred.

This type of dive profile may occur on a relatively shallow dive where the diver decides to ascend to the surface to check their bearings or possibly to find their buddy if they have been separated. This type of profile is also typical for diving instructors and certain types of commercial divers such as shellfish fisherman. In all of these cases the divers are often in shallow water and perform multiple ascents and descents during the day. As the diver is in shallow water and doing relatively short dives they assume that they have no risk of decompression illness. However multiple ascents have been shown to be a contributing factor to decompression illness during dives in as little as 5m of water.

For most divers a yo-yo profile with one or more intermediate ascents to the surface is not a normal occurrence. However saw-tooth profiles are much more common. A saw-tooth profile is a profile where the diver repeatedly ascends a certain way from the maximum depth and then descends again.

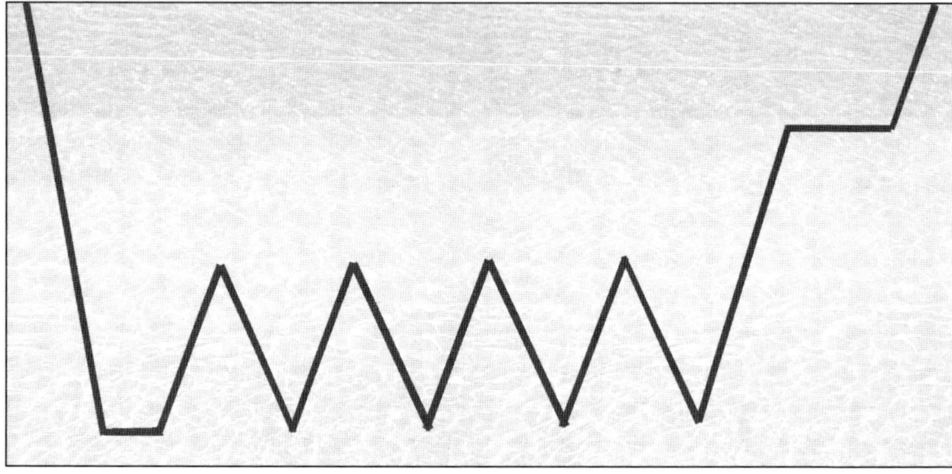

Figure 40: *Saw tooth profile*

Saw-tooth profiles can easily occur on a wreck dive where a diver swims up and over large sections of wreckage before dropping back down to the sea bed. It may also occur on a reef dive where a diver is varying up and down the reef wall without keeping a close eye on their depth.

Although less extreme than a yo-yo profile the reason for the increased risk of decompression illness is exactly the same. Each ascent is reducing the ambient pressure and risking the formation of silent bubbles. The risk increases as the dive gets longer and more compartments reach saturation. If a tissue compartment is saturated then *any* ascent will result in a decrease in ambient pressure which means that the tissue will be supersaturated.

Some modern decompression computers will penalise a diver who has performed a saw-tooth profile during their dive. This may lead them to think that their computer is giving them unnecessarily long decompression obligation when compared to their buddy's less conservative computer.

Repetitive Diving

It is worth bearing in mind that most of the impetus for decompression theory research and dive table generation came originally from the military and commercial areas. In both of these areas divers would typically dive until they had completed their allocated task or had reached their predetermined bottom time. Repetitive diving did not feature at all in their early diving operations. Even with the advent of SCUBA in the 1950's repetitive diving amongst commercial and military divers was the exception rather than the rule. As a result comparatively little research was done on this aspect of decompression theory. For recreational divers however, repetitive diving is much more common, especially during diving holidays where carrying out multiple dives per day over several days is very common.

Dive tables or calculations will tell us when we can surface without exceeding critical supersaturation in any of our tissues. However this still means that on surfacing we will have a significant amount of nitrogen dissolved in our tissues and we will remain in a state of supersaturation for some time after the dive. It may take more than 24 or even 48 hours for us to reach desaturate completely.

This can cause problems with a second dive which occurs following a relatively short surface interval after the first dive. It can also cause problems during diving holidays where you are doing multiple dives per day for several days at a time. On the second and subsequent diving days the slower tissues may still have residual nitrogen present at the start of the first day which can build up over the course of the holiday. Research from the Divers Alert Network (DAN) has shown that divers who make multiple dives per day over several days have a higher than average risk of decompression illness.

If a repetitive dive is carried out then this prior loading of nitrogen must be taken into account. Diving tables take this into account by allocating a penalty based on the previous dive and the surface interval which must be added to the bottom time of the subsequent dive. This penalty is meant to represent the prior nitrogen loading of the tissues.

The same situation can occur for professional instructors and dive guides who are diving day after day. This is the reason for the 'seventh day off' rule which states that after six days of diving the seventh day should be a rest day as it allows the body to desaturate fully. Some agencies recommend taking every fourth day off, especially if involved in repetitive decompression diving.

Temperature

Temperature affects decompression as changes in temperature will affect the circulation within the body which will change the regular pattern of on-gassing and off-gassing.

As the body cools down the circulation to the extremities is reduced. When the skin temperature starts to drop the body will reduce the circulation in your limbs, this is known as vasoconstriction. Reduced blood flow to the extremities reduces overall heat loss. Unlike the blood vessels in the other extremities, the blood vessels in the skin of your head do not constrict. As a result, in cold conditions the head will loose a great deal of heat as the blood flows close to the surface.

A constant body temperature throughout the dive, whether it is constantly higher or lower than average, does not seem to cause as many problems as changing temperature. Of the two a dive where the diver is constantly at a colder temperature seems to result in lower risk of DCS. However, several studies have noted an apparent increase in the risk of decompression illness risk with surface decompression diving in warm water or with hot water suits. Surface decompression divers who are warm at depth face an increased risk of DCS. Vasodilatation in warm divers may result in more rapid on-gassing of tissues with short time constants. For recreational or sports divers without access to surface decompression facilities or hot water suits this is not a major concern.

For sports divers a bigger problem is the effect of becoming progressively colder during a dive. During a decompression dive in cold water the diver will start the dive comparatively warm. This means that there is a good blood flow to all parts of the body and so on-gassing will occur across all the bodies tissues. As the dive continues the diver will become colder which may trigger the body to reduce circulation to those extremities. During a decompression stop, where the diver is moving less, they may become even colder, which causes the body to further restrict the flow of blood to the extremities. This reduced blood flow results in a reduced ability to off-gas by the tissues in the extremities. This reduced ability to off-gas means that there is more dissolved inert gas in the tissues than would be predicted and this may be enough to exceed the supersaturation ratio in these tissues and cause bubbles to form.

Obesity

There is a long history of empirical observation that obesity can increase the risk of DCS. The article following Haldane, Boycott, Damant and Lister's 1908 article in the *Journal of Hygiene* was an article by Damant describing how overweight sailors had shown an increased risk of DCS. Hyperbaric specialists from the early days of tunnel and caisson workers right through to modern scuba divers have noticed an increase in decompression cases amongst overweight, out of shape divers. Others, however, have found no correlation.

Nitrogen is five times more soluble in fat tissue than muscle. This means that an increase in fatty tissue leads to an increase in nitrogen loading in the body. Fatty tissues are usually poorly supplied with blood vessels which, combined with the high affinity of fat for Nitrogen can lead to problems in off-gassing from fatty tissues. Some researchers have suggested that this can cause the fatty tissues to act as bubbles reservoirs.

As well as fatty tissues below the skin obese people tend to have higher blood lipid levels. This can also lead to an increases risk of decompression illness as blood lipids have been suggested as triggers for bubble formation when the supersaturation ration is exceeded.

The majority of empirical observations, research and scientific papers support the view the obesity is a predisposing factor for decompression illness. However, some researchers have argued that obesity in itself is not a major contributor to decompression illness but that overweight divers tend to be unfit and out of condition and that it is these secondary factors that increase the risk of decompression illness rather than the obesity itself.

The long-term implications of obesity are well known. Heart disease, stroke, cancer, high blood pressure, osteoarthritis, gall bladder problems, adult onset diabetes, sleep apnea and fatty deposits blocking the circulatory vessels are all likely results of obesity. Many of the conditions related to obesity such as coronary artery disease are also believed to be DCS risk factors and many are contra indications to diving in their own right.

On the other hand obese divers tend to suffer less with the cold, whereas very thin divers will tend to get cold much quicker. As we have seen the cold is also a risk factor for decompression illness so in this particular case the overweight or obese diver may have an advantage over his skinnier buddy but it seems obvious that this potential advantage is outweighed by the many disadvantages.

Exercise

All decompression researchers agree that fit, healthy individuals are less likely to suffer from most medical conditions, including decompression illness, than unfit individuals. As a result, exercise as part of a healthy lifestyle is recommended as a way to reduce the risks of decompression illness. Regular, moderate exercise is known to improve blood circulation in muscle tissue and increases cardiopulmonary function which should help to increase the rate of nitrogen off-gassing from the body.

Dr. Bill Hamilton summarised this view in *Alert Diver*, May/June 2000, pg. 42: *"There is no doubt that fitness needs to be emphasised more and for divers of all levels. In addition to the obvious benefits of enhanced aerobic ability and athletic performance, a good level of fitness helps in decompression. A diver who is extremely fit can decompress more aggressively than someone who isn't fit. An overweight diver may have more problems off-gassing because of less efficient circulation and because of the way fat takes up gas."*

So while exercise as part of your daily routine has a positive impact on reducing decompression risk what impact does it have immediately before during and after decompression?

The views on exercise during diving initially focused on the impact of increased blood flow during diving. It seems intuitively obvious that increased exercise during the bottom portion of the dive which increases blood flow to the tissues will also increase the rate off on-gassing. This results in a higher loading of Nitrogen and of course a higher risk of decompression illness. The opposite effect was assumed for exercise during decompression. Increased exercise during decompression would result in increased blood flow to the tissues which results in more effective off-gassing.

This view dates back to the earliest days of decompression research. During the period that Haldane's work on decompression was being implemented by the Royal Navy and later by the US Navy these organisations insisted on divers exercising during decompression. The idea was that the exercise would accelerate the blood flow and hence the rate of decompression. However, over time, a number of experiments showed that excessive exercise during decompression could increase the risk of decompression illness.

For many years exercise during decompression was discouraged as there was a view that strenuous exercise immediately before, during or after a dive could trigger decompression illness. It has been suggested that strenuous exercise causes the formation in the body of tiny gas bubbles called 'micronuclei'. It takes several hours for these bubbles to disperse and although no absolute link has been established between the existence of micronuclei and decompression illness, Divers Alert Network (DAN) recommend that strenuous exercise be avoided for four hours before SCUBA diving.

Dr. Mike Powell before retiring from NASA has done a significant amount of research in the affects of exercise during decompression. He discovered that resistance to decompression illness can be increased by complete bed rest for several hours to days prior to decompression. It is also shown that even doing a few stair steps can increase the chances of decompression illness. However it has also been shown that MILD exercise during decompression decreases

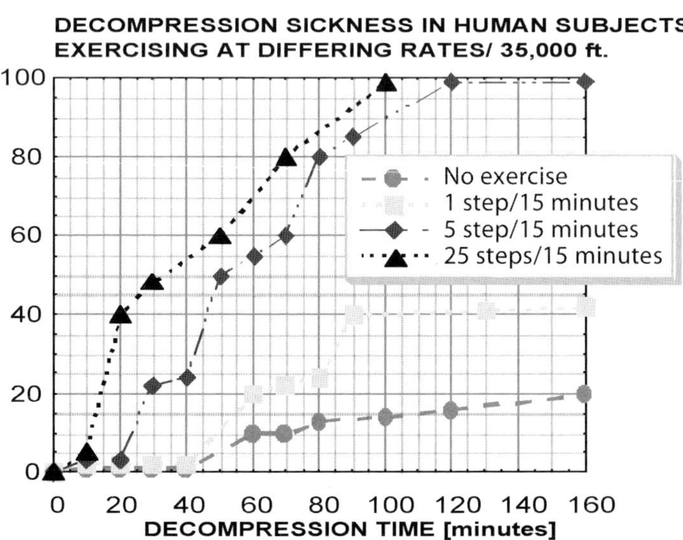

Decompression sickness in human subjects exercising at differing rates / 35,000 ft

the risk of the bends by increasing the removal of gas from the tissues. Dr Powell refers to research carried out during World War II on exercise at altitude when high altitude bombing made understanding aviation decompression illness a strategic priority.

So does that mean that exercise increases our risk of decompression illness or does it reduce the risk? The current view is that the desirability of exercise is dependant on the timing and intensity of the exercise. Aerobic exercise in advance of diving is generally considered to reduce the risk if performed between 10 and 48 hours before the dive. Exercise more than 48 hours in advance of the dive seems to have no benefit and exercise less then 10 hours before the dive seems to counteract any benefits by potentially creating more gas nuclei. Intense or strenuous exercise before a dive should also be avoided.

Exercise should also be avoided during the bottom part of the dive to avoid increasing the rate of on-gassing. During the decompression phase of the dive and immediately after surfacing excessive exercise should be avoided as this can significantly increase the risk of bubble formation. However gentle exercise during decompression can promote blood flow and hence increase the rate of off-gassing.

Smoking

The respiratory system is one of the key links in the chain of effective decompression. Any interference in lung function is going to affect the decompression process. For this reason the effects of smoking can have a considerable affect when diving.

Most of the risks of smoking and diving are related to long term usage: the chronic obstructive pulmonary disease that smoking produces over many years. This obstruction is in the terminal alveoli and the emphysema that's caused can (and does) produce air-filled dilations that can significantly increase your chances of pulmonary barotrauma and arterial gas embolism. Smoking also causes an increase in bronchial mucous production together with paralysis of the cilia, the fine ‘hairs’ that serve to move mucus, dust and other unwanted contaminants out of the lungs. Mucous plugs then become dangerous to the diver, setting the stage for air-filled sacs that lead to rupture upon ascent.

Most smokers also have nasal and sinus drainage problems. This markedly increases their chances of middle ear and sinus blocks and squeezes. There have been studies that have shown that stopping smoking prior to surgery actually increased the amount of mucous production for about a week. Applying this information to diving it means that if you are going to gain any benefit from stopping then you need to have stopped at least one week in advance of diving.

Longer term problems include chronic obstructive pulmonary disease (COPD) which leads to reduced oxygen availability and an increase in carbon dioxide (CO_2) retention in the body. This has been implicated as a factor in CNS oxygen toxicity. Smokers are also generally less healthy and are more prone to develop circulatory problems.

Cigarette smoke contains nicotine, which acts as a vasoconstrictor and may theoretically increase the risk of DCS due to altered blood perfusion.

Cigarette smoke also contains high levels of carbon monoxide (CO), which is a poison. This increased level reduces the ability of the red blood cells to carry oxygen. The CO combines with the haemoglobin in the red blood cells. Haemoglobin binds more closely with CO than with oxygen and so the CO reduces the capacity of the haemoglobin to carry oxygen. The effects of partial pressure on CO concentration in inhaled cigarette smoke would be the same as if the CO had come from some other source, such as from the atmosphere or from an oil lubricated compressors.

Your carbon monoxide level varies with the number of cigarettes you have already smoked that day, the length of time since your last cigarette, how the cigarette was smoked and your level of activity on the day of the reading.

Typical end-of-day readings are as follows:
0 - 10 ppm of carbon monoxide-non-smoker
11 - 20 ppm of carbon monoxide-light smoker
21 - 100 ppm of carbon monoxide-heavy smoker

CO binds with hemoglobin 220-290 times greater than O_2 and so as CO increases, the ability of the blood to carry Oxygen is diminished. To work out the approximate percentage of oxygen being replaced by carbon monoxide in your blood, divide your reading by 6. For example: 18 ppm of carbon monoxide is 18/6 = 3%. That is 3% of the oxygen in your blood is being replaced by carbon monoxide. If you are a heavy smoker, up to 15% of your oxygen is possibly being replaced by carbon monoxide.

Age

The majority of research literature suggests that ageing divers are at a higher risk of DCS although the evidence is by no means conclusive. Differences in the studies mean that there is no clear indication as to when this risk begins. One of the problems is that much of this research has been carried out by the military who are primarily interested in divers in their 20s and 30s whereas sport divers routinely dive into their 40, 50s, 60s, 70s and even later.

What is clear is that ageing divers are more likely to suffer from additional medical problems which are likely to increase their risk of DCS. Age manifests itself in degenerative joint disease, changes in heart and lung function which impairs circulation. It has also been found that older people in general are more likely to have gas nuclei present in their joints and especially in their spines.

Flying after diving

Atmospheric pressure is a result of the air above us. The 1 bar of pressure we feel at the surface is caused by the weight of all the molecules above us. Because there are fewer molecules of gas at higher altitude, there is less pressure and therefore a lower partial pressure of each gas in the air, which means there is less oxygen available. This hypobaric effect is the opposite of hyperbaric pressure.

Feet	Meters	psia	Atm	Bar (a)	Mm Hg
0	0	14.7	1.00	1.013	760
500	150	14.4	0.98	0.994	747
1000	300	14.2	0.96	0.976	734
1500	450	13.9	0.94	0.956	719
2000	600	13.7	0.93	0.939	706
2500	750	13.4	0.91	0.923	694
3000	900	13.2	0.89	0.906	681
3500	1070	12.9	0.88	0.888	668
4000	1220	12.7	0.86	0.871	655
4500	1370	12.4	0.85	0.858	645
5000	1520	12.2	0.83	0.842	633
5500	1680	12.0	0.81	0.825	620

Table 11: *The effect of elevation on ambient air pressure*

This concept is familiar to most people since aircraft flying at high altitudes must have pressurised cabins to support life. All commercial passengers are reminded during their safety briefing that in the event of sudden cabin de-compression oxygen masks will drop down from above. However, even in normal operation, the cabin 'altitude' can be as high as 7,500 feet which results in an ambient pressure of only 0.8 bar.

Although reducing the available amount of oxygen to the body can lead to hypoxic conditions, most healthy people will not experience symptoms during a normal commercial flight. The main risk to divers from flying is not the reduction in oxygen partial pressure but the reduction in atmospheric pressure itself.

As can be seen on the graph below, as pressure decreases with increasing altitude, the volume of a gas will increase. Although the degree of change in a hypobaric atmosphere is less pronounced than in a hyperbaric atmosphere, pre-existing nitrogen bubbles in the body will grow larger and may exacerbate or even cause DCS. Divers who have had no signs of DCS before boarding a plan may start to experience signs of DCS once the aircraft has climbed to altitude. Decompression chambers near airports frequently report admitting divers who developed signs and symptoms of DCS on board an aircraft after a diving holiday. Larger gas spaces, such as a pneumothorax, will also grow.

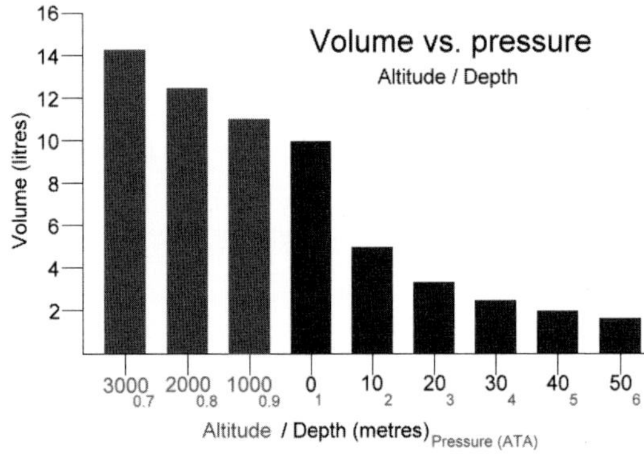

The length of time required between a dive and flying depends on many factors, including the depth, duration and number of dives, therefore it is impossible to give a definitive pre-flying period. In the past, guidelines for flying after diving were quite varied. For example, for a single no-stop dive, the U.S. Navy recommended a 2-hour surface interval time, DAN recommended 12 hours surface interval, and the U.S. Air Force recommended 24 hours interval.

In order to provide for useful advice DAN undertook a study to investigate the rsks of flying after diving. The study was conducted from 1993 to 1999 for 802 exposures. There were 40 DCS (decompression sickness) incidents (5%), of which 21 were moderate DCS, 18 mild DCS, and 1 serious DCS.

The details of the study were presented at a Flying After Diving Workshop at DAN in May 2002 and the following guidelines were agreed. They apply to air dives followed by flights at cabin altitudes of 2,000 to 8,000 feet (610 to 2,438 meters) for divers who do not currently have symptoms of decompression sickness (DCS). The recommended preflight surface intervals do not guarantee that the diver will have no risk of DCS as in order to guarantee this for all cases the interval would have to be inordinately long. Instead the guidelines provide a level where the risk of DCS has been reduced to an acceptable level. Longer surface intervals will reduce the risk of DCS further. For a single no-decompression dive, a minimum preflight surface interval of 12 hours is suggested. For repetitive dives or multi day dives an interval of at least 18 hours is recommended. For dives requiring decompression stops, there was less evidence on which to base a recommendation and a preflight surface interval substantially longer than 18 hours was suggested with a 24 hour interval being widely adopted.

Reverse profile

A reverse profile dive is a repetitive dive to a depth greater than the previous dive. For example if we dive to 15m and then follow this with a dive to 30m then this second dive is a reverse profile dive. Until quite recently reverse profile dives have been viewed in recreational diving circles as extremely bad practice and high risk behaviour from a decompression point of view. Recent analysis of the issue has shown that this restriction on reverse profile diving has no real basis.

What is quite remarkable about the issue of reverse profiles is that nobody seems to know why this guideline is in place and where it came from. It appears that the rule against reverse profiles started for reasons of bottom time efficiency and then, over time, got distorted into a diving urban myth about diving safety. The earliest documented recommendation to perform the deepest dive first can be traced back to a manual published by PADI in 1972. In each subsequent PADI manual the rule is repeated in increasingly strong terms up to 1999 where it is clearly stated that reverse profile dives have a high incidence of decompression illness. The influence of the PADI system has meant that, over the course of time, other publications and training manuals picked up the recommendation and strengthened it to the point where it became almost a golden rule. Subsequently PADI have made it clear that there are no records within the organisation to support either the initial statement or the subsequent reinforcements.

In 1999 a workshop was held on reverse diving profiles with the intention of coming to a conclusion on the risks of reverse profile diving. The workshop was hosted by the

American Academy of Underwater Sciences (AAUS) and was attended by most of the leading decompression researchers and theorists. The conference started out by looking at the origins of the ruling against reverse profile diving and it quickly became clear that there was no clear or scientific basis for the ruling. Studies into the relative risks of reverse profile diving versus forward profile diving were then considered.

It was fairly obvious to all there that the diving data presented did not point to any particular problems with reverse dive profiles in recreational, commercial, military, or scientific diving. It was also apparent that, despite the strength of warnings against reverse profile diving, divers were carrying out these profiles dives on a relatively frequent basis without incident. When occasional incidences of DCS did occur with reverse profiles, it was at a statistically lower rate than for forward profiles. It appeared that decompression algorithms and dive computers are adequately handling the issue of reverse dive profiles in real life situations.

It became clear that there is no basis in diving experience to draw the conclusion that reverse profiles are inherently more dangerous than forward profiles. There was essentially unanimous agreement about this point among the participants. There was more disagreement when it came to composing a final conclusion or set of recommendations.

Several of the researchers involved with bubble model theories had serious reservations about a complete retraction of warnings against doing reverse dive profiles. According to these researchers, the bubble models show that you can really get into trouble on an improperly planned/executed reverse dive profile. Many were concerned that divers, especially inexperienced sport divers, would get the wrong message about reverse profiles and think that it was okay to do them without any special consideration.

A couple of key concessions were obtained by the bubble modellers. First, David Yount pointed out that practical diving experience showed that there had not been many problems with reverse profiles, but bubble models showed that there could be. A further argument was made that the present lack of data that reverse profiles are dangerous could be, in part, due to the arbitrary prohibition against them that has been in place for many years and has prevented many divers from carrying out these profiles. In other words as many divers were avoiding reverse profile dives they were avoiding potentially dangerous profiles and so the lack of incidents was not surprising as they had been avoiding the high risk procedures which might have caused the incidents. As a result, some wording was changed to make it clear that it was only in the diving experience that there were few problems, not that there's a lack of evidence of any kind that reverse profiles are/can be dangerous.

Bruce Wienke prevailed in his argument that the pressure differential of most of the safely executed reverse profiles was 12m / 40fsw or less between the repetitive dives. Accordingly, it was agreed that reverse dive profiles are reasonably safe as long as the depth difference between repetitive dives is 12m / 40fsw or less. A point of final agreement was that the sport diving limit of 40 msw/130 fsw should apply to any relaxation of current prohibitions on reverse profile diving.

So, the consensus from the Workshop was summarised into four findings and a conclusion;

Findings:

- Historically, neither the U.S. Navy nor the commercial sector has prohibited reverse dive profiles.
- Reverse dive profiles are being performed in recreational, scientific, commercial and military diving.
- The prohibition of reverse dive profiles by recreational training organizations cannot be traced to any definite diving experience that indicates an increased risk of DCS.
- No convincing evidence that reverse dive profiles within the no decompression limits lead to a measurable increase in the risk of DCS was presented.

Conclusion:
We find no reason for the diving communities to prohibit reverse dive profiles for no-decompression dive profiles less than 40msw/130fsw and depth differentials less than 12 msw/40fsw.

Previous injury

Divers who have suffered previous injury have shown a tendency to develop DCI in the injured areas. Injuries tend to result in changes in blood flow to those areas as well as the formation of scar tissue.

Areas of decreased and increased blood flow have been identified as potential cases leading to DCI. Clearly anything that affects the rate of perfusion to a tissue will affect the on-gassing and off-gassing in that tissue.

PFO

In recent years it has become clear that one of the most significant causes of 'unearned DCS' is a physical abnormality of the heart, commonly called a hole in the heart, but specifically known as a Patent Foramen Ovale (PFO). This is a small opening between the upper two chambers of the heart (atria). The first recorded description of a PFO was in 1877 when a German Doctor named J Cohnheim performed an autopsy on a young woman who had died from a stroke. He suggested that a clot passing through the PFO must have caused the stroke.

Before birth babies cannot receive Oxygen via their lungs and so depend on the flow of blood from their mother to oxygenate their tissues. This oxygen rich blood enters the venous circulation and flows to the right side of the heart. As the lungs are unusable until birth and the blood has already been oxygenated by the mother there is no point pumping this blood to the lungs. The oxygenated blood needs to get into the baby's arterial system and hence to the rest of the body. To do this the blood crosses from the right, or venous, side of the heart to the left, arterial side. The foramen ovale (Latin for oval hole) is a hole in the wall of the heart that allows the blood to flow from the right atrium to the left. The blood is pumped around the body, supplying oxygen to the baby's tissues before being returned to the mother's circulatory system where waste products are removed, and oxygen replenished.

The foramen ovale is not just a hole, but a flap of skin over the hole forming a valve - allowing flow in one direction only - from right to left. In the foetus the pressure is higher in the right side of the heart, so the flap valve opens and allows blood to pass from the right atrium to left. After birth, the lungs expand, blood rushes through, and the pressure in the right atria is much lower. The pressure in the left atria exceeds the pressure in the right, and the flap of tissue which covers the foramen ovale is pushed closed. There is no further flow through the foramen ovale, blood passing from right atrium to right ventricle, around the lungs and then left atria, ventricle and the body.

The opening usually seals up following birth. Once sealed, it will remain sealed and flow through the hole will not be possible. If it remains open (in Latin - patent) then it can cause a potential 'short circuit' of blood flow. If the pressure in the right side of the heart rises above that in the left, the flap valve can open and blood passes through allowing venous blood returning from the body to pass through the wall of the heart and get pumped back around the body. It has been estimated that PFO is present in about 25-30% of the general population and does not normally cause health problems. Wheras an Atrial Septal Defect (ASD) where the flap has hardly closed at all is a true embryonic development abnormality. This is likely to have already been diagnosed since the signs and symptoms are more obvious - usually from an early age. The symptoms include heart murmur, cyanosis and faintness.

A PFO will not normally cause health problems for the majority of sufferers. The pressure on the left side usually exceeds the pressure on the right and so no transfer occurs. If the pressure difference is reversed, which can occur if we are straining or lifting a heavy object, and the pressure on the right exceeds the pressure on the left then, if you have a PFO, blood can pass from left to right. For non divers this has no real impact. It does become much more important for divers, it affects up to 75% of divers with 'unexplained' DCI. Although PFO increases the risk of decompression illness, individuals with PFO do not necessarily develop symptoms. Also, even in the absence of any apparent cause, DCS is not always due to a PFO.

A PFO is a risk factor for divers as it allows blood containing bubbles to pass directly from the venous circulation to the brain through the heart, bypassing the filtering effect of the lungs. Figure 41 shows the situation for a normal heart. Venous blood returns from the body to the heart where it is pumped to the lungs to be re-oxygenated and where the lungs will also filter out any bubbles present in the venous blood. The Oxygenated blood then returns from the lungs and is pumped via the arterial system to the bodies tissues.

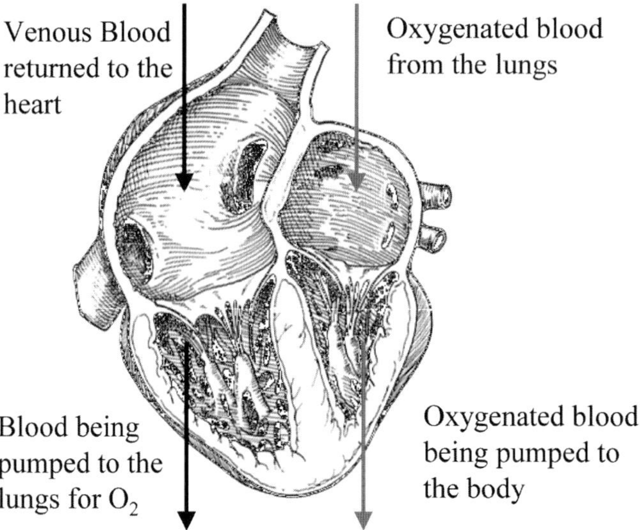

Figure 41: *Normal blood flow in the heart*

In the case where a PFO is present, as shown in Figure 42, the blood returning from the body bypasses the lungs and flows directly through the PFO from the right atrium into the left atrium where it is pumped into the left ventricle and from there back around the body. As this blood has not been filtered by the lungs it still contains inert gas bubbles which are now carried to the vital body tissues.

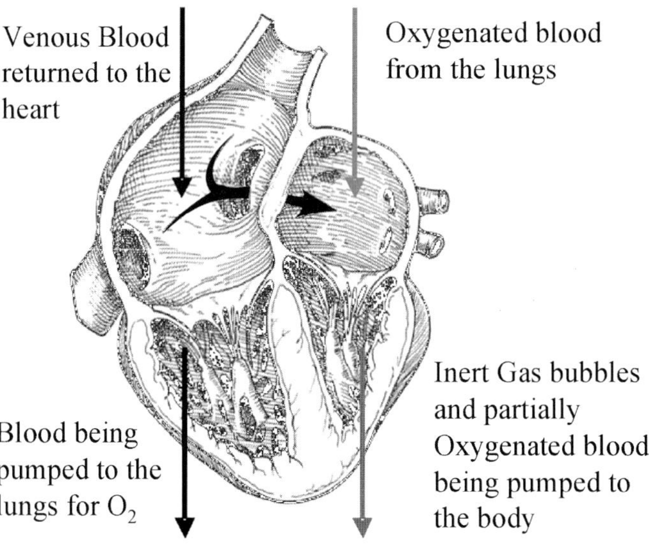

Figure 42: *Blood flow through the heart with a PFO*

A tendency to suffer from migraines has been identified as a possible indication of the presence of a PFO, however, as most people with a PFO show no obvious signs, diagnosis is usually only attempted following one or more unexplained incidences of DCS. Definitely a case of closing the stable door after the horse has bolted.

There are two methods to detect the presence of a PFO. The first method uses an echocardiograph machine to indicate the presence of blood flow between the two atria of the heart. A cardiologist, following referral by a specialist in hyperbaric medicine, normally carries out testing. This test gives a visual representation of the four chambers of the heart on a computer screen. A special solution of saline filled with tiny dissolved microbubbles is infused quickly into the venous circulation. This causes a sudden flow of small gas bubbles to pass through the right side of the heart - first through the right atrium and then immediately after, into the right ventricle. If a PFO is present, the bubbles will also be seen passing from the right atrium to the left atrium. The injection is repeated while the patient takes a deep breath, blows against a manometer to a given pressure and then exhales as these maneuvers may be required to "open" the PFO.

There are two procedures for carrying out an Echocardiogram with opinion divided as to which is the most effective. The first procedure is known as a Transesophageal Echocardiogram (TEE). With this procedure, an ultrasound probe is placed in the mouth and down the back of the throat. The ultrasound probe is then effectively looking out from inside the chest cavity. This test can be uncomfortable and a mild sedative is often used to relive the discomfort. The second type of Echocardiogram is known as a Trans-Thoracic Echocardiogram (TTE). In this procedure, the ultrasonic probe is passed over the patient's chest and is effectively looking in from outside the chest cavity.

The second method of detecting a PFO is by using Transcranial Doppler (TCD). A small ultrasound probe is placed on the temple just above the ear. Ultrasound waves locate the flow of blood in the arteries of the head. An intravenous connector is placed in the arm and a saline solution (sterile salt water) is injected. The saline solution is filled with tiny dissolved microbubbles. If there is no PFO, all the microbubbles are filtered by the lungs and no change is seen in the tracing of the blood flow. If there is a PFO, some of the microbubbles pass (unfiltered by the lungs) through the PFO and travel to the arteries in the head. The ultrasound waves are strongly reflected by even the smallest bubbles and are detected by the probe. They are displayed as sharp color lines on the display tracing. In the same way as for a TEE test the injection is repeated while the patient takes a deep breath, blows against a manometer to a given pressure and then exhales in order to "open" the PFO.

Studies vary but PFO incidence is generally given as 25% with Valsalva maneuver and 10% without any Valsalva maneuver, ie continuously open. This implies that 25% of divers will have a PFO. This doesn’t mean that they will automatically get DCS. Many divers with a PFO dive without ever getting DCS and others may carry out thousands of dives over a number of years before getting DCS. Clearly there is a link between PFO and DCS but it is not necessarily a simple relationship.

A PFO is only a risk if the venous system contains bubbles. Recreational sports divers following conservative profiles generate relatively few bubbles. Divers who push their bottom times close to the no-stop limits are at risk of generating more bubbles. Dives which require mandatory decompression stops can create even more bubbles. These bubbles cause no problems for most divers but are of significant risk to the diver with a PFO.

In 1998 Dr. Alfred Bove calculated the risk of a diver with a PFO developing DCS. This was based on data from 393 divers who had been screened for PFO. Of these 393 divers, 151 had suffered DCI (65/151 or 43% had a PFO). Dr. Bove determined that the risk of DCS was 1.9 times greater in a diver who had a PFO and the risk of type II DCS was 2.5 times greater than the expected incidence. He concluded that the risk of DCS in a diver who had a PFO was still too low to justify screening divers for PFO.

If a diver is diagnosed with a PFO then they may still be allowed to dive but under strict depth limitations designed to reduce the risk of further DCS incidents. Closure of the PFO is now possible without resorting to open heart surgery. A small umbrella like device known as a PFO Occluder is compressed inside a small catheter, placed at the desired location in the heart, and then opened, effectively sealing the hole. The procedure can be done with mild sedation and local anesthesia and usually takes about 30 minutes to complete. Once the PFO has been closed then the diver has no more risk of experiencing DCS than any other diver. Although this closure method is relatively safe and effective it is by no means risk free. Research by Moon and Bove has highlighted a number of cases where the treatment has lead to a number of serious health problems.

Lung Shunts

The fine capillary network of the lungs acts as an effective filter which traps intravascular bubbles. This prevents the bubbles being carried to key tissues by the arterial system. This is shown in Figure 45. The deoxygenated blood, shown as black, is carried to the lungs where it enters the fine capillaries surrounding the alveoli. As the capillaries become finer and finer the bubbles carried in the blood become trapped and are effectively filtered out. The oxygenated blood, shown as grey, which returns to the heart, is free of bubbles.

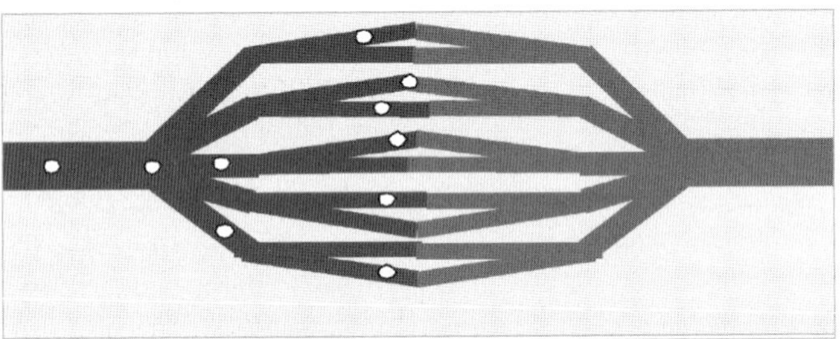

Figure 45: *Microbubbles being filtered in the capillaries of the lungs*

We have seen above that a PFO allows a potential bypass of this system by allowing blood to pass from one side of the heart to the other without first being sent to the lungs to be filtered. A pulmonary or lung shunt can result in a very similar situation. A lung shunt provides a route for the blood from the tissues to travel through the lungs without going through the fine capillaries. Without the filtering action of the capillaries the bubbles in the blood are allowed to return to the heart via the pulmonary vein where they are then pumped back out to the rest of the body. This is shown in Figure 46 where the lung shunt, represented by the larger blood vessel running through the middle of the capillary bed allows bubbles to pass through the lungs and return to the heart.

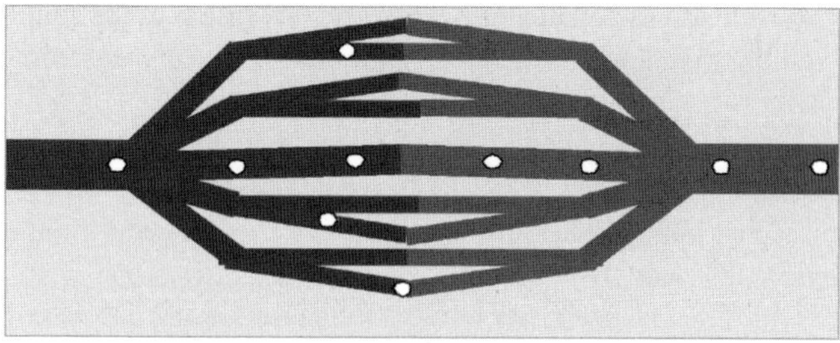

Figure 46: *A lung shunt allows bubbles to pass through the capillary network of the lungs and return to the heart*

The location of the bypass differs from a PFO and a lung shunt but the effect is exactly the same. Bubbles are not filtered out and are allowed to pass back into the arterial system where they can subsequently lodge in arteries supplying the brain and other key tissues.

Doppler Bubble Detection

Doppler bubble detection is a method where ultrasound is used to detect the presence of bubbles within the body. It uses the same phenomena that is used in police speed guns, astronomy and causes the shift in pitch when a train or ambulance goes past you. It was originally discovered by and named after the Austrian mathematician and physicist, Christian Doppler (1803-53).

The change in pitch results from a shift in the frequency of the sound waves. In the case of the change in pitch of an ambulance, as the ambulance approaches, the sound waves from its siren are compressed towards the observer. The intervals between waves gets shorter, which translates into an increase in frequency or pitch. As the ambulance recedes, the sound waves are stretched relative to the observer, causing the siren's pitch to decrease. By the change in pitch of the siren, you can determine if the ambulance is coming nearer or speeding away. If you could measure the **rate** of change of pitch, you could also estimate the ambulance's speed.

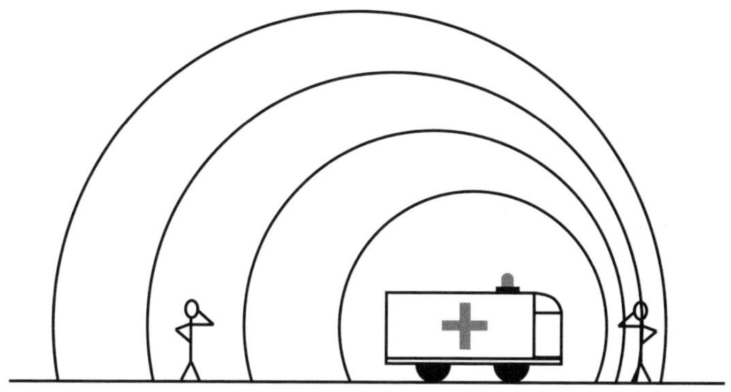

Figure 43: *The Doppler effect illustrated by an ambulance moving from left to right*

The effect can also be heard as a car speeds pasts you. The pitch of the sound is higher as it moves towards you but then drops as it passes and starts to move away from you.

Ultrasound systems use high frequency sound waves which are scattered and shifted in frequency by various moving parts of the body. Typically it is the blood cells in the body which scatter the signal but bubbles are very effective in scattering the ultrasound signal compared to blood cells, and so if bubbles are present in the blood stream a distinctive signal is returned which can be used to determine the presence and number of bubbles in the bloodstream.

The Doppler system uses headphones to listen to the blood flow. It sounds as though you were placing a microphone over the blood vessel but it is actually the ultrasound transducers that are placed on the body. The transducers are usually placed over the heart (known as the precordial region). Ideally the transducer is placed over the right ventricle, which is the lower right hand chamber where blood is pumped from the heart back to the lungs. Alternatively the transducer can be placed over the pulmonary artery. The veins in the shoulder, known as the subclavian veins, where blood from the arms and upper body return to the heart can also be used although these are not representative of blood flow in the whole body.

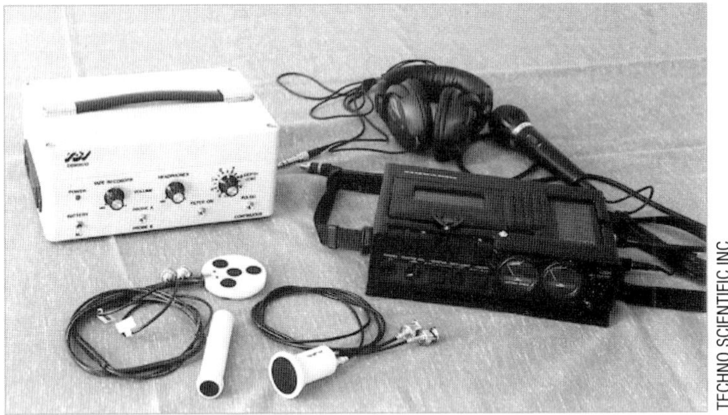

TECHNO SCIENTIFIC INC

Figure 44: *Doppler bubble detector.*

The flow sound is actually the Doppler-shifted ultrasound. The Doppler frequency shifts are typically in the audio range 2-100 kHz, which means that the signal can easily by monitored directly by human observers listening to the output. When gas bubbles are present, you hear what sounds like little "clicks" or "pops." Unfortunately these "bubble sounds" are not as always as distinguishable as one might hope for in the circulation near the heart as the flow of blood in each cardiac cycle (heart beat) also produces significant Doppler signals, and thus bubble detection requires significant training and experience.

Doppler bubbles testing was first used to detect bubbles caused by decompression in 1968. Dr Merrill Spencer and S.D. Campbell detected bubbles in sheep that had performed chamber dives to a depth of 60m/200ft. The following year the same technology was used to detect bubbles in humans after decompression. The first method to classify Doppler bubbles was developed by Dr Spencer. He graded the bubbles on a scale from 0 to 4 based on the number of bubbles detected in each cardiac cycle. This system is known as the Spencer scale.

Grade	Description
0	A complete lack of bubble signals
I	An occasional bubble signal discernable within the cardiac motion signal, with the great majority of cardiac periods free of bubbles
II	Many, but still less than half, of the cardiac periods contain bubble signals, singly or in groups.
III	All of the cardiac periods contain showers of single-bubble signals, but not dominating or overriding the cardiac motion signal.
IV	The maximum detectable bubble signal, sounding continuously throughout the systole and diastole of every cardiac period, and overriding the amplitude of the normal cardiac signals.

Table 12: *The Spencer scale for grading bubbles*

A variation of this code for laboratory studies with animals was developed by Dr Michael Powell with grade IVa (intense but discrete), grade IVb (numerous but not discrete) and grade V (flow sound louder than cardiac motion sounds).

An alternative method of classifying bubbles was developed, originally for computer grading by Kisman and Masurel and is known as the KM code. This system separates the bubble signal into three components; frequency, percentage of cardiac cycles with bubbles/duration of bubbles and amplitude. Each of these three components is graded on a scale of 0 to 4 with the results combined to give a global bubble grade from 0 – 4 similar to the Spencer system. Unlike the Spencer system the grades are further subdivided to give a greater granularity of values. For example grade 1 is further subdivided into 1-, 1, 1+. The advantage of the KM code is that it allows for greater scope for classifying bubble signals. Although it may appear more complicated than the Spencer code it is considered to be easier to learn because classification of the bubble signals is done in a step by step manner.

Doppler bubble detection may seem an ideal tool for investigating decompression illness. Unfortunately this approach has a number of drawbacks. There is no direct evidence of a link between the number of bubbles found using this method and the occurrence of DCS. Divers can have large numbers of bubbles detected and yet show no signs or symptoms of DSC. Similarly divers can suffer serious bends and get have a very low or even zero score the on the Doppler bubble scale. The reason for this discrepancy is that the Doppler system does not detect the same type of bubbles that are believed to cause DCS. The Doppler system detects moving bubbles in the blood stream but DCS is believed to be caused by stationary bubbles in the tissues or in the capillary beds. In addition the sites used to detect bubbles are all at points in the circulatory system prior to the lungs; in the veins leading to the heart, in the right hand side of the heart or in the pulmonary artery leading from the heart to the lungs. It is believed that bubbles in this area are not responsible for DCS as they are filtered out of the blood when it reaches the lungs. For all of these reasons it is impossible to extrapolate directly from the Doppler bubble codes to a likelihood of DCS.

Despite there being no direct correlation between Doppler bubble scores and incidences of DCS it has been assumed that the presence of bubbles in the venous blood is at least indicative of bubbles in other areas. The term decompression stress has been used to indicate a level of bubble formation that is not directly related to an incidence of decompression illness. For this reason Doppler detection is still used as a tool for assessing the likelihood of decompression illness. Doppler testing in the 1970's resulted in a reduction in no-decompression limits for a range of tables including the US Navy tables. This testing showed a high level of bubbles in divers who were diving to the edge of the tables and as a result the no stop times were made more conservative. More recent research has also used Doppler testing as a proxy for quantifying decompression risk.

Medical implications of DCI

When a bubble of inert gas forms in the body as a result of DCI it can block blood vessels and starve surrounding tissues of oxygen. It can also press on nerves and cause damage to the nerves and other tissues. These are the purely mechanical effects of a bubble trapped within a closed system and are analogous to an air lock within your central heating system. In addition to these mechanical effects there are a number of other side effects which contribute to DCI that are caused by the body's reaction to the bubble.

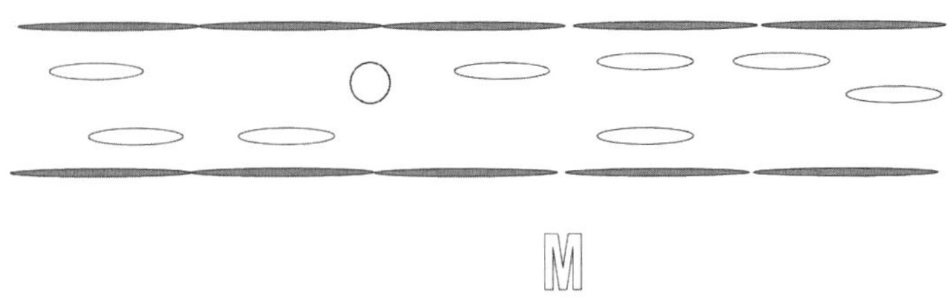

Figure 45: *Initial situation on bubble formation*

Bubbles that form in a blood vessel will attract blood proteins. Contact with the bubble will change the protein in a process known as denaturation. This means a change in the shape of the molecule and usually this means reduced solubility. The changes also trigger the body's immune system as the denatured proteins are now considered a foreign substance. The immune system sends white blood cells to the location to attack the foreign body.

Mast cells, which normally live in the surrounding tissues, are also sent into the blood vessel where they release histamines. Histamines cause inflammation of the area and also dilate the blood vessel to increase blood flow. They also cause the walls of the blood vessel to become 'sticky'. This is so that the white blood cells which have surrounded the foreign body can stick to the walls of the capillary in a process known as margination.

Margination also causes the cells in the wall of the blood vessel, known as the endothelium cells, to start to separate from each other which allows fluids, white blood cells and parts of the foreign body to leak from the blood vessel into the surrounding tissues. The reduction in fluid from the blood vessels can cause sludging of the red blood cells and can also cause shock.

Separation of the endothelium cells is viewed by the body as damage and so platelets are sent to the damaged areas. They combine with collagen to form a clot around the damaged areas. Platelets also release serotonin which constricts the blood vessel in order to reduce blood flow and loss of fluids. Combined with the white blood cells clumped around the foreign body and the sludging of the blood this tends to cause further blockage of the blood vessel as well as further swelling and inflammation.

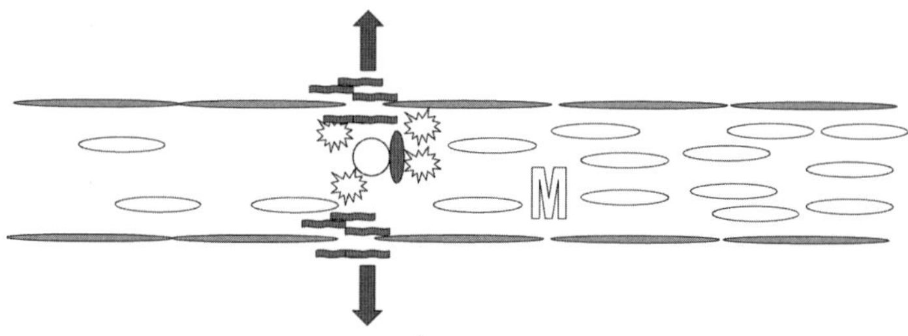

Figure 46: *The body's reaction to a bubble*

If bubbles get into the lymph system they can end up anywhere in the body. If they get into the nerve tissues they can cause permanent nerve damage and if they get through one of the capillaries on the blood-brain barrier this can result in focal swelling and the cerebral features of DCS.

Blood chemistry changes as described above do not happen instantaneously. They can take some time. Recompression within 2 hours to reduce the size and number of bubbles can help to reduce the blood chemistry changes and prevent long term tissue damage.

First Aid

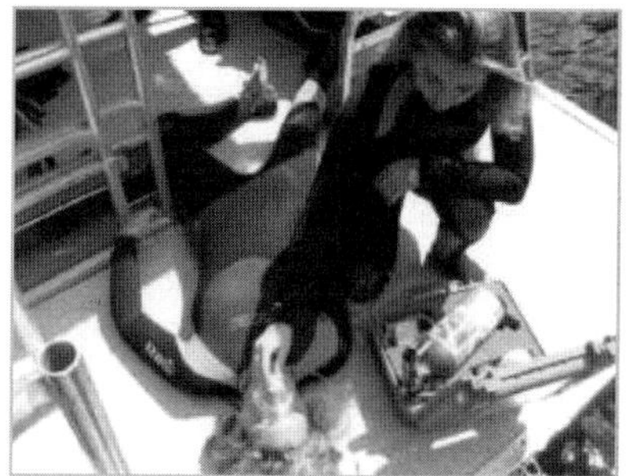

If a diver suffers from decompression illness (DCI), whether DCS or AGE, there is a well defined first aid treatment. First ensure that there is no danger to the casualty or the rescuers. If immediate danger is still present then remove the danger or remove the casualty from the danger. This will normally mean getting the casualty onto shore or a boat as there is little we can do while in the water. The ABC of first aid is always the priority. **A**irway, **B**reathing and **C**irculation should be checked and responded to as appropriate. Casualties suspected of suffering from DCI should be laid down, kept warm, administered still fluids and most importantly given Oxygen. The casualty should then be evacuated to specialist medical care as soon as possible. Whether the casualty is suffering from DCS or AGE is largely irrelevant as the signs, symptoms, first aid and need for immediate specialist medical care are identical in both cases.

A casualty suspected of suffering from DCI should be laid down in the horizontal position and not allowed to sit-up or stand. This is for a number of reasons. If the causalty is suffering problems with balance or paralasis then if they are standing up or walking around on a moving boat they may end up falling and causing further injuries. The other reason is that standing up may allow bubbles to travel from the left ventricle and aorta to the brain. Although this sitaution is rare the result can be very serious and so is considered a worthwhile precaution.

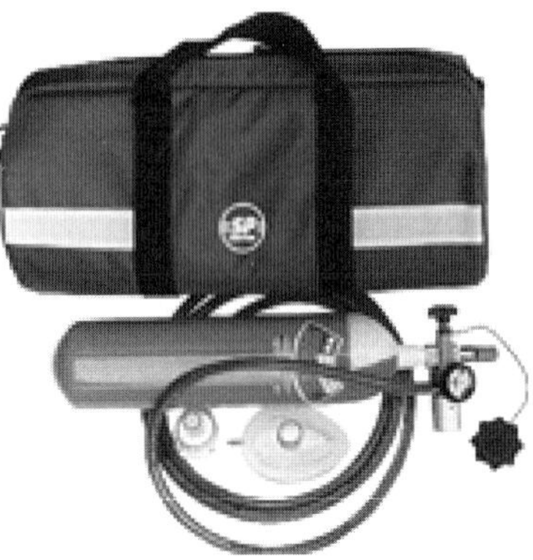

A horizontal position should be maintained until the injured diver begins recompression treatment or is cleared by a hyperbaric doctor. A head-down and legs raised position (the Trendelenburg position) is no longer advised as it may increase the risk of bubbles traveling to the arterial side of the circulation. It also makes it more difficult to perform resuscitation and assessment if required and in animal-model studies it was found to be less effective in promoting the recovery of brain function than the horizontal posture.

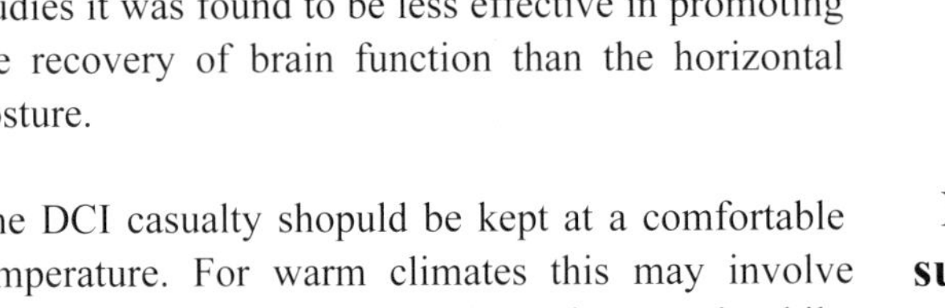

Never give Entonox to suspected DCI casualties

The DCI casualty shopuld be kept at a comfortable temperature. For warm climates this may involve keeping them in the shade to keep them cool, whilst in colder climates this may involve moving them out of the wind or using a blanket to keep them warm.

If the diver is conscious and doesn't feel nauseous then they should rehydrate with non alcoholic still fluids at a rate of 1 litre each hour. Tea and coffe should be avoided and still water is the best option.

Entonox is an anesthetic gas often called "gas and air". It is widely carried by paramedics and is a mild but effective painkiller. Entonox is a gas made up of 50 per cent oxygen and 50 per cent nitrous oxide. Despite the fact that it contains 50% Oxygen, Entonox should never be administered to casualties suspected of suffering from decompression illness or gas embolism. The nitrous oxide in Entonox worsens symptoms of both conditions by increasing bubble size. This occurs because Nitrous Oxide is a very fast diffusing molecule. As it is absorbed into the blood stream and travels around the tissues, it will diffuse into the bubbles formed in the blood or tissues. This causes the bubbles to grow and so quickly increases any symptoms of DCI. As a result, rather than acting as a painkiller it can in fact worsen the symptoms of decompression illness.

Oxygen

By far the most effective first aid treatment we can give a diver suspected of DCI is to provide 100% Oxygen. The prompt administration of Oxygen can, in some cases, prevent the onset of decompression; reduce the symptoms of mild decompression or reduce the impact of serous decompression. In all cases the use of Oxygen in cases of decompression illness or arterial gas embolism can only help.

Oxygen helps in a number of ways. Firstly by reducing the amount of Nitrogen in the gas we are breathing this accelerates the speed at which Nitrogen is off-gassed from the body. Secondly breathing pure Oxygen can reduce the size of bubbles that have been formed and finally the increased amount of Oxygen in the bloodstream helps to offset the damage caused by bubbles blocking the capillaries and preventing Oxygen reaching the tissues. Each of these advantages are described in more detail below.

If we are in a state of critical supersaturation, i.e. the difference between the pressure of the inert gas in our bodies and the ambient pressure is greater then the allowed supersaturation ratio or M-Value, bubbles will start to form within the body. However, bubbles do not always form immediately in these situations. If we can reduce the level of inert gas pressure in the tissues then we may be able to prevent bubbles forming or at least prevent additional bubbles from forming. When we breathe pure Oxygen we reduce the amount of Nitrogen being inhaled to 0%. This has the effect of maximising the inert gas gradient between the pressure of Nitrogen in the tissues and the pressure of Nitrogen in our inspired gas. The rate of off-gassing is determined by this inert gas gradient, and so by increasing the gradient to its maximum level, we will maximise the rate at which Nitrogen is off-gassed from the body. If Nitrogen is off-gassing faster then the tissue will get to the point where it is no longer in a state of critical supersaturation faster. This may mean that fewer bubbles are formed.
A related benefit to this is that high levels of Oxygen in our inspired gas will result in much lower levels of Nitrogen in the blood stream and surrounding tissues. This will cause Nitrogen in bubbles that have formed in the bloodstream and tissues to diffuse out of the bubbles and back into the blood or surrounding tissues. However there is a downside to this effect in that initially Oxygen may diffuse into the bubbles and may cause the bubbles to increase in size. This may result in the symptoms initially becoming worse. It is important not to suspend treatment at this point but to continue administering oxygen.

The final benefit of the use of Oxygen is in providing additional Oxygen to the tissues surrounding the site of a bubble. The previous advantages have been based on the physical results of lowering the inert gas gradient. The fact that the gas in use was Oxygen was of secondary importance, we were primarily interested in the fact that it was not an inert gas. However this final benefit is derived from the biological results of getting Oxygen to tissues that are 'downstream' of a bubble.

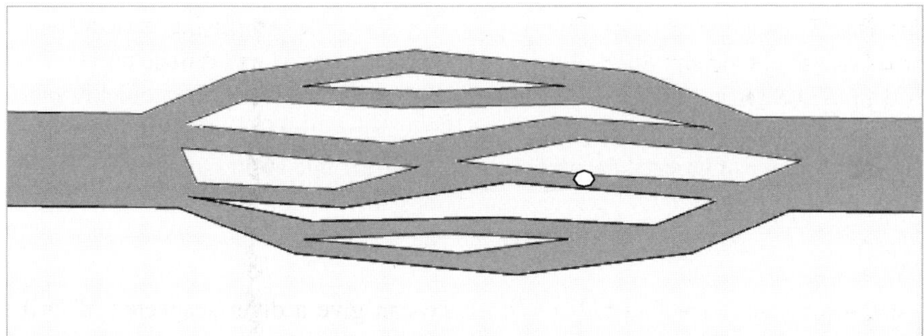

Figure 48: *Bubble in capillary bed*

If a bubble forms in a capillary bed as shown in Figure 48 the tissues beyond that point within that capillary will receive a reduced blood flow and will become starved of Oxygen. This can cause additional damage over and above any pressure damage caused by the bubble.
If pure Oxygen is administered then in addition to carrying Oxygen bound to haemoglobin the blood will also carry Oxygen dissolved in solution. The dissolved Oxygen in capillaries surrounding the blocked capillary can diffuse through neighbouring tissues to allow the blocked tissues to receive Oxygen. An increase in Oxygen partial pressure causes oxygen to diffuse further from the active capillaries. When breathing air at normal atmospheric pressure,

Oxygen diffuses about 64 micrometers from the capillary; this is about the thickness of a sheet of paper. Tissue oxygen content depends on 3 factors:

1. Distance from the functioning capillaries
2. Oxygen demand of the tissue
3. The oxygen tension of the capillary

During oxygen breathing at 3 ATA, oxygen diffuses about 250 micrometers (about the thickness of 3 sheets of paper).

If no Oxygen is available or your Oxygen runs out before the casualty can be evacuated then the next best option is to use the richest decompression mix that is available. The richest mix will give the most benefit but any Nitrox mix is going to provide a benefit when compared to the casualty breathing normal air. Any mixture which provides an increased percentage of Oxygen will increase the inert gas gradient and allow inert gas to off-gas faster. It will also provide an increased level of Oxygen to tissues that may be starved of Oxygen.

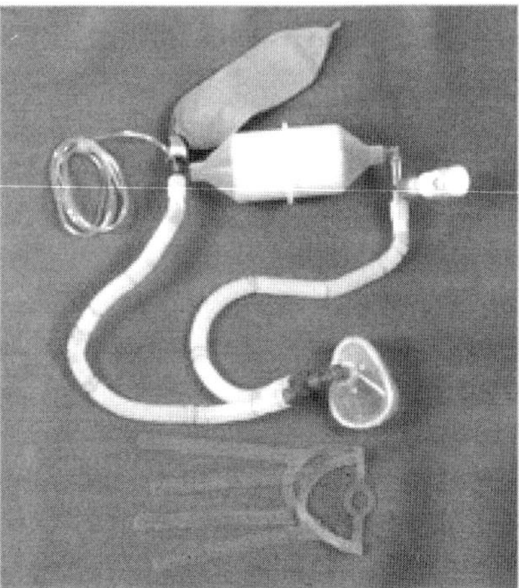

Figure 49: *A rebreather kit suitable for use with a surface Oxygen therapy kit*

A rebreather can be used to prolonging your supply of Oxygen as it will recycle the Oxygen breathed out by the casualty. With the increasing popularity of rebreathers for technical and also recreational diving this is now becoming a practical option in the case of suspected DCI. DAN now produces a medical Oxygen rebreather which is designed for surface use only. The unit can be attached to a medical Oxygen kit to allow the carbon dioxide to be scrubbed from the casualty's breath while allowing the Oxygen to be re-circulated. This can extend the life of an Oxygen cylinder by up to eight times.

Whatever the source of Oxygen, be it a first aid Oxygen kit, decompression gas or a rebreather, the key point is to provide Oxygen as soon as possible for as long as possible. Providing Oxygen will never make a situation worse and can only help the casualty.

Patients with Type I or mild Type II DCS can have dramatic improvement when Oxygen is administered and may appear to have a complete recovery. However, the casualty should still be referred to a hyperbaric expert as this may only be a temporary recovery and symptoms may return if not fully treated.

5 Minute Neurological Exam

If you are ever in the situation where you suspect someone may have a bend then the 5 minute neurological exam is designed to spot any potential problems and also take a baseline of their condition should they need treatment.

Information regarding the injured diver's neurological status will be useful to the chamber in not only deciding the initial course of treatment but also in the effectiveness of treatment.

The 5 Minute Neurological Exam is easy to learn and can be done by individuals with no medical experience. Perform as much of the exam as possible, but do not let it interfere with evacuation to medical treatment.

Perform the following steps in order, and record the time and results.

1. Orientation

- Does the diver know his/her own name and age?
- Does the diver know the present location?
- Does the diver know what time, day, year it is?

Note: Even though a diver appears alert, the answers to these questions may reveal confusion. Do not omit them.

2. Eyes

- Have the diver count the number of fingers you display, using two or three different numbers.
- Check each eye separately and then together.
- Have the diver identify a distant object.
- Tell the diver to hold head still, or you gently hold it still, while placing your other hand about 18 inches/0.5 meters in front of the face. Ask the diver to follow your hand. Now move your hand up and down, then side to side. The diver's eyes should follow your hand and should not jerk to one side and return.
- Check that the pupils are equal in size.

3. Face

- Ask the diver to purse their lips. Look carefully to see that both sides of the face have the same expression.
- Ask the diver to grit the teeth. Feel the jaw muscles to confirm that they are contracted equally.
- Instruct the diver to close the eyes while you lightly touch your fingertips across the forehead and face to be sure sensation is present and the same everywhere.

4. Hearing

- Hearing can be evaluated by holding your hand about 2 feet/0.6 meters from the diver's ear and rubbing your thumb and finger together.
- Check both ears moving your hand closer until the diver hears it.
- Check several times and compare with your own hearing.

Note: If the surroundings are noisy, the test is difficult to evaluate. Ask bystanders to be quiet and to turn off unneeded machinery.

5. Swallowing Reflex

- Instruct the diver to swallow while you watch the "Adam's apple" to be sure it moves up and down.

6. Tongue

- Instruct the diver to stick out the tongue. It should come out straight in the middle of the mouth without deviating to either side.

7. Muscle Strength

- Instruct the diver to shrug shoulders while you bear down on them to observe for equal muscle strength.
- Check diver's arms by bringing the elbows up level with the shoulders, hands level with the arms and touching the chest. Instruct the diver to resist while you pull the arms away, push them back, up and down. The strength should be approximately equal in both arms in each direction.
- Check leg strength by having the diver lie flat and raise and lower the legs while you resist the movement.

8. Sensory Perception

- Check on both sides by touching lightly as was done on the face. Start at the top of the body and compare sides while moving downwards to cover the entire body.

Note: The diver's eyes should be closed during this procedure. The diver should confirm the sensation in each area before you move to another area.

9. Balance and Coordination

Note: Be prepared to protect the diver from injury when performing this test.

- First, have the diver walk heel to toe along a straight line while looking straight ahead.
- Have her walk both forward and backward for 10 feet or so. Note whether her movements are smooth and if she can maintain her balance without having to look down or hold onto something.
- Next, have the diver stand up with feet together and close eyes and hold the arms straight out in front of her with the palms up. The diver should be able to maintain balance if the platform is stable. Your arms should be around, but not touching, the diver. Be prepared to catch the diver who starts to fall.
- Check coordination by having the diver move an index finger back and forth rapidly between the diver's nose and your finger held approximately 18 inches/0.5 meters from the diver's face. The diver should be able to do this, even if you move your finger to different positions.
- Have the diver lie down and instruct him to slide the heel of one foot down the shin of his other leg, while keeping his eyes closed. The diver should be able to move his foot smoothly along his shin, without jagged, side-to-side movements.
- Check these tests on both right and left sides and observe carefully for unusual clumsiness on either side.

Important Notes:
Tests 1,7, and 9 are the most important and should be given priority if not all tests can be performed.

The diver's condition may prevent the performance of one or more of these tests. Record any omitted test and the reason. If any of the tests are not normal, injury to the central nervous system should be suspected.

The tests should be repeated at 30- to 60-minute intervals while awaiting assistance in order to determine if any change occurs. Report the results to the emergency medical personnel responding to the call.

Good diving safety habits would include practicing this examination on normal divers in order to become proficient in performing the test.

Recompression

The definitive treatment for any form of decompression illness is recompression in a hyperbaric chamber. The main purpose of this is to reduce the size of any existing bubbles.

In addition, 100% oxygen is given in order to encourage the off-gassing of nitrogen from the body. Getting a casualty suffering from decompression sickness to a hyperbaric chamber is the priority, as rapid recompression can improve the chances of a complete recovery. Any delays in recompression will reduce the chances of a full recovery.

Hyperbaric recompression treatment has had a controversial history. It began in 1662, when Henshaw, a British doctor and clergyman, used it to treat respiratory ailments. His first chamber was called the "Domicilium". Ambient pressure in the chamber was either raised or lowered with organ bellows. The idea of the circulatory system was not in common usage so Henshaw believed that recompression would "cool the fires of the heart". Many spas opened up all around European spas offering hyperbaric facilities and promising all sorts of wondrous cures. After the discovery of oxygen, these spas began enriching the air with oxygen and many more benefits were claimed, but none of these claims were based on any scientific basis.

Modern hyperbaric oxygen therapy is based on the work of physicians and researchers who dealt with compressed air workers and divers in the mid 1800's. As we saw in Chapter 1, no one initially understood the connection between Caisson's disease and the pressure and amount of time spent in the Caisson but physicians Pol and Watelle returned the victims of the disease to pressure within the caisson and found that this alleviated their symptoms.

At the end of the 18th century, Paul Bert, the French physiologist presented his many discoveries about atmospheric pressure effects. One of these was the discovery that oxygen was poisonous at high pressure. This served to throw the whole idea of hyperbaric oxygen therapy into disrepute. As a result, virtually all the hyperbaric facilities at spas disappeared. The use of air or oxygen at increased pressure was actually banned by medical organisations. This was not what Bert had intended. He had also studied Caissons disease and, as we have seen, concluded it was due to Nitrogen bubbles caused by rapid decompression. Bert actually suggested the use of oxygen for decompression and for the treatment of the disease.

Despite the general medical ban on hyperbaric treatments, some individuals continued to champion their use, including an American physician named Orval Cunningham. In 1918 Cunningham was professor of anaesthesiology at Kansas University Medical School in Kansas City. After getting approval from the medical school to carry out experiments on animals, he started treating patients with pneumonia from the 1918-1919 influenza

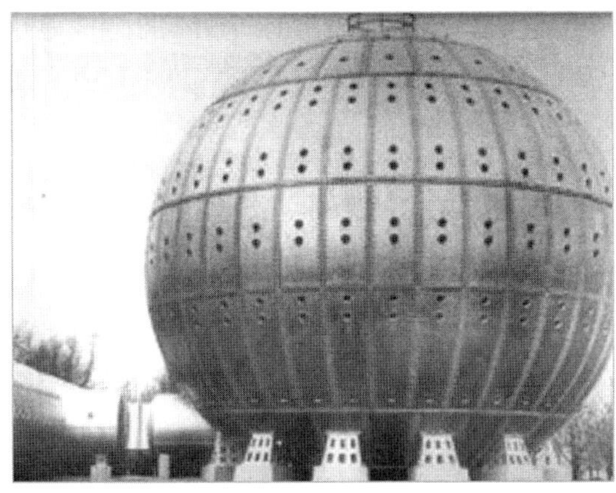

pandemic. Cunningham successfully treated many of these patients with hyperbaric air. His first chamber was based on the design of a caisson chamber. It was 10 feet in diameter and 30 feet long. With his initial success, he raised funds and built a second chamber. This was 10 feet in diameter and 80 feet long. The 36 patients it could house could move about freely and use the toilet and shower facilities inside. In 1923 the interior of the chamber caught fire. This was due to the open gas burners used to heat the chambers. Fortunately, no one was injured. The chamber was repaired and the heating system altered. Cunningham had so many patients that he had to buy a house to accommodate them, and soon after built an additional chamber.

After Cunningham treated ball-bearing king (of Timken Roller Bearings) Henry Timken, Timken offered to build Cunningham a multi-story hyperbaric hospital. This was built in Cleveland, Ohio and was in the shape of a sphere, 64 feet in diameter with 5 floors. The hospital was an impressive facility with 36 double bedrooms, a dining room on the ground floor and a game and recreation room on the top floor.

Cunningham's career began to falter in 1925. Kansas University asked him to resign due to concerns that he was spending his time promoting his hyperbaric treatments and an investigation into his treatments by the American Medical Association concluded that there was no evidence to support his claims. By this time the Cleveland chamber sponsored by Henry Timkin had been completed and, in 1928, Cunningham closed down the Kansas chambers and moved to Cleveland. Initially the chamber flourished but the economic crash of 1929 meant that many patients could no longer afford treatment. Cunningham's health was also failing so he turned the day-to-day operations of the hospital over to his assistant. One year later the hospital was closed and in 1937 Cunningham died. The steel sphere remained unused for several years until it was dismantled in 1942 in order for the scrap material to be used in the war effort.

Distinguished decompression researcher Dr. Albert Behnke performed a number of experiments in the 1930s using oxygen to increase the efficiency of decompression for divers and also to treat decompression sickness. He found that the toxic effects of oxygen were related to the pressure and length of exposure. A subject could be given oxygen at high pressure for an 'envelope' of pressure and time. At the same time Dr. Edgar End in Milwaukee,Wisconsin treated carbon monoxide poisoning victims with hyperbaric oxygen therapy with good results. It took over 20 years before this work was widely recognised. During the Second World War, there was little work carried out on hyperbaric research. However, considerable work on oxygen toxicity was done , redefining the pressure and time doses that were likely to cause Oxygen toxicity.

The growing popularity of SCUBA equipment in the 1950s together with the Navy and commercial diving use of SCUBA prompted a renewal in research into hyperbaric treatment.

Modern chambers can be classified into two types. Recompression chambers are used to treat diving injuries such as decompression sickness and arterial gas embolism as well as various other medical conditions. Decompression chambers are used to complete surface decompression so that divers can be removed from the water and complete decompression in the safe, dry conditions of a deck mounted decompression chamber. Both types of chamber can be referred to as a hyperbaric chamber as they work on the basis of increasing the pressure in the chamber to a level higher than normal atmospheric pressure. The pressure can be expressed as a depth corresponding to a depth of water. So for example chamber operators may talk of blowing the chamber down to 10m. This just means that they are increasing the pressure in the chamber to 2 Bar which is equivalent to the ambient pressure at 10m.

There are several types of hyperbaric recompression chambers, which range from small monoplace (single person) chambers to complex multiple place, multiple lock-out chambers large enough for multiple patients and medical or hyperbaric attendants.

Monoplace chambers are designed for a single patient and do not allow an attendant to be present during the treatment. The patient is placed in the chamber and is alone in the chamber until the treatment is completed. Monoplace chambers may be portable and can be used in remote locations where there is no access to a larger chamber.
Larger, multi place chambers allow more than one person in the chamber. Multiple lock chambers contain two or more pressured compartments with sealed hatches between each chamber. These chambers provide more facilities for treatment. A multi place chamber can allow up to 12 patients plus a medical attendant. This is important if there is more than one casualty or if the casualty has a serious condition and needs medical attention in addition to hyperbaric recompression. A multi lock chamber allows each compartment to be pressurised separately, like an air lock in a space craft or submarine. This allows medical staff or additional casualties to enter the chamber as the outer chamber can be depressurised to allow entry into the outer chamber then pressurised to the same pressure as the inner chamber thus allowing the medical staff or casualty to enter the inner chamber.

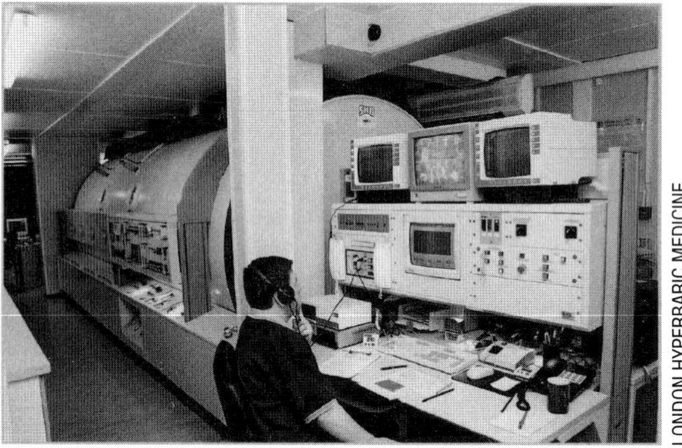

LONDON HYPERBARIC MEDICINE

Whilst in the chamber the patient will be breathing pure Oxygen to aid treatment. In order to avoid the pressure of Oxygen in the chamber rising to levels where it may cause a fire hazard the patient will breathe though a Built-In Breathing System (BIBS). This is a face mask which provides pure Oxygen to the patient and also removes the Oxygen rich exhaled breath to be released outside of the chamber. If the casualty were to breath out into the chamber then over time the Oxygen rich mixture being breathed out would cause the Oxygen pressure in the chamber to rise to dangerous levels and to become a fire risk. Even with the BIBS system some Oxygen will leak out of the mask and the Oxygen pressure will slowly creep up. The chamber operators will monitor the Oxygen pressure in the chamber and if it reaches a certain level they will flush the chamber with air to reduce the Oxygen pressure.

The combination of recompression to depth combined with breathing Oxygen at high pressure is known as Hyperbaric Oxygen therapy (HBO). The basic theory behind HBO therapy is to first recompress the patient to a depth where the bubbles from nitrogen or air are compressed and subsequently re-dissolved back into the body tissues and fluids. Then, by breathing higher concentrations of oxygen, a larger diffusion gradient is established allowing a faster rate of off-gassing. The patient is slowly brought back to atmospheric pressure, which combined with the Oxygen, allows the dissolved inert gases to diffuse gradually out of the lungs and body without reforming bubbles.

Finally the higher pressure of Oxygen affects the way that the Oxygen is carried by the blood and allows more effective supply of it to damaged tissues. Oxygen is carried in the blood by two distinct methods: Bio-chemically bound to haemoglobin, and physically dissolved in plasma, the liquid part of blood. At sea level with a pressure of 1 ATA and an Oxygen partial pressure of 0.21 Bar haemoglobin is already 97% saturated with Oxygen. Oxygen dissolved in the plasma of the blood does not play a big part in Oxygen transport at this pressure, only 1.5% of the Oxygen being carried at sea level is dissolved in the plasma.

As the haemoglobin is already 97% saturated with Oxygen it only takes a slight increase in the partial pressure of Oxygen for the haemoglobin to become completely saturated. Once this happens it cannot bind with any more Oxygen and any additional Oxygen can only be carried dissolved in the plasma. As the partial pressure of Oxygen is increased past this saturation point the amount of Oxygen carried by the blood is determined by Henry's law. This means that the amount of Oxygen dissolved in the blood increases linearly as the partial pressure increases.

The dissolved Oxygen in the plasma can help to supply tissues blocked by gas bubbles as the Oxygen can diffuse from the blood into surrounding tissues thus helping to maintain a supply to the tissues.

When a patient arrives at a hyperbaric facility the attending doctor will assess their condition and determine the best course of treatment. They will administer intravenous fluids for re-hydration and perform a neurological exam. This does not give a definitive diagnosis as there may be other factors which are causing the symptoms, however if there is any signs or symptoms that may be attributable to decompression illness the doctor will almost certainly recommend recompression. Recompression is the only definite way to identify decompression illness. If recompression alleviates the symptoms to any extent within the first 10 minutes then this confirms decompression illness as the diagnosis. This is known as the test of pressure. If the symptoms are not relieved then this indicates that decompression illness may not be the cause.

The exact combination of timing and depths used to treat a patient will be determined by the hyperbaric doctor. There are a number of standard recompression tables which are used depending on the seriousness of the incident. These were developed primarily by the British and American Military. The best known treatment tables ere developed by the US Navy with some minor modifications by the US Air Force. The US Navy developed a range of standard treatment tables designed for use after dives to varying depths and designed to treat various conditions. The most commonly used tables are Table 5 and Table 6. Table 5 involves a two hour fifteen minute treatment at 18m/60fsw. This was intended for less serious, pain only bends. However as it became clear that pain-only bends frequently masked or distracted from the more severe but less obvious neurological bends it has become more common for chamber operators to go directly to Table 6 treatments. Table 6 involves a four hour forty five minute treatment at 18m/60fsw. During the treatment the patient breathes Oxygen for a given period (shown in green in Figure 50) followed by five minutes breathing air (shown in blue) before returning to breathing Oxygen. These 'Air breaks' are introduced in order to reduce the risks of the casualty developing symptoms of Oxygen toxicity.

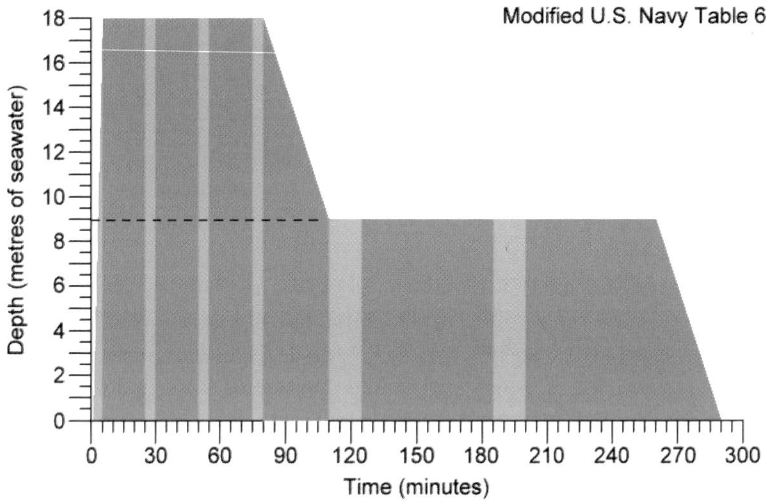

Figure 50: *US Navy Treatment Table 6*

In the UK some hyperbaric facilities will also make use of tables devised by the Royal Navy. The most common Royal Navy table is called Table 62. This is similar to the US Navy Table 6 and involves a four and a half hour treatment at 18m/60fsw.

The treatment for deeper dives is still often to use Table 6. This is primarily due to the greatly increased risk of Oxygen toxicity if the patient is breathing Oxygen at depths in excess of 18m/60fsw. The increased pressure of a recompression deeper than this must be balanced against the need to use a gas other than pure Oxygen. Table 6 is also the common choice for hyperbaric therapy following Trimix dives. As the Helium in Trimix is a fast gas this means that in the majority of cases the Helium has already off-gassed from the body and it is the slower Nitrogen that is causing the decompression illness.

For cases where the hyperbaric doctor decides that recompression to a greater depth is required there are again a number of treatment tables available. US Navy Treatment Tables 6a, 8 or 9 or Royal Navy Treatment Table 63 are all designed to treat decompression sickness following deep dives or dives with significant missed decompression obligations. However, the most common treatment for this type of situation is the Comex 30 table.

This treatment involves the patent breathing a mixture of 50% Oxygen and 50% Helium while being recompressed to 30m/100fsw. The patient is then kept at this depth for an hour before beginning a slow ascent, taking 30 minutes, up to 24 m. They will remain at 24m for 30m minutes before beginning another 30 minute ascent up to 18m/60fsw. At this point the patient is switched to pure Oxygen and begins a treatment similar to a standard Table 6 treatment. This results in a total treatment time of seven and a half hours.

In Figure 51 the red portion represents the time spent breathing Heliox; the green portion is Oxygen and the blue portion air.

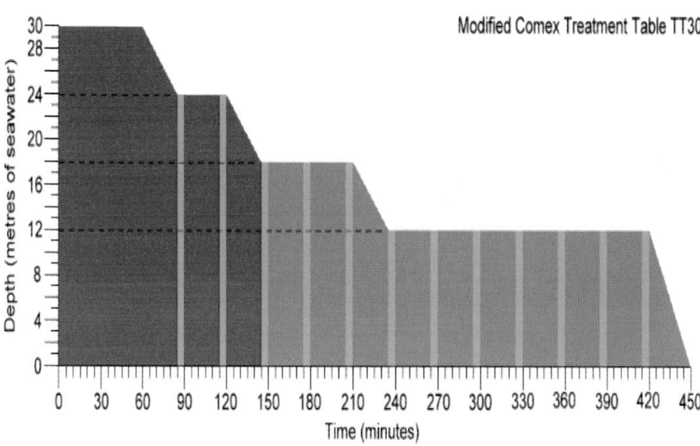

Figure 51: *Comex Heliox Treatment Table 30*

With early recognition and treatment over 75% of patients improve. However not all symptoms will be resolved on the first treatment and some symptoms may return following treatment. In this case repeat treatments will be required. Repeat treatments will continue on a daily basis until all symptoms are resolved or until treatments are producing no further improvement. These repeat treatments may involve shorter or shallower tables than the initial treatment.

In Water Recompression

In water recompression (IWR) is a highly controversial subject – one of the most controversial subjects in field which has its fair share of controversial subjects. IWR involves treating a diver who is already showing signs or symptoms of suffering from the bends by re-descending and following a treatment profile in the water rather then in a recompression chamber. In most areas of the world the practice is completely counterproductive and has serious safety consequences.

The time involved in a recompression treatment is of the order of one or more hours. This introduces a number of logistic problems into the process. For all but the most tropical regions several hours of recompression in water can result in the casualty becoming extremely cold and even hypothermic. As well as the normal dangers from hypothermia the cold will also reduce the effectiveness of the treatment as the cold will slow the rate of off-gassing from the peripheral areas of the body.

Supplying enough gas for the casualty and support diver to spend am hour or more in the water is also a challenge. The procedure will need a large number of support divers and attendants to ensure that enough gas is available. Of course if the support divers were also involved in the dives then these repeat dives may potentially put them at risk from subsequent decompression illness.

For IWR treatment to be effective, the casualty needs to be breathing pure Oxygen. This is in order to ensure the maximum inert gas gradient which will give the fastest rate of off-gassing. Pure Oxygen will also help by saturating the blood and tissues with dissolved Oxygen which will help to oxygenate the hypoxic areas caused by the bubbles in the capillary beds or tissues. Unless significant pre-planning for IWR has been carried out, there may not be sufficient supplies of Oxygen to complete the treatment. Even if enough Oxygen is available the risk of central nervous system toxicity is extremely high. In a recompression chamber a patient may breathe Oxygen at a partial pressure of 2.8 Bar for extended periods of time. However it has been shown that the body can tolerate higher partial pressures of Oxygen whilst in a warm, dry, comfortable recompression chamber then it can whilst immersed in water. For this reason the depth to which the casualty can be returned and hence the effectiveness of the recompression is reduced. If the casualty suffers a CNS toxicity hit whilst in a chamber then the treatment is simply suspended until the casualty recovers. A CNS hit underwater is much more serious and may result in drowning or other injuries unless suitable precautions have been taken.

Communications between the casualty and their support diver(s) as well as between the support divers and surface crew is very limited. In addition the facilities for additional treatment such as intravenous (IV) re-hydration are simply not possible underwater. If the casualty deteriorates whilst underwater then further treatment may be difficult. Identifying the extent and progression of symptoms whilst underwater is also difficult. Many of the tests used to detect decompression illness, such as a 5 minute neurological exam, are difficult if not impossible to perform underwater. Balance cannot be tested, touch and sensation cannot be established and it will not be possible to estimate limb strength.

The location of the dive site is also a major variable. If a convenient sandy sea bed at 9m with no current is easily available then this is ideal. However, if an incident occurs on a live aboard anchored over a deep wreck while the current is starting to turn then the conditions in the water; no convenient bottom and strong tides, introduce a number of problems into the treatment procedure.

In the UK, US and many other popular diving locations the presence of excellent emergency services and easy access to recompression chambers, combined with the logistical problems associated with IWR make this procedure completely unnecessary. For these reasons almost all diving physicians, chamber operators and training agencies maintain that IWR recompression should not be attempted. DAN's advice is clear:

"In-water recompression should never be attempted".

Whilst this is the standard advice there are times when IWR may need to be considered. If you are diving in very remote areas where the nearest recompression chamber is 24 or 48 hours away then IWR may be the only option. In situations such as these experienced divers will greatly extend their safety margin to try and ensure that they do not get into this position but despite the most cautious planning there is always the chance that an unearned decompression illness hit will occur.

To deal with these extreme cases a number of IWR protocols have been developed. In Diving and Subaquatic Medicine by Edmonds and Pennefather a method for performing IWR, which has also become known as the Australian method, is described. This involves the diver re-descending to 9m while breathing pure Oxygen. They stay at this depth for 30 minutes in the case of a mild bend or 60 minutes for a severe bend. If symptoms persist then these times can be extended to 60 and 90 minutes respectively. The patient then ascends at the rate of 1 meter every 12 minutes. This results in a total treatment time of 126 to 156 minutes for a mild case and 156 to 186 minutes for a serious case.

Depth (Metres)	Elapsed Time (minutes) Mild	Elapsed Time (minutes) Serious
9	30-60	60-90
8	42-72	72-102
7	54-84	84-114
6	66-96	96-126
5	78-108	108-138
4	90-120	120-150
3	102-132	132-162
2	114-144	144-174
1	126-156	156-186

Table 13: *Australian In Water Recompression Table*

It is recommended that, to carry out this treatment, a shotline with at least 10m of line is rigged and if possible a seat or harness is used to attach the casualty to the shotline. Furthermore the casualty should be wearing a full face mask in case of Oxygen toxicity. If the casualty suffers an Oxygen toxicity hit whilst wearing a standard scuba regulator they may loose the regulator and be at risk of drowning. With a full face mask they will still be able to breathe safely.

If insufficient Oxygen is available to complete the treatment then the casualty should be returned to the surface rather than continue the treatment on air. After surfacing this procedure specifies that the casualty should breathe pure Oxygen on a one hour on, one hour off basis, for a further 12 hours. The support divers accompanying the casualty should be replaced on a regular basis.

The *US Navy Diving Manual* also includes a procedure for conducting IWR. Although designed for use with an Oxygen rebreather it can also be used with an open circuit or surface supply source of pure Oxygen. This procedure involves the casualty descending to 9m whilst breathing pure Oxygen. The casualty then remains at 9m for 60 minutes for mild symptoms and 90 minutes for serious symptoms. The casualty then ascends to 6m and spends a further 60 minutes at this depth followed by another 60 minutes at 3m. This results in a treatment time of 180 minutes for a mild bend and 210 minutes for a serious bend.

Depth (Metres)	Elapsed Time (minutes) Mild	Elapsed Time (minutes) Serious
9	60	90
6	120	150
3	180	210

Table 14: *US Navy In Water Recompression Table*

After surfacing the US Navy treatment specifies that the casualty should breathe Oxygen on the surface for an additional 3 hours.

It is clear that IWR recompression is a process that can only be carried out after considerable pre-planning and preparation. The provision of sufficient supplies of Oxygen together with a full face mask delivery system is not something that will be available for an ad-hoc treatment. As such IWR can only be considered a last resort treatment in situations where evacuation to a recompression chamber is not an option.

Omitted Decompression

Omitted or missed decompression protocols are often confused with In Water Recompression. The key difference is that IWR involves recompression at depth to treat signs or symptoms of decompression illness *that have already been observed,* in other words treating an already bent diver. Missed decompression protocols are used for divers who have missed one or more decompression stops *but show no signs or symptoms of decompression illness*. Many hyperbaric experts consider the distinction to be irrelevant and maintain that if decompression stops are missed the safest place to be is on the boat breathing pure Oxygen and, if signs or symptoms of decompression illness do present themselves, awaiting evacuation to a recompression chamber. In this case the argument is that the danger of re-descending outweighs any potential benefit from going back down to carry out missed decompression stops.

The other side of this argument is that decompression sickness does not occur immediately on surfacing, signs and symptoms may take several hours to appear. So if a diver has missed decompression stops and surfaces without any signs or symptoms they may be able to re-descend quickly enough to prevent decompression sickness from occurring. To many it seems preferable to try and prevent decompression sickness rather than sitting on the boat waiting for it to hit.

It has been argued that even if no signs or symptoms of DCS are detectable bubbles may already have started to form. This can be taken as an argument for or against re-descending to complete missed decompression. It can be argued that as bubbles are already forming it is likely that symptoms of DCS will occur during the decompression. However it is also possible to argue that bubbles continue to grow for hours after their initial formation and so by recompressing them it is possible to stop the bubbles reaching a point where they start to cause DCS.

A study by Farm, Hayashi, and Beckman on diving and decompression sickness treatment practices among Hawaii's diving fishermen suggests that immediate recompression within less than 5 minutes is effective in reducing bubble size. If bubble size can be immediately reduced through recompression, blood circulation may be restored and permanent tissue damage may be avoided. Rapid reduction in the size of the bubble can prevent permanent damage as irreversible injury to nerve tissue can occur within just 10 minutes of the nerve tissues being starved of Oxygen.

The US Navy's procedure for omitted decompression is shown below.

If the diver has missed stops 6m or shallower; is showing no signs or symptoms of decompression sickness and can return to the water in less than a minute - descend to the required stop depth and continue with the planned decompression.

If the diver has missed stops 6m or shallower and is not able to return to the water in less than a minute but is showing no signs or symptoms of decompression sickness then the diver can return to the missed stop and multiply all remaining stop times by 1.5.

If the diver has missed stops at 6m or deeper; is showing no signs or symptoms of decompression sickness; a standby diver is available and the water conditions allow then the diver can return to the depth of the first stop and repeat the decompression schedule for any stops greater than 12m. Stops at 9, 6 and 3m should be multiplied by 1.5.

On completion of omitted decompression the diver should be placed on Oxygen for at least 30 minutes and if any signs or symptoms of decompression sickness are detected should be evacuated to a recompression chamber for treatment.

Figure 52: *US Navy Procedure for Omitted Decompression*

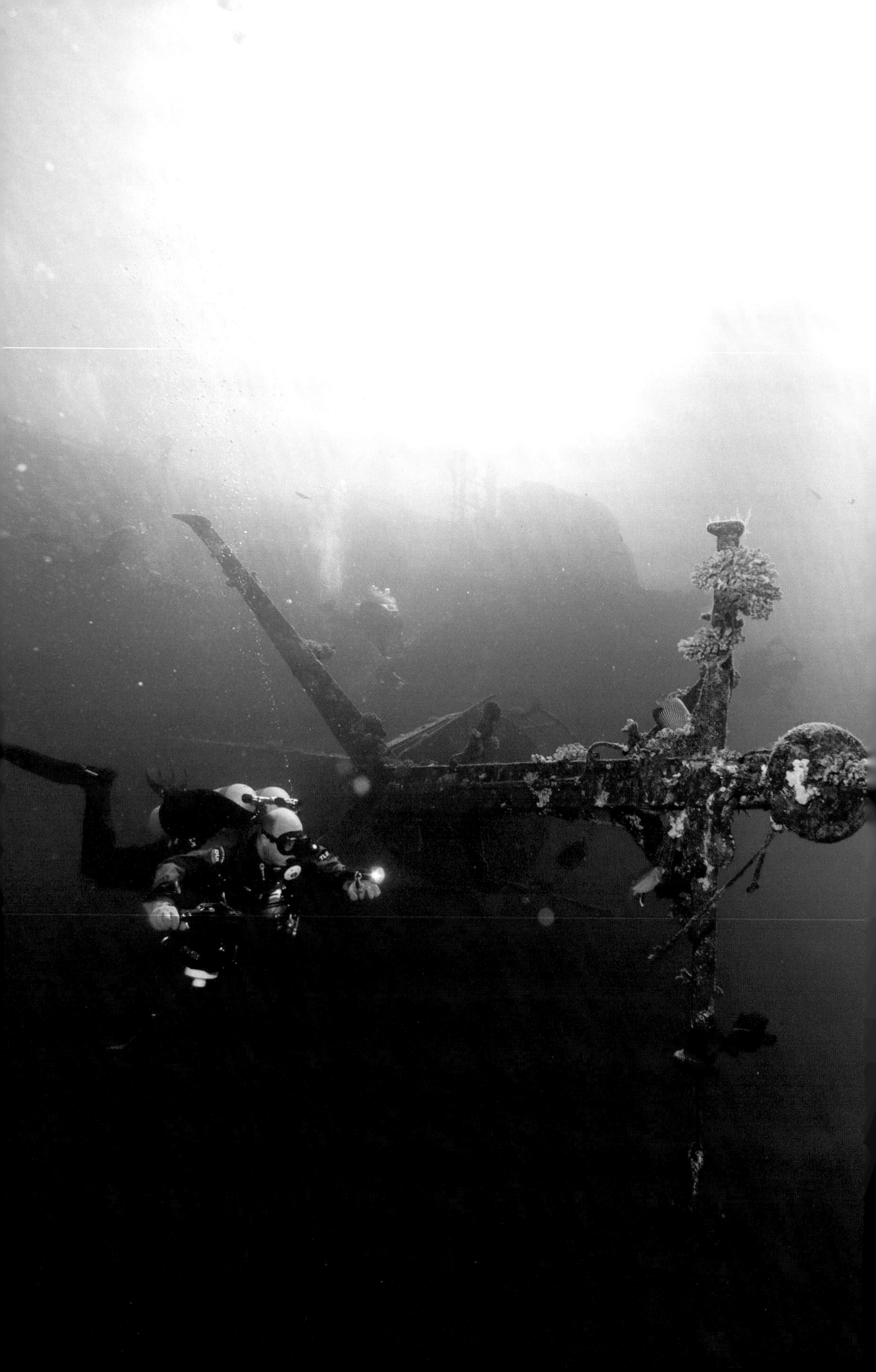

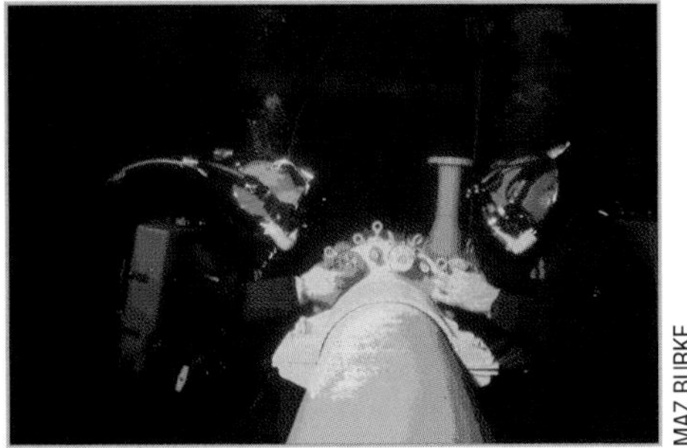

MAZ BURKE

A saturation decompression profile for a given depth will always be the same no matter what the duration of the dive was

4 Saturation Diving

For many dives the time spent in decompression is longer, often much longer, than the bottom or working part of the dive. For commercial diving where a specific task must be completed this ratio of diver work time to decompression time becomes a critical factor in determining the feasibility of a project.

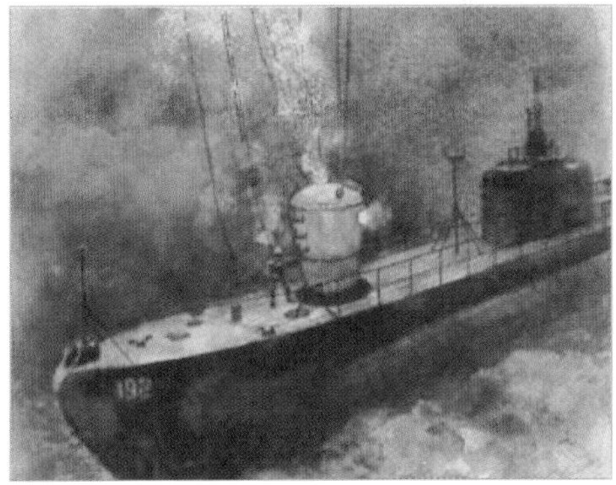

Figure 53: *The Salvage of USS Squalus*

An example of the high cost of working at depth using traditional 'bounce' decompression dives is the salvage of the *USS Squalus* which sank in May 1939 in the North Atlantic in a depth of 243 ft. Salvage operations carried out by the US Navy from May to September of that year involved over 600 dives but because of the time required for decompression each dive was limited to just 10 minutes bottom time. This greatly restricted the amount of work that could be done on each dive and slowed down progress on the salvage. Had saturation diving techniques been available for this project then it is likely that the work could have been completed in weeks rather than months by divers living and working in an underwater habitat.

Saturation diving is used in the commercial diving world for dives of extended periods at depth. In Haldane's original 1908 paper he pointed out that if a body stays at a particular depth for long enough then all of the tissue compartment will become saturated.

In all the discussion about decompression principles in previous sections the length of decompression required is related to the amount of inert gas dissolved in the tissue. The

Left: A diver using Nitrox to extend no-stop times

decompression obligation will continue to increase as the amount of inert gas dissolved in the tissues increases. However once all tissues have become saturated then no more inert gas will be absorbed into the tissues and the decompression obligation will no longer increase. This means that the diver can stay at that depth indefinitely without incurring any further decompression obligation.

Our fastest tissues may become saturated on normal recreational dives but the slowest tissues take much longer to saturate than even the longest recreational dive. For example if we consider the Bühlmann set of compartments then our slowest tissue will have a half time of 720 minutes. We consider the tissue to be effectively saturated after 6 half times which is 4320 minutes or 72 hours. Clearly for recreational or even technical diving we will never come close to reaching saturation.

Development Of Saturation Diving

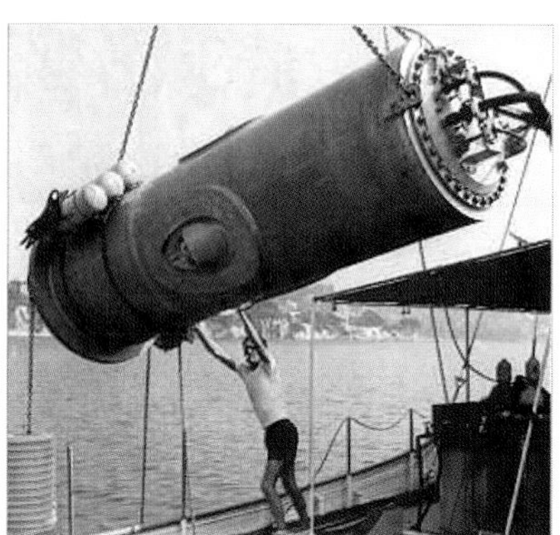

Captain George F Bond of the US Navy is considered the father of saturation diving, In 1957, as head of the Naval Medical Research Laboratory, he began investigating the possibility that after an extended period at depth a diver would become saturated and would not incur any further decompression penalty. Together with Capt Walter F Mazzone and Capt Robert D Workmann he carried out numerous tank experiments on various animals which confirmed Haldane's theory of saturation diving. By 1962 Bond was ready to test out his work on divers. Two US Medical Officers, John Bull and Albert Fisher spent six days in a helium-oxygen atmosphere at a pressure of one atmosphere at the US Medical Research Institute at Bethesda MD. The experiment was a success and the US Navy had finally proved the theory of saturation diving on humans.

In April 1963 three volunteers, spent six days at a depth of 30m in a chamber at the Naval Experimental Diving Unit in Washington. They were breathing a mixture of 7% oxygen, 7% Nitrogen and 86% Helium. In August to September of 1964 three volunteers spent 12 days at a depth of 60m.

Research into saturation diving was then taken up by American millionaire Edwin A Link. Link was a very successful businessman who also saw the potential for applications of new technology. He was the first man to design a flight simulator for training pilots while on the ground. Link organised the first saturation dive in the open sea. He designed a cylindrical saturation chamber 11ft x 3ft called Trial Link and in August 1962, at the age of 58, he tested it himself by spending 8 hours at 20m followed by 6 hours of decompression. One month later Robert Stenuit made the first open water saturation dive in the same cylinder, now renamed Man-in-the-sea, at 60m for 24 hours breathing an oxygen helium mix. After 24 hours on the bottom Stenuit required 66 hours of decompression, 8 hours in water and a further 58 hours while back on board the support vessel.

Jacques-Yves Cousteau, the pioneer of scuba diving equipment, had originally collaborated with Link but they had gone their separate ways as their aims were quite different. Link was primarily interested in researching deep saturation diving for use in commercial applications while Cousteau was more interested in experiments at shallower depths which although less technically challenging were likely to generate more publicity. Cousteau launched his own underwater living project, named Conshelf One, which was based at Marseilles in the Mediterranean at a depth of 10m. The two divers, Albert Falco and Claude Wesly, successfully spent a week submerged in the chamber which had been named Diogenes.

Cousteau continued his experiments with Conshelf Two in 1963. Based in the Red Sea the Conshelf Two project involved seven aquanauts spending a month at 36ft. As well as the main habitat, named Starhouse, Raymond Kientzy and Andre Portelatine spent a week in a mini habitat called Deep Cabin at 90 fsw from which they carried out excursion dives to as deep as 360ft. In 1965 Conshelf III was the most ambitious of Cousteau's underwater habitats. Based again in the south of France near Cap Ferrat it featured two stories. The upper storey included a dinning area, communication and data gathering facilities while the lower floor included areas for sleeping, sanitation and diving. Six divers spent 22 days at a depth of 110m.

Meanwhile Edwin Link was also continuing his experiments in the US. In 1963 he began his Man in the Sea II project. The habitat for the Man in the Sea II project was known as SPID (Submersible Portable Inflatable Dwelling) and was an 8ft x 4ft inflatable bag on a steel frame. In the Bahamas in July 1964 Robert Stenuit and marine biologist Jon Lindbergh (son of the aviator Charles Lindbergh) spent 48 hours at 432fsw on an oxygen helium mix.

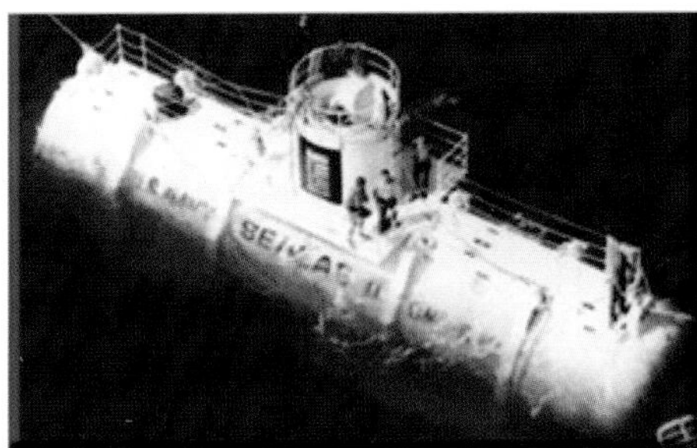

Figure 54: *Sealab II*

The US Navy wanted to ensure it kept at the leading edge of saturation diving research and in July 1964 launched it's own Sealab I project. Rather than simply extending the limits of saturation diving or gaining publicity, Sealab I was designed to scientifically study human physiology underwater. Divers were based at 193 ft breathing an oxygen helium mix. Ultimately they only spent 11 days at depth instead of the planned 21 due to weather conditions. In 1965 Sealab II, based in La Jolla California, was the most ambitious saturation diving experiment to date. Three teams spent 10-16 days each at 205ft. Experiments were carried out in a wide range of areas including new methods of salvage, the testing of new tools, porpoise training and various behavioural studies.

Although largely the preserve of commercial or military divers the development of saturation also involved inspired, or some might say eccentric, amateurs. In 1965 members of Bournemouth BSAC undertook their own saturation diving experiment. Colin Irwin and John Heath spent a week in a small cylinder named Glaucus at a depth of 12m in Plymouth Sound.

The British Navy were also very active in saturation diving research. The Royal Naval Physiological Laboratory (RNPL) carried out several research projects and in 1970 divers

John Bevan and Peter Sharphouse spent 10 hours at 1500ft. Between 1972 and 1974 Royal Navy divers carried out more than 28 saturation dives to depths in excess of 800ft.

French commercial diving company Comex were also developing the techniques of saturation diving for use in commercial diving operations. In 1970 Patrick Chemin and Bernard Reuillier were lowered in stages down to a depth of 1706ft. The dive took a total of 14 days and of that time 5 days were spent at a depth greater than 1000ft with 38 hours spent below 1500ft. Comex's achievements signified a change in saturation diving where individuals and even the naval research institutes of the US and the UK were overtaken by commercial companies who were interested in the commercial opportunities of saturation diving.

Comex continued a range of research programmes through the 1980s and 90s. The Hydra project investigated the use of Hydrogen based breathing gases for depths in excess of 500m. In 1988 the Hydra 8 project involved six divers descending to 534m and in 1992 the Hydra 10 project reached a a depth of 701m.

.

Year	Project	Site	Depth	Duration	No of Divers
1962	Man-in-Sea I (Link)	Mediterranean	200 ft 60m	24 hours	1
1962	Conshelf I (Cousteau)	Mediterranean	33 ft 10m	7 days	2
1963	Conshelf II (Cousteau)	Red Sea	36ft 11m	30 days	5
			90ft 27m	7 days	2
1964	Man-in-Sea II (Link)	Bahamas	432 ft 130m	49 hours	2
1964	Sealab I	Bermuda	193 ft 59m	11 days	4
1965	Conshelf III (Cousteau)	Mediterranean	330 ft 100m	22 days	6
1965	Sealab II	California	205 ft 62m	45 days (15 days per team)	3 teams of 10
1969	Tektite I	Virgin Islands	50 ft 15m	60 days	4
1970	Makai Range	Hawaii	520 ft 157 m	5 days	6
1970	Tektite II	Virgin Islands	50 ft 15m	12-30 days each team	11 teams of 5
1971-72	Makai Range	Hawaii	200 ft 60m	10 days	6
1988	Hydra 8	Cassis	534 m		6
1992	Hydra 10	France	701m		

Table 15: *Significant milestones in saturation diving*

Commercial Saturation Diving

The 1970 saw the maturing of saturation diving techniques at the same time as an increased demand for working underwater as a result primarily of the offshore oil industry. The 1970's and 80's were a boom time for commercial diving in the oil industry.

Saturation divers usually make use of an underwater habitat where they live and rest between dives. In addition to the underwater habitat a full saturation diving system has a number of other components including a deck decompression chamber (DDC) and a personal transfer chamber (PTC). A saturation diving support vessel is used to carry the saturation system as well as diving supervisor, chamber operators and medical personnel.

The saturation diver is compressed to depth in the deck decompression chamber which is fixed to the deck of the diving support vessel. The DDC is a warm and dry environment which allows for a reasonable amount of space, hot meals, toilets and showers. Medical help is also available if required. Once the divers have been compressed to the relevant diving depth they are transfer to the personnel transfer chamber (PTC) for the descent to depth. The PTC is lowered to the required depth and is locked onto the habitat. The divers can then move from the PTC into the habitat.

Once the divers are living in the habitat they can exit the habitat to work and as long as they stay at the same depth they avoid any further decompression obligation. Divers may stay in the surface supplied habitat for weeks, making daily excursions of eight hours or more to accomplish their underwater. Theoretically it would be possible to ascend or descend to any depth from the habitat and decompress accordingly. For practical reasons and because of a lack of reliable decompression tables at deeper depths, this is usually not done.

When a diver needs to surface they move into the PTC, which is compressed to the same depth as the habitat. The PTC is then raised to the surface while still compressed and, once back on the support vessel, it is locked onto the DDC. The diver can spend several days decompressing in the safety of the DDC. If the task has been completed, the support vessel can be underway whilst the divers decompress – a process that can take several days. Decompression rates for saturation dives are very slow, approximately one hour for every meter of saturation depth. A 2000 fsw dive might require nearly a month for decompression! By increasing the inhaled O_2 content to 0.5 ATA some time can be eliminated from the decompression obligation, but it is still a lengthy process.

Saturation Decompression

From a theoretical point of view saturation decompression is quite straightforward. As all of the tissues are, by definition, fully saturated the very slowest tissue is always the controlling tissue. The ascent profile is simply the profile required to safely decompress the slowest tissue.

Bounce Dives
In commercial diving terms a 'bounce dive' is any dive that is not a saturation dive. So an 8 hour dive would still be a bounce dive as it is not a saturation dive.

Unlike a bounce dive, where the length of the bottom time is key in determining the required decompression schedule, the decompression schedule for a saturation dive is the same no matter how long the dive was. Once saturation is reached the decompression obligation doesn't increase any further and so a saturation decompression profile for a given depth will always be the same no matter what the duration of the dive was.

The US Navy saturation diving procedure uses an ascent rate of 6 fsw/h (1.84 msw/h) for depths from 1,600 to 200 fsw (488 -61 msw) and then 5 fsw/h (1.54 msw/h) from 200 to 100 fsw (61 to 31 msw). 4 fsw/h (1.23 msw/h) from 100 to 50 fsw (31 to 15.4 msw) and then 3 fsw (0.92 msw/h) to the surface. This is shown in metric units in Table 16 as well as imperial units in Table 17.

Depth	Rate
488 – 61 msw	1.84 m per hour
61 – 31 msw	1.54 m per hour
31 – 15.4 msw	1.23 m per hour
15.5 – 0 msw	0.92 m per hour

Table 16: *USN Saturation decompression schedule (Metric). Source USN Diving Manual*

Depth	Rate
1,600 – 200 fsw	6 feet per hour
200 – 100 fsw	5 feet per hour
100 – 50 fsw	4 feet per hour
50 – 0 fsw	3 feet per hour

Table 17: *USN Saturation decompression schedule (Imperial). Source USN Diving Manual*

In practice, saturation decompression is usually carried out by decompressing the DDC in 1-foot or 2-foot increments when indicated in the dive protocol. For example, when using an ascent rate of 6 feet per hour the operator will decompress the chamber 1 foot every 10 minutes. Decompression is often conducted for only 16 hours in each 24-hour period. A 16-hour daily travel/rest outline example consistent with a normal day/night cycle is shown in Table 18.

Time	Activity
2400–0600	Rest Stop
0600–1400	Travel
1400–1600	Rest Stop
1600–2400	Travel

Table 18: *Daily decompression schedule*

This type of schedule minimises travel when the divers are normally sleeping. However, this specific daily routine is not mandatory. Other 16-hour periods of travel per 24- hour routines are acceptable, although they usually include at least two stop periods dispersed throughout the 24-hour period and may continue decompression while the divers are asleep.

After surfacing from a saturation dive, the divers are still at risk from decompression illness as the slowest tissue is still close to critical supersaturation. As a result saturation divers will remain in the immediate vicinity of a chamber for 2 hours after completion of decompression and stay within 30 minutes travel of a chamber for a further 48 hours. Saturation divers should not fly for 72 hours after the completion of a dive.

Other than adjusting the ascent rate the only other factor that can be used to affect saturation decompression is the partial pressure of Oxygen breathed in the DDC. A higher partial pressure of Oxygen means a lower fraction of inert gas than would otherwise be present. This allows the inert gas in the body to off-gas faster.

The maximum ascent rate is directly related to the Oxygen partial pressure. However the long duration of saturation dives and decompression means that a partial pressure of 0.5 bar or above is likely to lead to problems with Oxygen toxicity. To balance out the benefit of faster off-gassing with the risk of pulmonary Oxygen toxicity a partial pressure of between 0.4 and 0.5 Bar is often used. Some commercial companies use slower ascent rates coupled with a higher partial pressure to try and increase the safety of decompression. In a series of experimental dives carried out to determine the benefits of higher partial pressures of Oxygen it was shown that raising the inspired oxygen partial pressure from 0.22 atm to 0.4 atm reduced the incidence of DCS from 52% (14 incidents in 27 dives) to zero (no incidents in 42 dives.

Despite significant research into saturation decompression, most saturation decompression rates were based on trial and error rather then any specific decompression theory. A simple model relating the rate of ascent from a saturation dive to the inspired oxygen partial pressure assumes that ascent rate is a linear function of oxygen partial pressure. This can be expressed as

$$\text{rate} = k\ PO_2$$

where rate is ascent rate, PO_2 is oxygen partial pressure and k is an empirically determined constant. To develop a saturation decompression procedure, the value of k and the resulting ascent rate is adjusted in successive dives until the incidence of DCS becomes acceptably low.

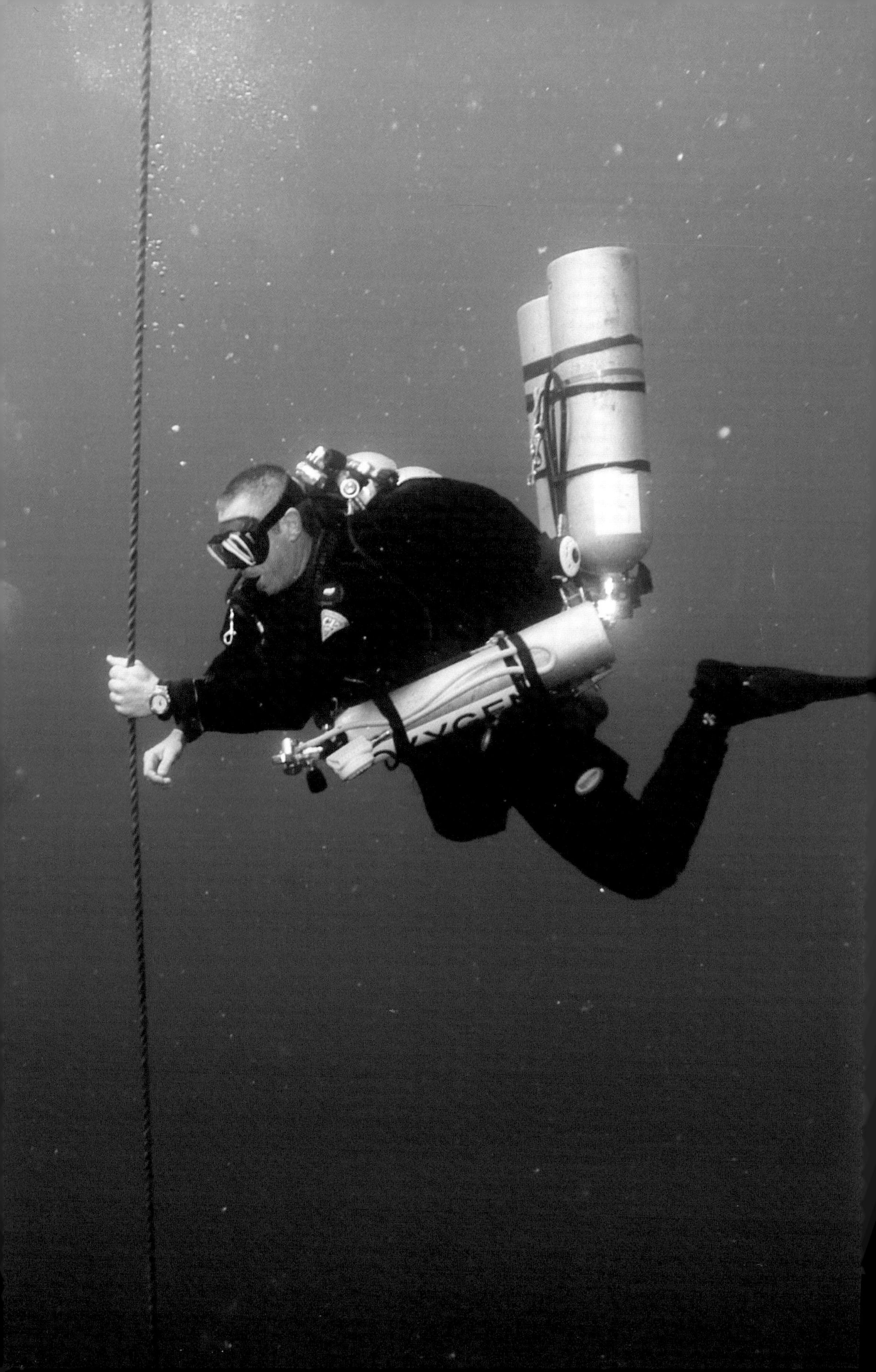

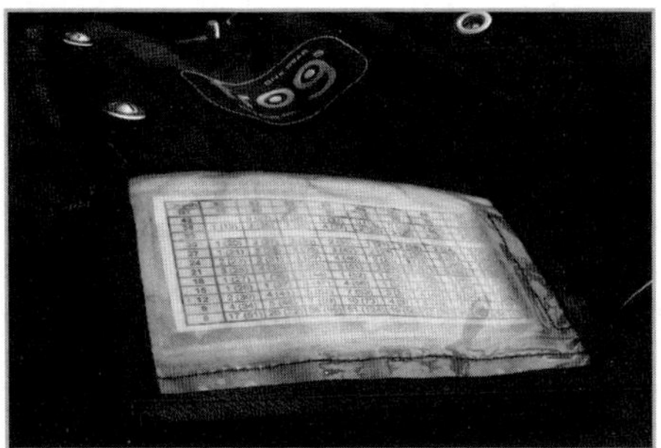

By reducing the amount of nitogen in the gas we breathe we can reduce the partial pressure of nitrogen at depth and so reduce our decompression obligation

5 Nitrox

During basic SCUBA training instructors tell trainees that decompression is related to depth and time. If we look at air decompression tables then the only variables are the depth and time. To work out our no-stop time we just need to know our depth. Similarly, if we know the depth that we are diving to and the time we are going to stay there then we can work out our tissue loading, or residual nitrogen group as it is called in some tables. So when instructors say that decompression is related to depth and time it appears that they are telling the truth. By now we can see that this is an over simplification, but for air diving it is effectively true.

As we have seen in previous chapters, a diver's decompression obligation is actually determined by the partial pressure of nitrogen in the gas being breathed along with the amount of time that gas is breathed. With air, the partial pressure of Nitrogen is always the same at a given depth, and so the depth is used as a proxy for the partial pressure of Nitrogen. By reducing the amount of nitrogen in the gas we breathe we can reduce the partial pressure of nitrogen at depth and so reduce our decompression obligation. This is the reason why divers use Nitrox.

Nitrox is any combination of Nitrogen and Oxygen. This means that even normal air is a form of Nitrox and can be referred to as Nitrox 21, EAN21 or even, if you want to make it sound complicated, Normoxic Nitrox. However for diving, when we refer to Nitrox we usually mean a mixture with a higher level of Oxygen, and correspondingly lower level of Nitrogen. Nitrox mixes always focus on the Oxygen content of the mixture and are referred to by their Oxygen content. For example EAN32 contains 32% Oxygen, but the fact that it also contains 68% Nitrogen is not mentioned. In fact we are not really looking to increase the Oxygen percentage in our Nitrox mix; rather we are looking to reduce the Nitrogen percentage. However, without adding a third gas the only way to reduce the percentage of

Left: Rich nitrox mixes can be used accelerate decompression

Nitrogen is to increase the percentage of Oxygen. We therefore refer to Oxygen Enriched Air Nitrox or EAN. Nitrox is also referred to as EANx where 'x' is the percentage of Oxygen in the particular mix, so EAN32 contains 32% Oxygen, EAN50 contains 50% oxygen. As there are only two gasses present the Nitrogen content can be inferred, i.e. EAN36 contains 36% Oxygen and so the Nitrogen percentage is 100-36 = 64.

The first evidence of a dive using oxygen enriched air was in 1879 by Henry Fleuss, who was Master Diver for Siebe, Gorman & Co. of London. Fleuss was breathing a mixture with an estimated 50-60% Oxygen and completed an hour long dive in a large tank. A week later, he completed an open water dive using the same equipment. In 1912 Robert Davis and Leonard Hill developed a diving helmet that used a 50% oxygen-nitrogen mixture. This diving helmet was used under the guidance of J.S. Haldane and was used to complete dives to 30m (100 fsw).

Siebe Gorman continued research into nitrox mixes and between the two World Wars introduced the technique of using different concentrations of Oxygen mixed with Nitrogen. This was used to great effect by British commandos during World War Two who used oxygen-enriched air re-breathers. Their rebreathers used mixtures of 45-60% Oxygen which had a greater maximum operating depth than their opponents whose pure oxygen rebreathers were limited to 6-10m. The British used this to their advantage and their simple but effective strategy was to simply pull their opponents to deeper depths until convulsions overwhelmed the enemy diver.

Prior to 1970 Nitrox was used by commercial and military divers but was relatively unknown amongst recreational divers. During the 1970's scientific divers working for the US National Oceanic and Atmospheric Administration (NOAA) began to use Nitrox for scientific dives. This was largely driven by Dr Morgan Wells, Chief Diving Officer for NOAA, who has subsequently become known as the godfather of Nitrox diving. In 1978 NOAA introduced a full set of diving procedures and tables for Nitrox use. These were published in 1978 in the NOAA Diving Manual. The main mix used was EAN32 (32% Oxygen and 68% Nitrogen) which was known as NOAA I. Tables and procedures were also published for EAN36 which was known as NOAA II. EAN32 is still the most common Nitrox mix in use and is occasionally still referred to as NOAA I.

Initially the recreational agencies resisted the use of Nitrox for recreational divers. The training agencies and many so called experts maintained that Nitrox was for too dangerous for recreational divers. The main arguments were that the increased oxygen levels would increase the risk of CNS oxygen toxicity and that by breathing Nitrox the diver was more likely to suffer pulmonary Oxygen toxicity if they subsequently needed to be recompressed. This meant that divers wanting to safely use Nitrox were unable to get comprehensive training on how to use this mysterious gas. The introduction of Nitrox to recreational diving was brought about largely through the efforts of two men. Dick Rutkowski was the ex-deputy diving director for NOAA and the founder of the International Association for Nitrox Diving (IAND). In latter years this was modified to become International Association of Nitrox and Technical Divers (IANTD). Rutkowski published the first recreational Nitrox manual and set up one of the first nitrox mixing stations in Florida.

Ed Betts was a commercial diver who had owned and run a number of dive shops on Long Island on the North East Coast of the US. Betts founded American Nitrox Divers Inc (ANDI). In order to play down the association with technical diving ANDI refers to EAN32 (NOAA I) as "Safe-Air". They aimed their program at entry level divers using air tables or air diving computers as a way to increase the safety margin.

The arguments over the use of Nitrox reached a climax when the organisers of DEMA 1991 were pressured into banning all suppliers, trainers and any other exhibitors related to the use of Nitrox. Following an outcry over the decision the organizers relented and allowed Nitrox exhibitors to attend. In addition a parallel two day conference on the use of Nitrox was arranged to run alongside DEMA. This was chaired by renowned decompression researcher R. W "Bill" Hamilton. Hamilton co-ordinated a wide range of training agencies, manufacturers, instructors, speakers and experts who proceeded to dispel many of the myths and misconceptions over the use of Nitrox. The argument that divers had an increased risk of CNS Oxygen toxicity was shown to be less of a risk provided each diver stayed within the operating limits of the gas they were breathing. In addition the assertion that a diver who had been breathing Nitrox would be more at risk of pulmonary Oxygen toxicity if they subsequently needed to be recompressed was also shown to be unfounded.

As the momentum for the use of Nitrox increased the recreational training agencies were forced to reconsider their position on Nitrox. One of the first agencies to recognise the use of Nitrox for recreational diving was the UK Sub Aqua Association (SAA) who recognised Nitrox use in 1994. The following year they were followed by the British Sub Aqua Club (BSAC) and the Professional Association of Diving Instructors (PADI). Now all recreational diving agencies not only recognise the use of Nitrox for recreational diving but have also developed their own Nitrox training programmes. Many agencies are now taking a step further allow the use of Nitrox for entry level divers on their very first open water dives.

Using Nitrox

A diver breathing Nitrox is breathing a gas containing less Nitrogen then Air. For example a diver breathing EAN32 at the surface will be breathing a mixture with 68% Nitrogen rather than the 79% Nitrogen in normal air. As the diver descends the lower Nitrogen content results in a lower partial pressure of Nitrogen compared to breathing air.

Depth (m)	Partial Pressure of Nitrogen (Bar)	
	Air (79% Nitrogen)	EAN32 (68% Nitrogen)
0	0.79	0.68
10	1.58	1.36
20	2.37	2.04
30	3.16	2.72
40	3.95	3.40

Table 19: Partial pressure of Nitrogen in Air and EAN32

As we can see in Table 19 a diver breathing air at 10m would have a partial pressure of nitrogen of 1.58 Bar. At the same depth a diver breathing EAN32 would only have a partial pressure of Nitrogen of 1.36. At 30m the partial pressure of Nitrogen if breathing air would be 3.16 whereas the partial pressure of Nitrogen if breathing EAN32 would be 2.72.

If we remind ourselves of Henry's Law, which says that the amount of gas that can be dissolved in a liquid is proportional to the partial pressure of the gas in contact with the liquid, then we can start to see why we get such a benefit from using Nitrox. As the partial pressure of Nitrogen is lower when using Nitrox then less Nitrogen is absorbed into the blood and is carried to the tissues. The tissues absorb less Nitrogen and so for the same dive a diver on Nitrox will on-gas less Nitrogen than a diver on air. Of course if the diver has on-gassed less Nitrogen then they subsequently have less Nitrogen to off-gas and so have a greater margin before critical supersaturation is reached.

This effect can be seen in Figure 55. This compares the amount of on-gassing for a single tissue compartment with a half time of 5 minutes for a dive to 30m using air with the same dive using EAN32.

For the air dive the partial pressure of Nitrogen during the dive is 4 x 0.79 = 3.16. If we are breathing Nitrox with a 32% Oxygen content (and 68% Nitrogen) then the partial pressure of Nitrogen is 4 x 0.68 = 2.72 Bar.

As the inspired partial pressure is lower when breathing EAN32, the tissues will on-gas slower and at any point the same tissue will contain less Nitrogen then if the diver had been breathing air.

For a tissue with a 5 minute half time as shown here the tissue will be effectively saturated after 6 half time periods or in this case 30 minutes. This is shown in the graph as the dark line, representing the air dive, which converges on an inert gas tissue tension of 3.16 at 30 minutes. The grey line, representing the EAN32 dive has converged on 2.72 bar. So if we are breathing EAN32 then, for this tissue compartment at least, it doesn't matter how long we stay at 30m the tissue will never become as saturated as it would be if we were diving on air.

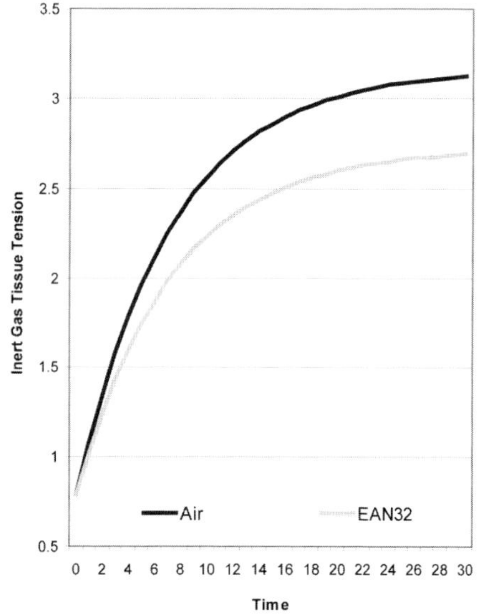

Figure 55: *Comparison of on-gassing rates with air and EAN32 for a 30m dive for 30 minutes*

At any point during a dive the reduced partial pressure of Nitrogen in a Nitrox mix will be the same as for an air mixture at a shallower depth. As we saw in the example above; if we are breathing EAN32 at 30m then the partial pressure of Nitrogen is 0.68 x 4 = 2.72. If we were breathing air at 25m then the partial pressure of Nitrogen would be 0.79 x 3.5 = 2.76. In other words we are breathing almost the same partial pressure of Nitrogen whether we are diving on air at 25m or EAN32 at 30m. As our on-gassing and hence our decompression obligation is determined by the partial pressure of Nitrogen then a dive to 30m on EAN32 will have the same decompression obligation and the same no-stop time as an air dive to 25m.

Another way of saying this is that a dive to 30m on EAN32 has an Equivalent Air Depth (EAD) of 25m.

The equivalent air depth for any depth and any mixture can be calculated using a simple formula.

$$\mathbf{EAD = \left[\frac{(1-FO_2)}{0.79} * (Depth + 10)\right] - 10}$$

Figure 56: *Equivalent Air Depth Formula*

By stepping through an example of using the EAD formula we can get a view of how the formula works.

$1\text{-}F0_2 = 1\text{-}0.34$ $= 0.66$	First we calculate $1\text{-}FO_2$, this is to work out the fraction of Nitrogen in the mix. Assuming we are breathing EAN34 then the FO_2 is 0.34 and so the fraction of Nitrogen is 0.66
$0.66/0.79 = 0.84$	Next we divide the fraction of Nitrogen by 0.79, which is the fraction of Nitrogen in normal air. This gives us the ratio of Nitrogen in the Nitrogen in the Nitrox mix we are breathing compared to normal air. In other words we are only getting 84% of the nitrogen that we would get if we were breathing air.
$Depth + 10 = 31 + 10$ $= 41$	Next we take our actual depth, say 31 metres and add 10. This is to convert from gauge pressure which doesn't include the presence of the atmosphere to absolute pressure which does include the pressure of the atmosphere. Adding 10msw is like adding the 1 bar of pressure for the atmosphere.
$0.84 * 41 = 34.4$	Then we multiply the ratio of nitrogen by the absolute pressure to give the equivalent depth in absolute pressure. We can see that 34.4m is deeper than our actual depth but remember this is in absolute pressure and includes 10m to account for the pressure of the atmosphere.
$34.4 - 10 = 24.4$	Finally we subtract 10m to convert from absolute pressure back to gauge pressure. So we can see that for a dive to 31 metres breathing EAN34 our equivalent air depth is 24.4 metres. From this we could then use an air table and use 24.4m (25m) as the depth to plan our dive.

If we breathe Nitrox during our dive we can gain significant bottom time before we reach our no-stop time. The exact amount of extra bottom time will depend on the depth that we are diving to and the Nitrox mix that we are breathing. For a decompression dive then a diver will be able to spend longer on the bottom before they reach the no-stop time and go into decompression. Once the diver has passed their no-stop time and has to perform decompression stops then the amount of decompression they need to do will increase more slowly when using Nitrox than when using Air.

Nitrox can also be used to introduce an additional safety margin by breathing nitrox but using air tables or an air computer. By working out our decompression obligation based on breathing air when we are in fact breathing Nitrox we will overestimate the Nitrogen take up and loading in our tissues.

If we use the EAD concept and stay to the end of our bottom time then we will have the same level of Nitrogen loading as an air dive to the shallower EAD depth. Nitrox continues to give us an advantage during the ascent in that we are continuing to breathe a reduced partial pressure of nitrogen during this part of the dive whereas for the air dive we would be breathing a slightly higher partial pressure of nitrogen. The lower partial pressure of Nitrogen in the Nitrox mix means that we will be off-gassing slightly faster during the ascent when we breathe Nitrox when compared to breathing air. So even though our loading was the same at the start of the ascent the loading will be lower at the end of the ascent if we have been breathing Nitrox compared to air.

The lower partial pressure of Nitrogen and the increased rate of off-gassing also results in less silent bubbles being formed during the ascent. This has been suggested as one of the reasons why divers often claim that they feel less tired when diving on Nitrox rather than on air. We know that silent bubbles or micro bubbles are routinely formed after dives even if there are no signs of clinical decompression sickness. The immune system reacts to the micro bubbles as they are effectively 'foreign bodies'. See Chapter 2 for more information on the body's reaction to the formation of bubbles.

The immune system's response results in the lymphatic system having to carry off the excess dead white cells produced to mount the attack. The immune system's response, as well as the lymphatic aftermath, both serve to create fatigue, stiffness, sore muscles, etc. By avoiding subclinical DCI, the stress on the body is avoided and there is an absence of tiredness or fatigue. Similar benefits have been reported by divers who added deep stops to their profiles.

Research by Harris et al (2003) supports the idea that the reduction in fatigue experienced when using Nitrox is solely due to the reduction in sub clinical DCS rather than any inherent property of Nitrox. In their double blinded, randomized controlled study 11 divers breathed either air or EAN36 during an 18m dry chamber dive for a bottom time of 40 minutes. Two periods of exercise were performed during the dive. Divers were assessed before and after each dive using a range of performance measuring tests. Diving to 18m produced no measurable difference in fatigue, attention levels or ability to concentrate following dives using either breathing gas. As a result of this and other research the current thinking at this time is that there is no difference in terms of fatigue between diving air and Nitrox.

Using Nitrox as a Decompression Gas

We have seen that there is a significant benefit from a decompression point of view from using Nitrox as a back gas (ie. the primary source of gas worn on the divers back). The reduced partial pressure of Nitrogen means that Nitrogen is absorbed more slowly then if we were breathing air. Nitrox, and especially rich Nitrox mixes, can also be of great benefit during decompression.

The benefits of using a rich Nitrox mix as a decompression gas can be seen in Figure 57. This shows a dive to 45m for a bottom time of 20 minutes. If the diver breathes his back gas during the entire ascent then his decompression scheduled is shown by the grey line. This schedule involves a total run time of almost 100 minutes with a 50 minute decompression stop at 6m. If the diver breathes their back gas until reaching 9m and then switches to a mixture of 80% Oxygen (and 20% Nitrogen) then the 9m decompression stop is greatly reduced as is the 6m stop which drops from 50 minutes to only 12 minutes. The overall run time for the dive is reduced from 98 minutes to only 53 minutes – a reduction of 45 minutes - just from switching to another gas for the 9m and 6m decompression stops. This is known as accelerated decompression.

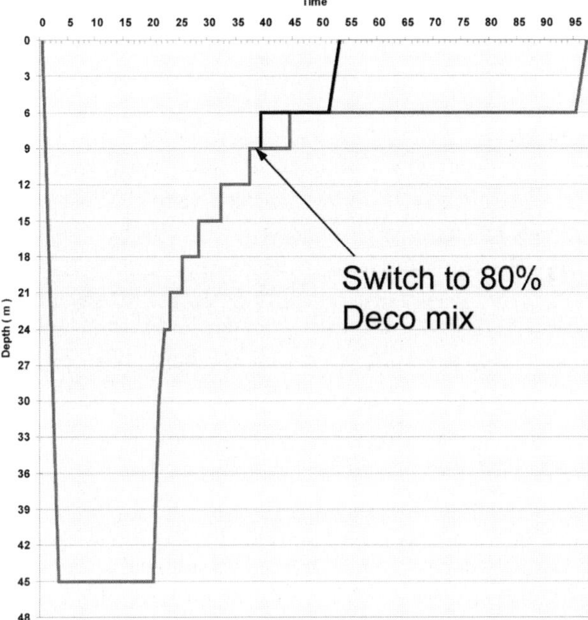

Figure 57: *Accelerated decompression using rich a Nitrox mix*

On the face of it, this significant reduction from using nitrox as a decompression gas is less obvious then the benefits of using Nitrox as a back gas. At the end of the bottom time the body has already become highly loaded with Nitrogen. For most of the ascent we are still breathing our back gas and only switch to a decompression gas during the later part of the ascent. So why would switching to rich Nitrox gas so late in the dive make such a significant difference?

The rate of off gassing is related to the partial pressure within the tissues of the body and the partial pressure of the gas being breathed. If we only have a single gas then the only way to reduce the partial pressure of the gas we are breathing is to reduce the ambient pressure by ascending to a shallower depth.

In Figure 58 below we are breathing a single mix throughout the dive. As we descend at the start of the dive the partial pressure of both the Nitrogen and Oxygen increases with depth. Once we reach 30m the partial pressure of Nitrogen is 3.16 bar. Nitrogen is absorbed by the tissues as they are at a lower partial pressure. By the end of the dive it is likely that at least the fastest tissue compartment is saturated and so it is at the same partial pressure as the Nitrogen in the breathing mix. As the diver ascends the partial pressure of Nitrogen in the breathing mix is reduced along with ambient pressure. Off gassing occurs as the inspired partial pressure is now lower than the tissue partial pressure.

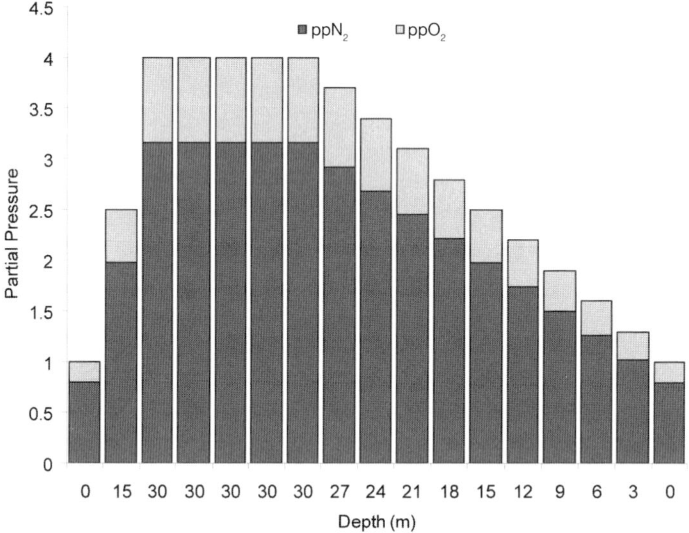

Figure 58: *Breathing air during the whole dive*

However the depth to which we can ascend is governed by the M-Value. We cannot reduce the ambient pressure too much as the difference between the tissue tension and the ambient pressure will exceed the M-Value.

Bubbling is controlled by the difference between the tissue tension and the ambient pressure – however off-gassing is controlled by the difference between the tissue tension and the inspired inert gas pressure. This difference, which is known as the inert gas gradient, determines the amount of off-gassing. If this tissue compartment has a 5 minute half time then the tissue will go 50% of the way from the current tissue tension to the inspired inert gas pressure in 5 minutes. It will then go a further 50%, for a total of 75%, in a further 5 minutes.

This three way relationship is shown in Figure 59. The arrow along the bottom shows the level of pressure or tension for each of the three main factors. The tissue tension is higher then the inspired inert gas pressure. This means that there is an inert gas gradient between the tissues and the inspired gas and so the tissues will be off-gassing. This is represented by the black dotted arrow. The 50% mark shows the point 50% between the current tissue tension and the current inspired inert gas pressure. We have already seen that this 50% mark is the point which the tissue tension will reach in one half time period. Clearly a bigger gap or distance between the tissue tension and the inspired gas pressure means that 50% of that gap will be further and so the tissue will off-gas further.

The tissue tension is also higher than the ambient pressure and so the tissue is supersaturated. As the inspired inert gas pressure is tied to the ambient pressure, as shown by the solid black line between them, we can only reduce the inspired inert gas pressure by reducing the ambient pressure. The problem is that if we reduce the ambient pressure too much the difference between the tissue tension and ambient pressure, shown by the grey dotted line, will exceed the M-Value limit as represented by the vertical line.

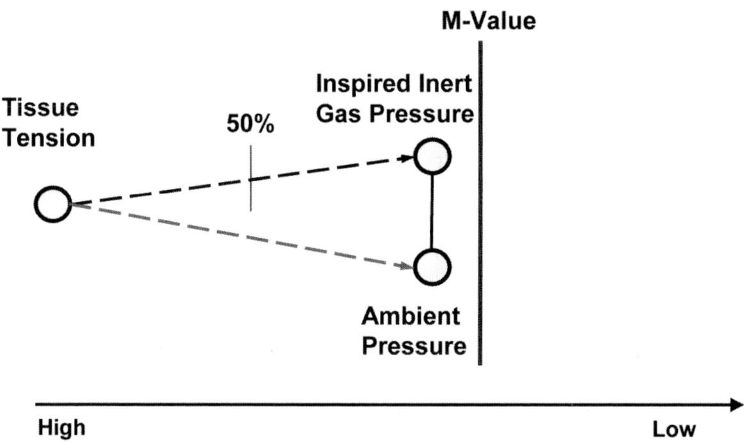

Figure 59: *The relationship between tissue tension, inspired inert gas pressure, ambient pressure and M-values.*

The challenge is to reduce the ambient pressure as much as possible so that the inspired inert gas pressure is also reduced in order to create the largest inert gas gradient. At the same time the ambient pressure cannot be reduced too much or we will exceed the M-value and trigger bubble formation. As long as the inspired inert gas pressure is linked to the ambient pressure this will always be the limit that controls the rate of off-gassing.

The only way to break the link between the inspired inert gas pressure and ambient pressure is to change the gas we are breathing. By reducing the partial pressure of Nitrogen within the breathing mixture used during decompression it is possible to greatly increase the inert gas gradient. By doing this we also increase the rate of off-gassing and subsequently reduce the amount of decompression required.

If we switch to a decompression gas during the ascent we get the situation shown in Figure 60. Here we switch from our back gas (air) to EAN50 at 21m. As you can see from the graph the decreased fraction of Nitrogen results in a drop in the partial pressure of the inspired gas.

The partial pressure of Nitrogen in the inspired gas is now much lower than that in the tissues and so the tissues start to off gas much faster.

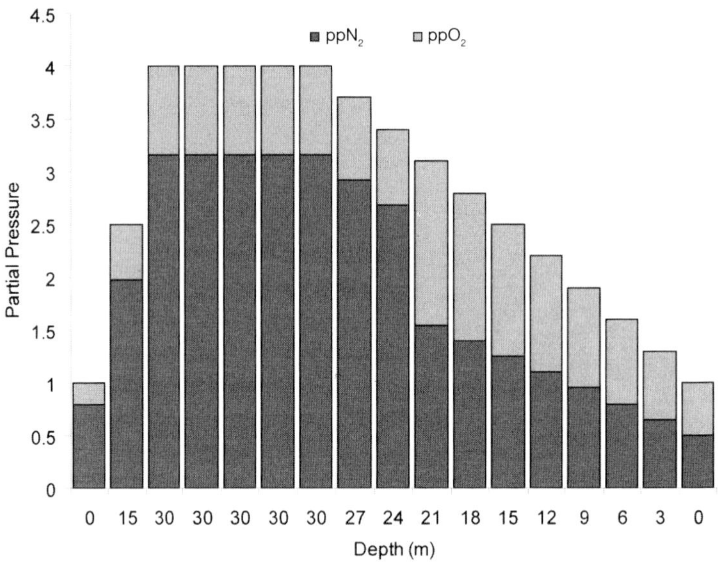

Figure 60: *Switching to EAN50 at 21m*

This is shown in Figure 61. Here we have broken the link between the inspired inert gas pressure and ambient pressure. By switching to a rich Nitrox mix we can greatly reduce the inspired inert gas pressure resulting in a much larger inert gas gradient. This can be done without changing the ambient pressure and so there is no additional risk of exceeding the M-value.

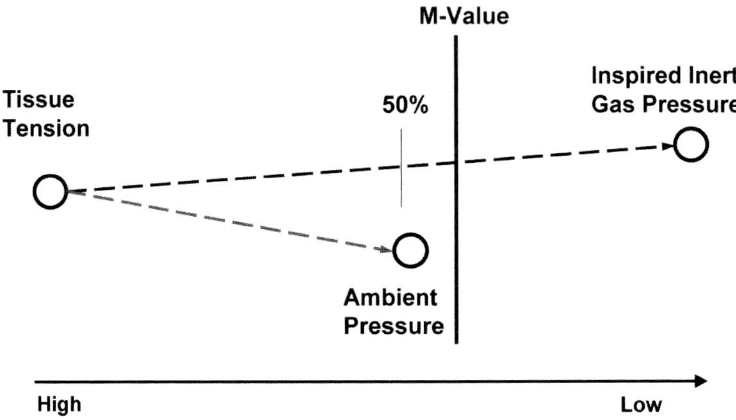

Figure 61: *Accelerated decompression breaks the link between inspired inert gas pressure and ambient pressure.*

The larger inert gas gradient means that the difference between the tissue tension and the inspired inert gas pressure is much larger. If our tissue has a 5 minute half life then it will still only go 50% of the way in 5 minutes but now it is going 50% of a much larger distance and as such will off-gas faster. We can see this by comparing Figure 59 and Figure 61. In Figure 61 the larger inert gas gradient means that the 50% point is much further than in Figure 59.

By breaking the link between inspired inert gas pressure and ambient pressure we can achieve this greater inert gas gradient without changing the ambient pressure. We can see in Figure 61 that the ambient pressure is unchanged and so there is no additional risk of exceeding the M-value and triggering DCS. This is only possible due to the fact that off-gassing is related to the relationship between tissue tension and inspired inert gas pressure whereas bubble formation is related to the relationship between tissue tension and ambient pressure.

A simple analogy would be to imagine a balloon at 30m which has a hole in it, if you bring it up to the surface the air in the balloon will expand but it will also leak out of the hole. If you bring it up too fast the balloon will expand and burst, despite the leak. This is because the internal gas pressure is sufficiently higher than the ambient pressure. Now if you increase the size of the hole then the air will leak out of the balloon faster and it won't burst. By using a decompression gas with a lower fraction of Nitrogen you let the gas diffuse out of the tissues faster – in other words you have a bigger hole in your balloon.

If pure oxygen is used as a decompression gas then the change is even more significant. Figure 62 shows switching to 100% oxygen at 6m. As we are breathing pure oxygen we no longer have any Nitrogen in the breathing gas and so the inspired partial pressure of Nitrogen is zero. The gradient between the tissue tension of Nitrogen and the inspired partial pressure of Nitrogen is now at its maximum and the tissue will off gas at the fastest possible rate.

As Oxygen gives the largest inert gas gradient then it might appear that it is the best gas to use for decompression. However, as you might have guessed by now, decompression is seldom that straightforward. It is true that Oxygen gives the largest inert gas gradient but due to the risk of central nervous system oxygen toxicity we cannot breathe pure Oxygen any deeper than 6m. This means that we cannot start to accelerate our decompression until we get to 6m. If we use another decompression gas with a lower fraction of Oxygen then we can start using it sooner. For example we can start breathing EAN50 at our 21m stop, EAN70 at the 12m stop or EAN80 at our 9m stop.

By using a decompression gas with a lower fraction of Nitrogen you let the gas diffuse out of the tissues faster.

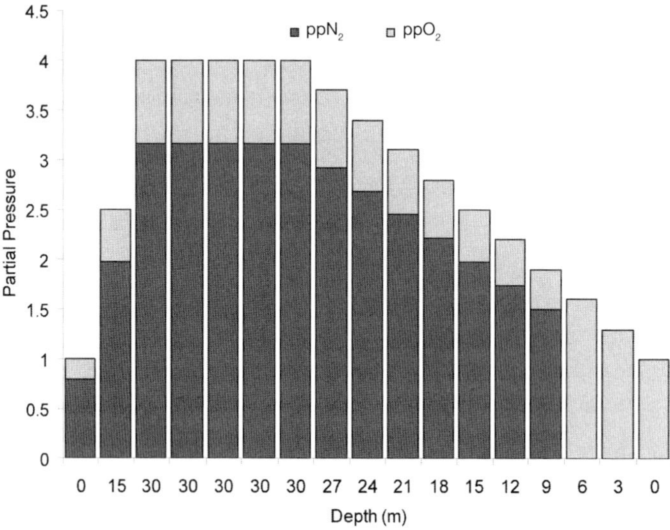

Figure 62: *Switching to 100% Oxygen at 6m*

So we have a choice we can use a leaner mix such as EAN50 and start to decompress on it sooner with a lower inert gas gradient or we can use a richer mix such as 100% Oxygen knowing that we can't start breathing it until 6m, but that when we do start breathing it we will have the maximum inert gas gradient. So which do we choose?

The choice of the most efficient decompression gas will, to a large extent, depend on the decompression profile we have. If our decompression profile only shows stops at 6m then we would not benefit from using a much leaner mix such as EAN50 as we can switch onto 100% for our decompression stop. If we have stops at 9m and 6m then there is no point picking a decompression gas which is leaner then EAN80 as we can switch onto EAN80 at our first stop and we would not have any real benefit from switching to a leaner gas earlier. The choice here is between EAN80 and EAN100.

Similarly if we have a dive which has the first decompression stop at 21m then we could switch to EAN50 at this stop or any richer mix at subsequent stops.

With a traditional Haldane based decompression schedule such as the Bühlmann model the decompression stops tend to be relatively shallow - 15m or shallower with the majority of the decompression time spent at 9m, 6m and 3m. We can see that an EAN50 decompression gas would give us less benefit for this type of dive as we can switch to it at 21m but will then continue to ascend to a shallower depth where we will not have as big an inert gas gradient as we would have if we waited until 9m and then switched to EAN80. We can therefore see why for decompression diving using Bühlmann based tables EAN80 became a popular decompression gas. With the introduction of deeper stops and bubble models it has become much more common for our first decompression stops to be at a depth of 21m or even deeper. Here the use of EAN50 as a decompression gas becomes more advantageous. By switching to EAN50 at 21m we can start to off-gas earlier.

The Oxygen Window Revisited

At the end of Chapter 2 we were introduced to the first usage of the term 'The Oxygen Window'. This was the drop in pressure between the arterial and venous side of the circulation. Well the section above has just introduced the second usage. By switching to a decompression mixture with a higher Oxygen fraction, and by implication a lower Nitrogen fraction, we increase the inert gas gradient. The inert gas gradient is also known as the Oxygen window and this increase in the inert gas gradient is sometimes referred to as "opening the Oxygen Window".

In Figure 63 the change in inspired inert gas pressure when switching from back gas to decompression gas is shown as opening the Oxygen window and is shown by the solid green arrow.

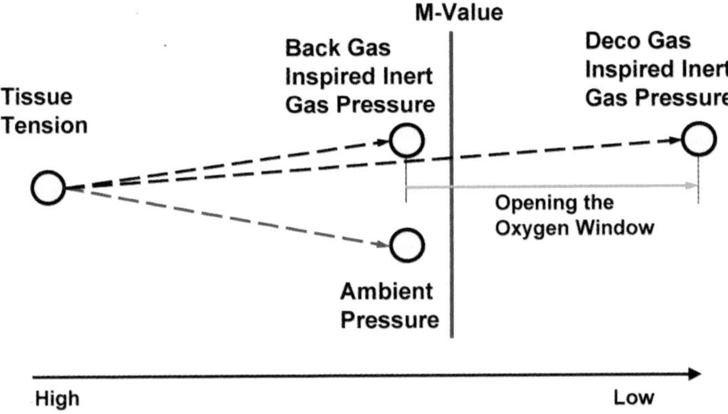

Figure 63: *Opening the oxygen window*

There is however a third usage of the term which is also caused by switching to a decompression gas but is closely related to the first definition of the Oxygen window. This third usage suggests that it is not just the reduction of Nitrogen in a rich Nitrox mix that provides an advantage but that the higher partial pressure of Oxygen in itself helps decompression by creating a greater drop in pressure between the venous and arterial sides of the body.

We know that Oxygen is transported around the body, from the lungs to the tissues by the blood. Oxygen is carried in the blood by two distinct methods: Bio-chemically bound to hemoglobin, and physically dissolved in plasma, which is the liquid part of blood. At sea level with a pressure of 1 ATA and an Oxygen partial pressure of 0.21 bar hemoglobin is already 97% saturated with Oxygen. At this saturation level the blood has an Oxygen content of about 19.8 ml of oxygen per dl of blood. Oxygen dissolved in the plasma of the blood does not play a big part in Oxygen transport at this pressure, only 1.5% of the Oxygen being carried at sea level is dissolved in the plasma.

As the hemoglobin is already 97% saturated with Oxygen it only takes a slight increase in the partial pressure of Oxygen for the hemoglobin to become completely saturated. Once this happens it cannot bind with any more Oxygen and from that point on additional Oxygen can only be carried dissolved in the plasma. As the partial pressure of Oxygen increases past this saturation point the amount of Oxygen carried by the blood is then determined by Henry's law. This means that the amount of Oxygen dissolved in the blood increases linearly as the partial pressure increases. It also means that Oxygen dissolved in the blood can be thought of in exactly the same way as an inert gas dissolved in the blood.

With increasing levels of partial pressure of Oxygen the amount of Oxygen carried in solution becomes increasingly important. This can be seen by comparing the two graphs below.

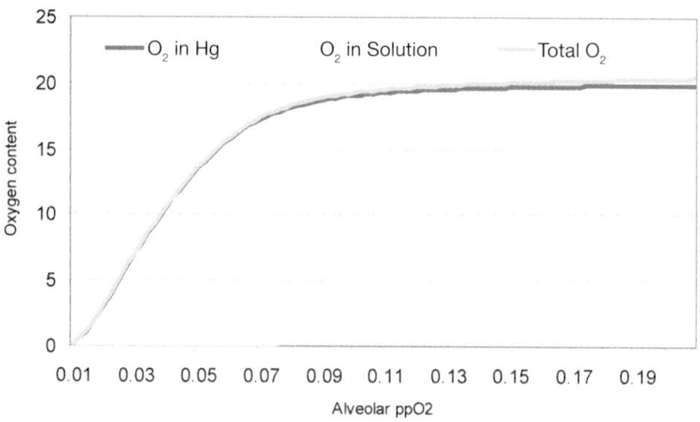

Figure 64: *Oxygen content of the blood at normal Oxygen partial pressure*

The only difference between these two graphs is the scale of the horizontal axis. In Figure 64 we are looking at a partial pressure of Oxygen up to 0.2 bar. This represents the situation when breathing air at the surface. As we can see dissolved Oxygen in the blood (represented by the yellow line) has almost no impact on the total Oxygen in the blood.

The situation is quite different when we increase the partial pressure of Oxygen. Figure 65 shows the Oxygen content of the blood when breathing an increased partial pressure of Oxygen. Here we can see that the Oxygen in solution (again represented by the yellow line) plays an increasingly important role. It is the shape of the graph in Figure 65 which gives us the third view of the Oxygen widow.

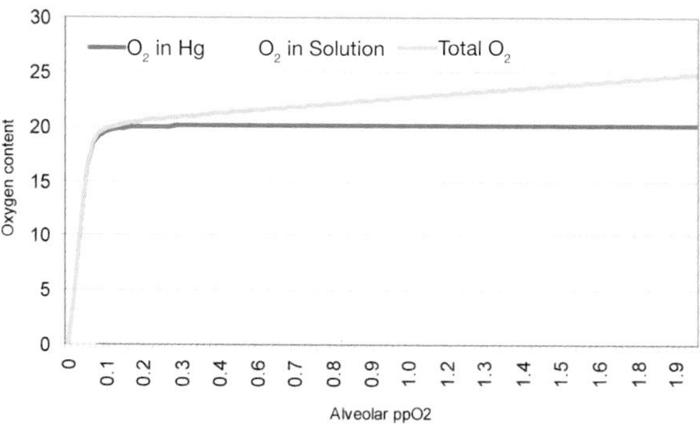

Figure 65: *Oxygen content of the blood at increases partial pressures of Oxygen*

Our tissues have a certain appetite for Oxygen. This will change depending on whether we are at rest or exercising vigorously but on average the tissues will use approximately 6 ml of

Oxygen per dl of blood. This means that the total Oxygen content of the blood (the light blue line) will drop by approx 6 ml between the arterial and venous side of the body.

The shape of the graph and the fact that it is not linear over its whole length means that in order to get a drop of 6ml on the left hand axis the change in the partial pressure will vary considerably depending on the starting point.

In Figure 66 we see the situation where a diver is breathing a mixture which gives an alveolar Oxygen partial pressure of 0.8 bar. This corresponds to a blood Oxygen content of approximately 22 ml. The tissues will consume 6 ml leaving 16ml of Oxygen in the venous system, this results in a partial pressure of 0.05 bar. A drop of 0.75 bar between the arterial and venous systems.

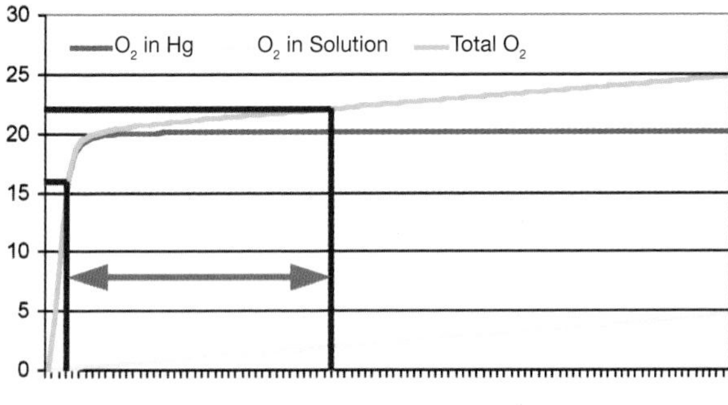

Figure 66: *The Oxygen Window*

If we now consider Figure 67. Here our diver is breathing a mixture which gives an alveolar Oxygen partial pressure of 1.5 bar. This corresponds to a blood Oxygen content of approximately 24 ml, that's only 2ml more than our previous example. Again the tissues will consume 6 ml which leaves 18ml of Oxygen in the venous system. This results in a partial pressure of 0.6 bar. In this case we see a drop of 0.9 bar between the arterial and venous systems as compared to a drop of only 0.3 bar in the previous example.

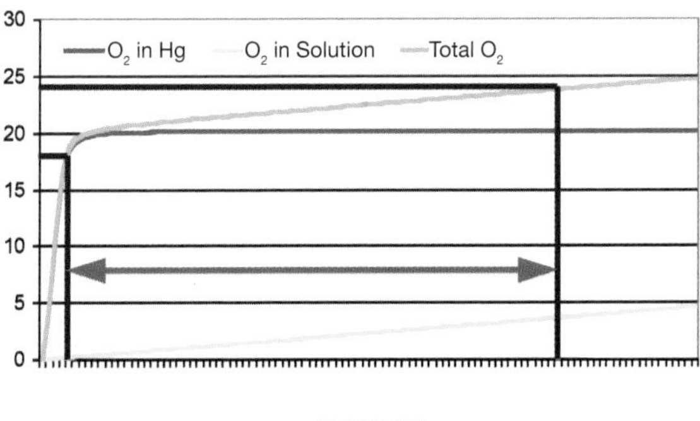

Figure 67: *Opening the Oxygen Window – Again*

This clearly shows that the pressure difference between the arterial and venous sides is much greater when breathing high partial pressures of Oxygen. Or in other words high partial pressures of Oxygen can be used to widen the Oxygen window.

If we look again at the graphs in Figure 66 and Figure 67 we can see that the large drop in overall pressure is due to the shallow slope of the line once the hemoglobin reaches saturation. The tissues require an average of 6ml of Oxygen which is represented by a drop on the vertical axis. In order to achieve this drop a large movement on the horizontal axis is required. However, once the line reaches the 'knee' point, where the dissolved Oxygen has been used up, it drops off quickly and a smaller reduction in pressure is required in order to satisfy the required oxygen content. If the initial Oxygen content of the blood is sufficiently high then it is possible for the tissues to use up the 6ml of Oxygen and still be above the 'knee' point of the graph. As the knee point is at approximately 20 ml then if the initial Oxygen content of the blood is 26 ml the tissues can remove 6ml and the line is still above the knee point. This occurs at an alveolar partial pressure of 2.5 bar which is equivalent to breathing a gas at a partial pressure of 2.7 bar. Above this pressure the drop in partial pressure for a 6ml drop in Oxygen content is linear and the Oxygen window is at its widest. This is shown in Figure 68. As we can see from this graph, if the alveolar partial pressure is increased further then all of the Oxygen required can be supplied by the dissolved Oxygen in the plasma and so the drop in partial pressure will always be approximately 2.4 bar.

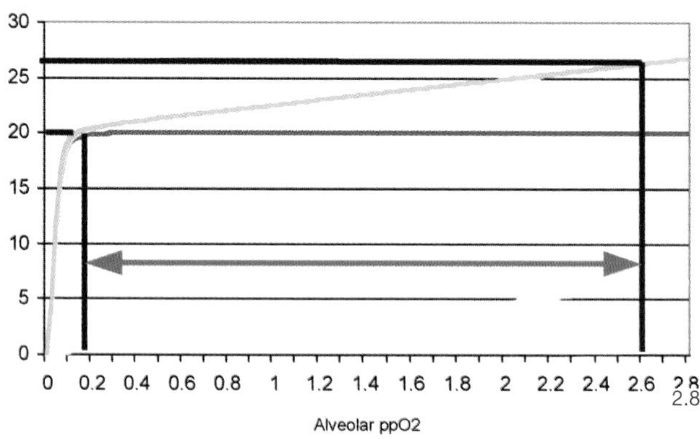

Figure 68: *The Oxygen Window is wide open*

Notice that we have not referred to the inert gas component of our breathing mix. This effect is independent of the inert gas and is solely dependant on the partial pressure of Oxygen. This means that we will get the same effect breathing pure Oxygen at 6m, EAN80 at 10m or EAN50 at 22m. In each case we are at a partial pressure of 1.6 bar.

This makes sense so far but how do all these clever graphs actually help decompression? Remember that our rate of off-gassing is controlled by the inert gas gradient and so it's only the difference between the inert gas tension in our tissues and the partial pressure of the inert gas in the blood that will affect off-gassing from the tissues. The fact that there is a lower partial pressure of Oxygen and hence a lower overall gas pressure in the venous system, will not influence this at all. So is this version of the Oxygen window a red herring that doesn't help us at all?

Whilst this version of the Oxygen window will not have an effect on our rate of off-gassing from the tissues it still does have a useful effect. It's true that off-gassing is related only to the relative inert gas gradients but bubble formation is related to the difference between the total gas tension and the ambient pressure. By reducing the Oxygen partial pressure we also reduce the total gas tension. So this use of the oxygen window does not mean that we will off-gas faster but it does mean that we are likely to get less bubbling.

It is clear that the term "The Oxygen Window" means different things to different people. Furthermore the benefit of the Oxygen window varies according to which version you are referring to. It should be no surprise that people have trouble agreeing on the concept when in fact they are talking about different concepts. Table 20 summarises the different definitions of the term together with the benefit of each version.

Definition	Benefit
Drop in partial pressure between arterial and venous systems	Reduces bubbling
Reduced inspired pressure of inert gas due to increased Oxygen content in the breathing mixture.	Greater inert gas gradient gives faster off-gassing
Increased drop in partial pressure between arterial and venous side as a result of breathing high partial pressure of Oxygen	Reduces bubbling to a greater degree

Table 20: *The different views of the Oxygen Window*

Of course high partial pressures of Oxygen can also introduce significant problems. Oxygen Toxicity is always a risk with higher partial pressures of Oxygen. In addition a slight complicating factor is that oxygen is a vasoconstrictor which means that it can reduce the size of blood vessels and hence the flow of blood to various tissues. As a result elevated oxygen partial pressures may actually decrease inert gas elimination as any reduction in perfusion will slow the rate of off-gassing.

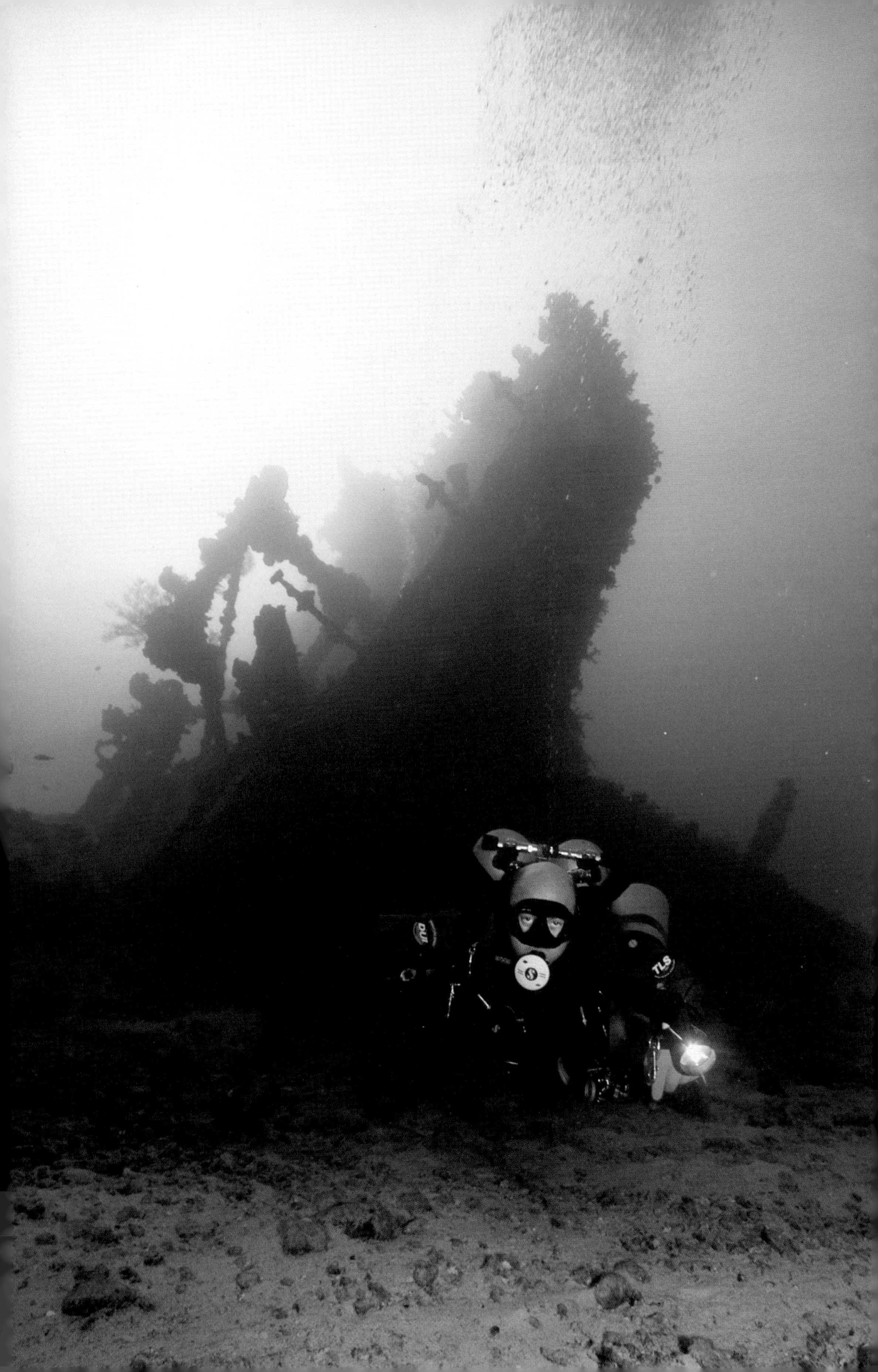
TLS

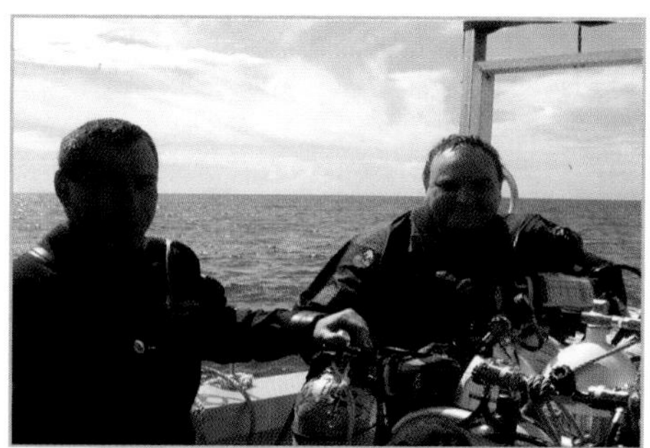

Deep stops were initially adopted by technical divers but the advantages are relevent for all divers

6 Deep Stops and Bubble Models

We saw in Chapter 2 that traditional decompression models as proposed by Haldane and subsequent generations such as Workman and Bühlmann's models have encouraged divers to ascend relatively quickly at the end of a dive from the maximum depth to a shallow first stop depth. This is based on the Haldanian or dissolved gas theory that by reducing the ambient pressure and increasing the inert gas gradient this will maximize the rate of off-gassing. This is combined with the theory that bubbles will only form in the bloodstream if the pressure gradient within the tissues exceeds the M-Value for that tissue. Haldane's paper states that 'liquids such as blood, will hold gas in a state of supersaturation, provided the supersaturation does not exceed a critical limit'. This model assumes that a relatively fast ascent from depth to a much shallower depth where the pressure gradient is just below the M-value will give the maximum rate of off-gassing while at the same time preventing bubbles forming and limiting the amount of additional nitrogen being absorbed into any currently unsaturated tissues.

So a traditional Bühlmann table would bring you as close to the surface as possible in order to get you as close to, but not exceeding, the M-Value and then keep you there until you could either move up to the next decompression stop or to the surface without exceeding the M-Value. This is reflected in profiles calculated from Bühlmann tables or using dive computers which use the Bühlmann algorithm which are characterized by fast initial ascents followed by long deco stops at shallow depths. The graph in Figure 69 shows a dive using a Bühlmann profile and shows the ascent continuing until we hit the M-Value and then stopping at this depth until we can ascend again without hitting the M-Value.

Left: The wreck of the Ulysses

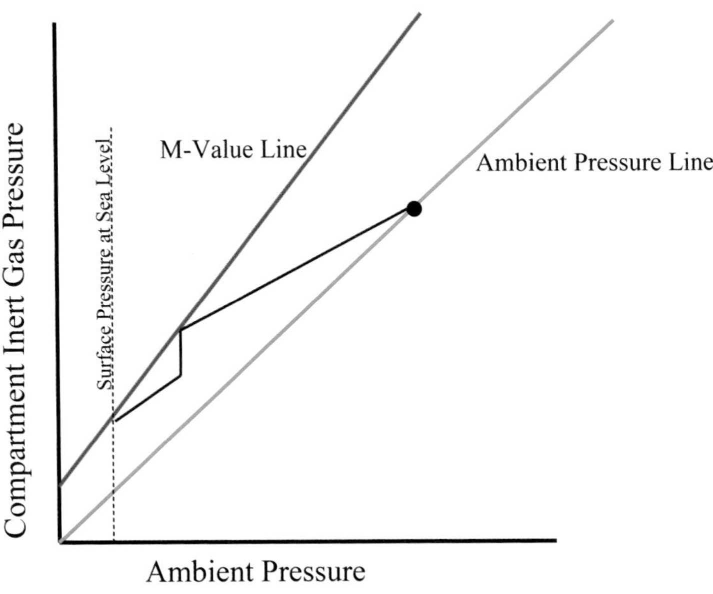

Figure 69: *Bühlmann type ascent profile*

However we saw that Doppler bubble detection has shown that bubbles form on a large number of dives. This includes dives where the diver does not approach critical supersaturation and where he shows no traditional signs or symptoms of decompression sickness. This was illustrated in the diagram reproduced below as Figure 70. This shows that our M-Value is, at best, an attempt to delineate a sensible limit where the number of bubbles produced is small enough to avoid the appearance of traditional signs and symptoms of decompression sickness.

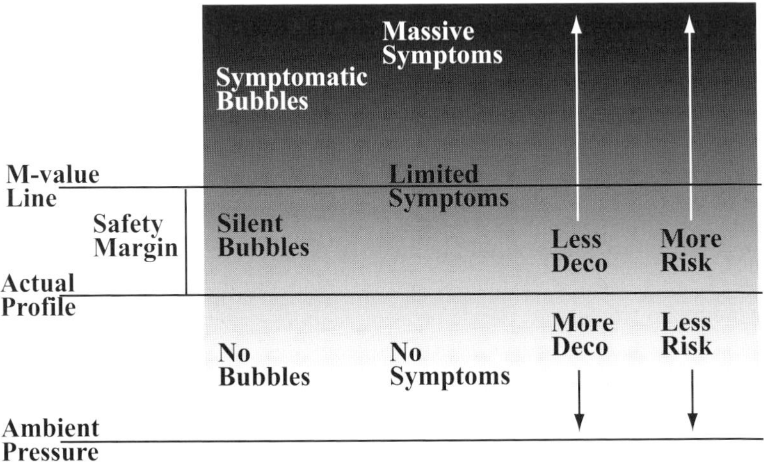

Figure 70: *An M-Value is a solid black line through the middle of a broad 'grey' area*

This provides a significant challenge to the traditional view of decompression theory. If bubbles are formed well within our M-Value limit then what use are M-Values? And if bubbles form, and yet there are no signs or symptoms of decompression sickness, then how can we say that bubble formation causes decompression sickness? If it is not bubble formation that causes decompression sickness then what does cause it?

Haldane himself goes on to state in his original paper that 'the volume (not the mass) of gas (measured at the existing pressure) which would be liberated if the whole excess of gas present in supersaturation were given off is the same whether the absolute pressure is reduced from two to one atmosphere, or from four to two, or from eight to four.' In subsequent developments of Haldane's theory attention has focused on the supersaturation ratio but it's interesting to notice that Haldane himself thought that the potential volume of released gas was an important factor rather then the supersaturation ration in isolation. However the ratio approach became established and it wasn't until 1951 that Albert Behnke proposed that 'It may well be that what appears to be a ratio of saturation tolerance is in reality an index of the degree of embolism that the body can tolerate.' In other words bubbles of inert gas are not the trigger for DCI as bubbles are routinely formed and a certain volume of these bubbles can be handled by the body but once the volume reaches a critical level DCI is the result. The overwhelming weight of established thought was in favour of the supersaturation ratio method and this meant that Behnke's work was not initially developed.

We can see that the discovery of silent bubbles threw quite a large spanner into the theoretical basis of traditional (dissolved gas) decompression theory. Two alternate views developed on how best to deal with this spanner. The first view was that the dissolved gas model has served us well for many years and many millions of dives have been conducted with an acceptable level of safety. As a result there is no need to completely reject the dissolved gas model. Instead a number of modifications can be made to the model to take into account the existence of silent bubbles. Models which include these modifications to the traditional dissolved gas approach are often called "modified Haldanian" or sometimes "neo-Haldanian" models.

The alternative view was that the discovery of silent bubbles highlighted such a fundamental flaw in the dissolved gas model that a mere tweak was not sufficient to solve the problem. Nothing less than a new theory which attempted to explain the formation of silent bubbles as well as the cause of decompression sickness was the only way forward. This approach led to the development of dual phase models or, as they are more commonly known, bubble models.

Deep Stops

Most of the 'tweaks' that have been applied to the traditional Haldanian approach result in the introduction of much deeper initial stops. As a result the term 'deep stops' has become a generic term for stops introduced to avoid the formation of silent bubbles whilst otherwise using a dissolved gas model. The best known flavour of deep stops is the approach developed by Richard Pyle and as a result the term 'Pyle stops' has been used almost as commonly as deep stops.

Pyle is an experienced diver and marine biologist. Specifically he is an ichthyologist, although he describes himself as a 'fish-nerd'. Pyle regularly dives to depths of 55-67 metres in order to study and collect specimens of the various fish species that live at these depths. During dives to these depths Pyle noticed that after some of his dives he felt overly tired and lethargic, a classic indication of asymtomatic DCI and silent bubbles, whereas after other dives there were no such indications. He realized that the feeling was related to decompression rather than just the physical exertion of the dive as a dive to 60m for a total time of an hour would give more of a feeling of tiredness than a dive of 4-6 hours at a much shallower depth.

Pyle tried to identify the factors that separated the dives on which he felt good from the ones in which he felt overly tired. He considered a whole range of factors including obvious ones such as the length of the dive, depth, current, hydration levels, whether he had felt seasick during the journey, extra time added to the last deco stop, water temperature, how well he has slept the night before, etc as well as less obvious factors such as the clarity of the water, days or dates of the month on which the dives were carried out, etc.

After looking for patterns in the dives which produced no signs he eventually realized the common factor was that on dives on which he was catching and raising fish specimens from depth he was much less likely to get signs of asymptomatic DCI than on dives where no specimens were collected. This was a surprising result as initially there seemed to be no explanation as to why these dives would produce less symptoms. The major difference in these dives was that, in order to prevent damage to the fish from the gas in their swim-bladders expanding upon ascent, he would use a hypodermic syringe to extract air from their swim bladders during the ascent. The pause in the ascent required to carry out this procedure was usually much deeper than his first prescribed decompression stop, for example on a 60 metre dive, the first decompression stop would usually be around 15m, but Pyle would pause to remove air from the swim-bladder at around 38m. So, whenever he was collecting fish, his ascent profile would include an extra 2-3 minute stop much deeper than the first decompression stop required by a traditional decompression model. Using a traditional decompression model this approach doesn't make sense as the traditional model predicts that by stopping deeper you are not providing the maximum off-gassing gradient possible for off-gassing of the faster tissues and are allowing additional gas loading in slower, under-saturated tissues. A traditional model would indicate that these stops should increase the symptoms of sub clinical DCI rather than reducing them.

Despite being at odds with traditional decompression theory Pyle concluded that it was these "deep stops" which were reducing the signs of lethargy. As a result he began to include these "deep stops" in all his deep dives with a subsequent reduction in signs of sub-clinical DCI.

Through an empirical process Pyle developed the following process for calculating deep stops.

Pyle deep stops process:

---

1. Take the distance between the depth when you start your ascent and the first required decompression stop, and find the mid point. This depth will be our first deep safety stop and should be 2-3 minutes in duration.

2. If the distance between your first deep safety stop and your first required stop is greater then 9m, then add an additional deep safety stop at the midpoint between the first deep safety stop and the first required decompression stop.

3. Repeat as necessary until there is less then 9m between your last deep safety stop and the first required stop.

Pyle used decompression planning software to calculate the dive plans and recommended that the decompression profile was recalculated between steps 1 and 2 on each iteration. Divers using a dive computer will find that the computer will recalculate the decompression stops and may add additional decompression time and even additional decompression stops. This can increase the overall length of the ascent as many current dive computers use a neo-Haldanian algorithm which penalises the additional time spent at depth during the deep stops by adding on additional decompression time to account for the additional on-gassing at depth. This additional time on the total dive can be considered an additional safety margin.

Pyle deep stops – an example

Using the standard Bühlmann tables a dive to 45m for 24 minutes would give stops at 9m, 6m and 3m. This means that a traditional ascent would involve an ascent from 45m to 9m. We then add in Pyle stops using the process described above.

Take the distance between the depth when you start your ascent	45m
and the first required decompression stop	9m
and find the mid point	(45+9)/2 = 27m
This depth will be our first deep safety stop and should be 2-3 minutes in duration	
If the distance between your first deep safety stop and your first required stop	27-9 = 18m
Is greater than 6m	Yes it is
then add an additional deep safety stop at the midpoint between the first deep safety stop	27m
and the first required decompression stop.	9m
Which is	(27+9)/2 = 18m
If the distance between your latest deep safety stop and your first required stop	18-9 = 9m
Is greater than 6m	Yes it is
then add an additional deep safety stop at the midpoint between the first deep safety stop	18m
and the first required decompression stop.	9m
Which is	(18+9)/2 = 13.5m (rounded up to 15m)
If the distance between your latest deep safety stop and your first required stop	15-9 = 6m
Is not greater than 6m	No it isn't
Then carry on to first traditional decompression stop	

So in this example we would end up with Pyle stops at 27m, 18m, 15m as well as traditional decompression stops at 9m, 6m and 3m.

Pyle met considerable skepticism when he initially discussed his approach. This is not surprising as his findings directly contradicted established decompression theory. However in 1989 Pyle attended a meeting of the American Academy of Underwater Sciences (AAUS) and saw a presentation by Dr David Yount who was discussing his work on the Variable Permeability Model (VPM) (see below). The VPM model also calls for initial decompression stops that are much deeper than those suggested by traditional neo-Haldanian decompression models. Although calculated in completely different ways they were very similar to the deep stops generated by Pyle's empirically derived method. This gave credence to the empirically derived method derived by Pyle. As the decompression modeling community as well as the growing ranks of technical divers began to appreciate the implications of VPM and other 'Dual Phase' or 'Bubble' models Pyle's empirical approach began to be acknowledged as having some scientific basis. Although an over-simplification in some cases it certainly provided the easiest way to incorporate deep stops in decompression practice and "Pyle Stops" has become a commonly used term.

Other divers have also developed empirical approaches to decompression that feature a similar approach to Pyle's deep stops. Divers involved in commercial fishing have often developed empirical approaches to reducing decompression. This is not based on any scientific interest in decompression theory but purely as an economic necessity for carrying out the maximum working bottom time for minimum overall decompression. Le Messurier and Hills studied Pearling fleets, operating in the deep tidal waters of the Torres Straits off northern Australia in an attempt to assess their decompression strategies. These pearling fleets employ Okinawan divers who dive to depths of 100m for as long as one hour, twice a day, six days per week, and ten months out of the year. In order to minimise the decompression times these divers developed optimised decompression schedules, this was done largely on the basis of trial and error. Their decompression profiles featured deeper decompression stops, but shorter overall decompression times, than required by traditional Haldane theory. Diving fishermen in Hawaii have also adopted similar profiles where multiple deep dives are carried out but with considerably less decompression than would be predicted by a Haldane decompression model.

In order to investigate the claimed benefits of deep stops DAN performed a series of dives to study the impact of ascent rates and deep stops on bubble formation. A series of dives were carried out to 25m for 25 minutes followed, after a surface interval of 3 hours and 30 minutes, by another dive to 25m for 20 minutes. Ascent rates of 18m, 10m and 3m were performed on each of the dives. Each ascent rate was combined with a direct ascent to the surface, a traditional safety stop of 5 minutes at 6m and finally a deep stop of 5 minutes at 15m combined with a traditional safety stop of 5 minutes at 6m. The only exception was that a direct ascent was not performed with an 18m/minute ascent rate as this was considered too risky. After each dive Doppler bubble detection was used to calculate a Bubble Score Index (BSI) for that dive. The results of the research are shown in Table 21.

Ascent Rate	Stops	Surfacing Saturation 5 Min	Surfacing Saturation 10 min	BSI	Total Time to Surface (min)
3m/min	None	48	75	8.78	8
3m/min	6m / 5 min	30	60	8.10	13
3m/min	15+6m / 5 min	22	49	3.50	18
10m/min	None	61	82	7.51	2.5
10m/min	6m / 5 min	43	65	5.39	7.5
10m/min	15+6m / 5 min	25	52	1.79	12.5
18m/min	6m / 5 min	42	60	7.41	6.5
18m/min	15+6m / 5 min	28	55	3.25	11.5

Table 21: *Results of DAN research on ascent rates and deep stops*

If we just look at the results for the BSI, as shown in Figure 71, we can see that the bubble score for the ascents with no stops was higher then than with a stop or 6m or a stop at 15m and 6m. The results for the ascents incorporating a deep stop at 15m as well as a stop at 6m clearly show a significantly lower BSI. This seems to confirm that the incorporation of a deep stop has a positive effect on bubble formation, even on recreational no-stop dives in the 25m depth range.

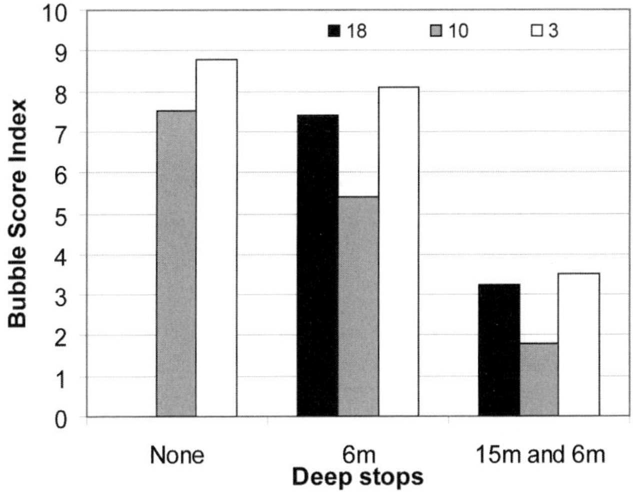

Figure 71: *Impact of deep stops on bubble score index*

From the graph we can also see that an ascent rate of 18m/min gives a higher bubble score (where carried out) than the 10m/min. Interestingly we can also see that the 3m/minute ascent rate gives a higher bubble score reading than either the 18m/minute or 10m/minute ascents. This shows that a slow ascent rate is beneficial but that there is such a thing as an ascent rate that is too slow. The best combination is a 10m/minute ascent rate combined with a deep stop at 15m and a traditional safety stop at 6m

Finally the surfacing saturation levels for the 5 minute and 10 minute tissue compartments were calculated. This is shown in Figure 72. This shows, as we might expect, that the surfacing saturation levels are lower with the inclusion of a 6m safety stop than with a direct ascent. Similarly the addition of a 15m deep stop further reduces surfacing saturation levels.

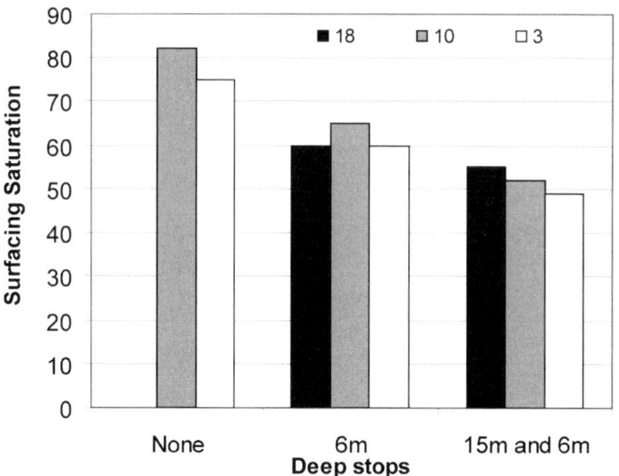

Figure 72: *Impact of deep stops on surfacing saturation in 10 minute tissue*

There has been a recent study by the US Navy which appeared to show the opposite conclusion to the DAN study in terms of the benefit of deep stops. This received a lot of publicity and was seen by many as evidence that deep stops were not such a good thing. However, if you look at the US Navy study you can see that they are testing something very different to what we have been calling deep stops and so their conclusions do not apply to this discussion.

The value of deep stops has been increasingly recognized in the recreational diving area. It would appear that deep stops can give an advantage when performing repetitive dives over multiple days, typical on a recreational diving holiday. A number of the most popular manufacturers of dive computers have recently introduced models that include some form of deep stop or micro bubble suppression algorithm and the Sub Aqua Association has recently introduced a set of deep stop tables designed for recreational club diving.

The inclusion of additional safety stops on recreational dives is likely to be more widely adopted in the future in an attempt to provide an additional safety margin and as a way of reducing post dive fatigue.

Gradient Factors

As we have seen, Pyle stops are an empirically derived method of introducing deep stops into a traditional dissolved gas decompression schedule. Although deep stops appear to have good physiological reasons for providing a benefit, Pyle stops do not claim to model or predict any physiological aspects of decompression and the calculation has no real basis in the underlying model.

Gradient factors on the other hand provide an approach which modifies the specific calculations of the dissolved gas model. They are an attempt to include a method of reducing asymptomatic DCS within the framework of the Bühlmann model. The basic concept behind gradient factors is that if there is a danger of bubbling even if we stay within the M-Value, then to increase safety we can simply stay further away from the M-Value. Gradient Factors are just a way of controlling how close we are prepared to get to the M-Value.

Gradient Factors are expressed as a percentage of the distance between saturation and critical supersaturation or in other words as a percentage of the way into the decompression zone. So a 0% GF is on the saturation or ambient pressure line while 100% is on the M-Value line. A gradient factor of 20% would be 20% of the way between the saturation line and the M-value line. From this explanation we can see that a higher gradient factor is closer to the M-value line and represents a higher level of supersaturation whereas a lower gradient factor is closer to the saturation line and so represents a lower level of supersaturation.

Gradient factors are used in pairs with a lower limit, known as the gradient factor low or GF(Lo), and a higher limit, known as gradient factor high or GF(Hi). The GF(Lo) and GF(Hi) can be thought of as an additional set of lines between the ambient pressure and M-Value lines. This is shown graphically in Figure 73.

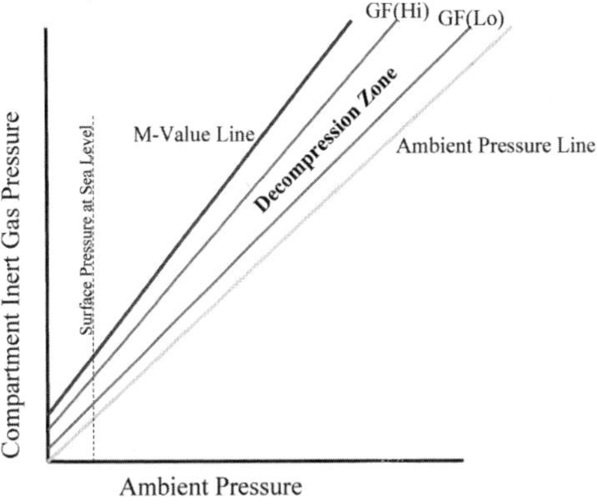

Figure 73: *Gradient factors shown graphically*

The GF adaptations to the Bühlmann model work by inserting a stop during the ascent when tissue supersaturation reaches the value for gradient factor low. So, for example, with GF(Lo) set to 30% a stop will be inserted when the leading compartment reaches 30% of the way to the M-Value line. Subsequent stops allow the maximum gradient factor to move from the low to high limit.

GF(Hi) determines the tissue tension on surfacing. You would stay at your final stop until you can ascend to the surface without any of the tissues exceeding Gradient Factor High or GF(Hi). The value of GF(Hi) determines the length of the final stop with a lower value resulting in a longer final stop and a higher value resulting in a shorter final stop.

So a GF ascent with GF(Lo) set to 30% and GF(Hi) set to 80% would let you an ascend until tissue supersaturation in your leading compartment reaches 30% of the M-Value for that compartment. This is shown in Figure 74. Once you reach the GF(Lo) limit, in this case 30% the model calculates the maximum gradient factor required to move from the GF(Lo) point to the GF(Hi) on reaching the surface. This is also shown in Figure 74 as the black line connecting the 30% and 80% lines.

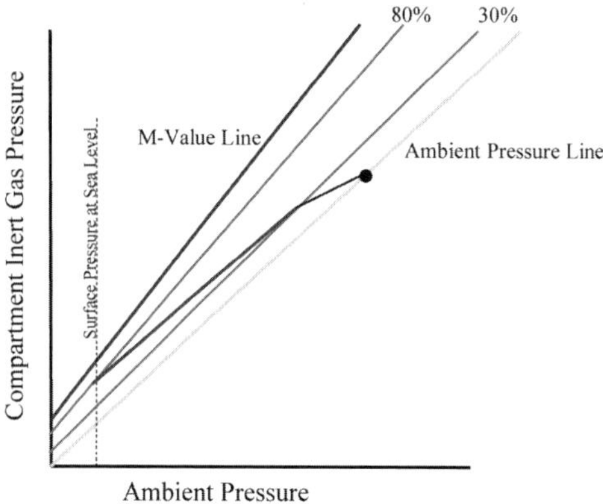

Figure 74: *Gradient factors applied to a Bühlmann model*

In this example a Gradient Factor ascent would then keep you at the first stop depth until your can move up to the next stop depth without any of your compartments exceeding the recalculated maximum gradient factor, i.e. without breaking the 80% line. The ascent continues with the maximum gradient factor and hence the maximum percentage of supersaturation moving from 30% towards 80%. On the last stop the model will keep you at the stop depth until you can ascend to the surface without any of your compartments exceeding 80% of their M-Value. The full ascent using these settings is shown in Figure 75.

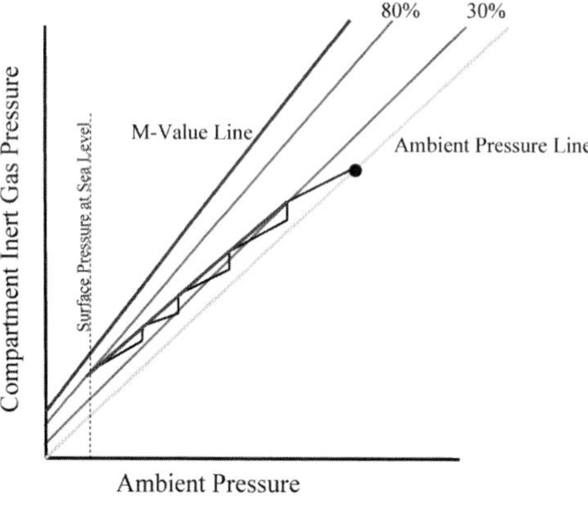

Figure 75: *A gradient factor based ascent*

The values used for GF(Lo) and GF(Hi) are not fixed. They can be chosen by the user and altered to produce a profile which suits their individual preference. The choice of settings for GF(Lo) and GF(Hi) will make significant changes to the decompression profile and the depth and length of decompression stops. The lower the value of GF(Lo) the deeper the first stop will be. For example if GF(Lo) is set to 1% then only a very slight ascent is required to reach this limit and so the first stop may only be a few metres above the bottom. On the other hand a higher setting for GF(Lo) will result in a much later or shallower first stop depth as the diver can ascend to a shallower depth before reaching the specified percentage of their leading tissue M-Value. Equally the setting for the GF(Hi) will determine the length of the last stop as the diver will have to stay at their last stop until their surfacing tissue tension is less then the value for GF(Hi). Lower values of GF(Hi) will result in longer final stops whereas higher values will result in shorter final stops.

Setting the value of GF(Lo) too low can cause problems as a certain level of supersaturation is required in order to allow off gassing. By setting it too low we will introduce stops at a depth where the leading compartments are not off-gassing to any great extent but at the same time the slower compartment are still on-gassing at a significant rate. This on-gassing in the slower compartments will need to be offset by longer decompression during the shallower stops, which can add significantly to the overall decompression time.

Setting both GF(Lo) and GF(Hi) to 100 gives us the same results as using a traditional Bühlmann model. In this case the ascent would involve the diver ascending until they reached 100% of the leading compartment M-Value. They would then stay there until they could move up to the next stop again without exceeding 100% of the M-Value and on again until they could ascend to the surface without exceeding 100% of their M-Value. This of course is exactly the same as the traditional Bühlmann model ascent. It is even possible to set the GF(Hi) to a value greater than 100 which gives us a shorter final stop than the traditional model would dictate. The reasoning behind this is that the initial deep stops serve to prevent bubbles forming during the initial part of the ascent or at least reduce the number and size of bubbles formed. As a result there is less reason to carry out extended shallow decompression stops to ensure these bubbles are allowed to shrink back down and so the latter part of the decompression can be more aggressive.

30/80 is a common set of Gradient Factor settings but there are many other popular combinations. Values of GF(Lo) from 5% to 35% are used together with values for GF(Hi) ranging from 70% up to 150%.

Dual Phase (Bubble) Models

Traditional decompression models were based on the assumption that inert gases are held in solution in the body until they form bubbles and it is these bubbles that cause decompression sickness. These models are known as dissolved gas models due to the assumption that the gas is held in solution or dissolved in the body. More recent research shows that bubbles can form within the body without traditional symptoms of decompression sickness. In fact it appears that a certain level of bubbles is formed on almost every dive.

Furthermore it is now believed that bubbles are present even in people who have never dived. As a result the emphasis of modern decompression theories is not focused on preventing the formation of bubbles as we know this is not possible. Instead they try to prevent bubbles from becoming large or numerous enough to cause problems.

In the late 1960 and early 1970's an Australian PhD student named Brian Hills started studying decompression theory based on the assumption that it was necessary to track gas dissolved in tissues as well as some gas in the form of bubbles. Hills referred to this as a 'thermodynamic and kinetic approach to decompression sickness'.

Hills was one of the leading researchers of the 1970's and contributed a chapter to the third edition of Bennett and Elliot's *Physiology and Medicine of Diving,* the standard textbook on diving physiology. Despite this, his theories were so far from mainstream decompression theory that his ideas did not receive much support and there was very little follow up on his research. The pioneering work carried out by Hills faded into academic obscurity until his ideas were rediscovered by later researchers.

In addition to Hills a number of other decompression researchers were considering alternative approaches to the traditional dissolved gas model. Val Hemplemann and Tom Hennessy suggested that the body could tolerate a certain level of bubble formation and that it was only when the total volume of free phase gas exceeded a certain critical limit that DCI was triggered. This idea is known as the critical volume hypothesis and was adopted by a number of subsequent bubble models.

In Hawaii David Yount and a group of other researchers, who became known as the tiny bubble group, were investigating the factors which influenced the formation and growth of bubbles.

Theories involving a combination of dissolved gas and gas in bubbles have been christened "Dual Phase" models. The first evidence that inert gas is present in dissolved form and as bubbles was discovered once ultra-sound techniques were developed. These techniques allowed scientists to detect the presence of gas emboli within the body's tissues. This technology showed that many dives produce asymptomatic or silent bubbles. These are bubbles that appear in the blood and tissues without the pressure gradient exceeding the M-value and without causing symptoms of DCI (hence the term asymptomatic). There is clearly a grey area either side of the M-Value line which can result in bubbling even well within the limits of a traditional neo-Haldane model.

A bubble model does not completely disregard the concept of dissolved gas held within the tissues. A bubble model will track the formation of bubbles (known as the free gas phase) but will also track the gas dissolved in the body (known as the dissolved gas phase). This is achieved in a similar way to a traditional Bühlmann model with a number of tissue compartments each with their own half time which determine the rate of uptake and release of inert gas in and out of the compartment. This is the reason why bubble models are often referred to as dual phase models. During the deeper stops introduced to control bubble growth many of the slower tissues will still be on-gassing. This means that a bubble model must deal with the advantages of deeper stops as well as dealing with the increased gas loading in some tissues. The model will produce a decompression schedule that maximises the advantages of one while minimising the disadvantages of the other.

Bubble models assume that there are bubbles present in the body even before a dive. In fact they assume that even non-divers may have bubbles present in their bodies having never been exposed to any compression and decompression. These bubbles are caused by movement and cavitation in the body. If you imagine a liquid moving through a clear pipe with tight corners and a number of valves then at the corners and valves the movement and turbulence in the liquid means that we would see bubbles being formed through cavitation.

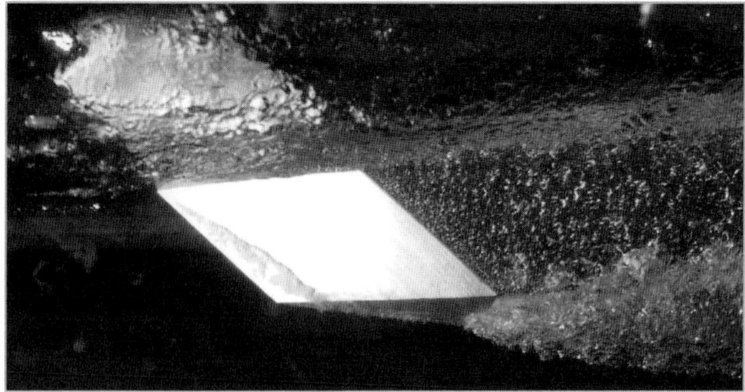

Figure 81: *Cavitation caused by a fin passing through water*

Exactly the same happens in our bodies. As blood moves through the circulatory system and travels through our muscles and other tissues, bubbles are formed by the turbulence caused. In addition, as blood is pumped through valves in the heart from one chamber to the next and then out through the arteries, the turbulence and cavitation causes more bubbles to form. These bubbles are completely normal and cause us no problems on the surface but for divers they can potentially be the trigger for decompression sickness.

Doppler studies have shown that additional bubbles are formed during almost all ascents. In contrast to the teachings of traditional models, these bubbles do not just form when we are close to or over our critical supersaturation limits. In fact bubbles start to form almost as soon as we exceed saturation and so comparatively small levels of supersaturation, well short of critical supersaturation, can still cause bubbles to form. In many cases these bubbles form in the bloodstream and are carried back to the lungs where they are 'scrubbed out' of the blood. However in some cases these bubbles can become serious enough to cause decompression sickness.

A bubble model attempts to stop these bubbles from expanding above a critical size during the ascent. There are two key aspects to bubble models. The first involves the behaviour of individual bubbles under different pressure situations and the second involves the behaviour of groups of bubbles.

Individual Bubble Behaviour

To understand how a bubble model works we first have to understand some of the pressures acting on an individual bubble. If a bubble in the body is stable, in other words it isn't growing and it isn't shrinking, then the pressures trying to make the bubble shrink must be equal to the pressures trying to make the bubble grow. If one is greater than the other then the bubble will shrink or grow depending on which is greater. When they are equal then the bubble is stable or in equilibrium.

There are usually three pressures acting on a bubble. The first is the pressure of the gas in the bubble which is pushing out and trying to make the bubble grow. The second is the ambient pressure which is squeezing the bubble and trying to shrink the bubble. The third pressure is the surface tension, known as the Laplace pressure which acts like a skin on the surface of the bubble and tries to squeeze the bubble down. If you think of a soap bubble the skin of the bubble constrains the gas in the bubble and the surface tension of the bubble causes the familiar spherical shape of the bubble. For a stable bubble these pressures are in equilibrium and so the pressure of gas in a bubble must be equal to the surrounding ambient pressure plus the surface tension. This is shown Figure 76 where the pressure of the bubbles is matched by the ambient pressure and the surface tension.

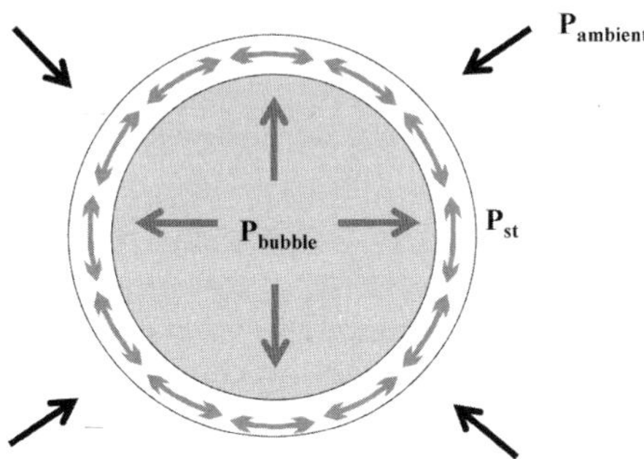

Figure 76: *The pressures acting on a bubble. The pressure in the bubble is equal to the ambient pressure plus the pressure caused by surface tension.*

If the ambient pressure is 2 bar, then the pressure within the bubble would be 2 bar plus the surface tension. A bubble about the size of a red blood cell (4 μm radius) has a surface tension of approximately 0.5 bar. Thus, the internal pressure inside the bubble is the sum of the ambient pressure (2 bar) and the surface tension (0.5 bar) which gives a total pressure of 2.5 bar. This means that due to the impact of surface tension, the pressure inside the bubble is always greater than the ambient pressure surrounding the bubble.

Ambient Pressure	2 bar
Surface Tension	0.5 bar
Bubble Pressure	2.5 bar

If the pressure of the gas inside the bubble is greater than the pressure of the inert gas dissolved in the surrounding tissue then the gas in the bubble will diffuse out of the bubble into the surrounding tissues and the bubble will shrink. Conversely if the pressure of the gas in the bubble is less than the pressure of the inert gas dissolved in the tissues then the gas will diffuse into the bubble which causes the bubble to grow. Notice that when we were looking at whether the bubble was stable we were concerned about the relationship between the pressure of the gas in the bubble and ambient pressure. Here we are concerned with the pressure of the gas in the bubble and the insert gas pressure in the tissue. The inert gas pressure can be quite different from the ambient pressure.

For example let's consider what happens to the bubble described above while we are at a depth of 10m. At this depth the ambient pressure is 2 bar. If we assume that the diver is saturated at this depth while breathing air then the dissolved nitrogen pressure in the surrounding tissues is

$$0.79 \quad x \quad 2 = 1.58 \text{ bar}$$

The pressure of the gas inside the bubble is the sum of the ambient pressure and the pressure due to surface tension so let's assume that the pressure inside the bubble is still 2.5 Bar. This pressure is therefore higher than the inert gas tissue tension of 1.58 Bar. This pressure gradient means that gas will diffuse out of the bubble and into the surrounding tissue, and so the bubble shrinks in size.

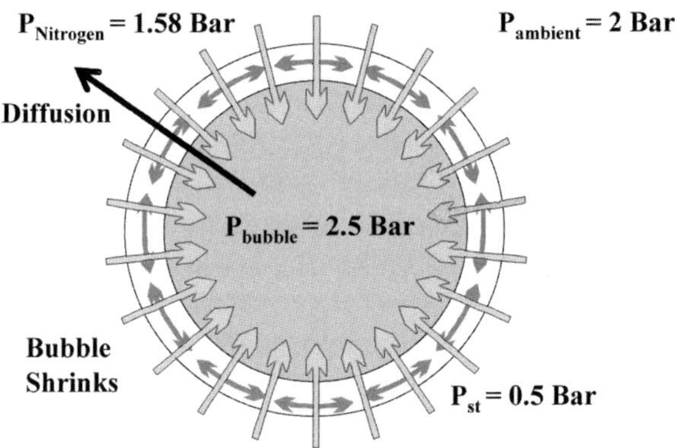

Figure 77: *If the bubble pressure is higher then the inert gas pressure surrounding the bubble then gas will diffuse out of the bubble and the bubble will shrink*

In order for the bubble to grow the dissolved gas pressure in the tissues must be higher than the combined ambient pressure plus surface tension effect. In other words, the dissolved gas pressure must be in a state of supersaturation. This could happen, for example, if a diver ascends to 10m (2 bar) from a depth of 30m where the ambient pressure is 4 bar. If the diver was saturated at 4 Bar then the inert gas tissue tension would be 4 x 0.79 = 3.16.

If the diver ascends rapidly then the tissue will not have time to off-gas and the tissue tension will still be at 3.16 even when the ambient pressure has dropped to 2 bar. This tissue is supersaturated but the inert tissue tension (3.16 bar) also exceeds the pressure inside the bubble (2.5 bar). In this situation gas will diffuses into the bubble, and as a result the bubble will grow.

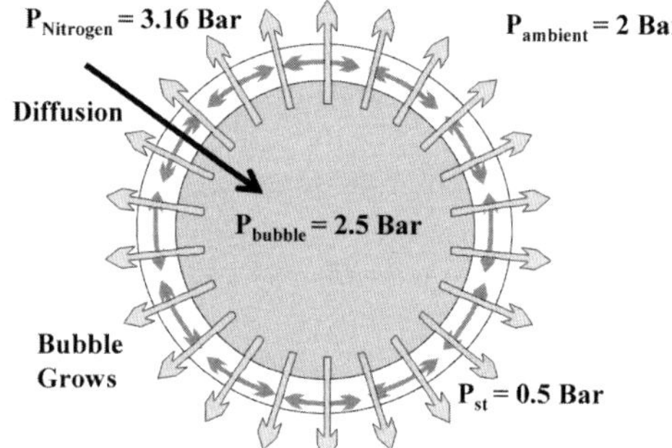

Figure 78 *If the bubble pressure is lower then the inert gas pressure surrounding the bubble then gas will diffuse into the bubble and the bubble will grow*

As the tissue off-gasses the inert gas tension will drop and at some point may drop lower than the bubble pressure. If this happens the gas will start to diffuse back out of the bubble and the bubble will start to shrink.

The surface tension of a bubble is related to the radius, i.e. the size of the bubble. Larger bubbles have a lower Laplace pressure from surface tension while smaller bubbles have a larger Laplace pressure from surface tension. As the bubble pressure is determined by adding up the ambient pressure and the surface tension pressure then, at any fixed ambient pressure, a smaller bubble with a larger Laplace pressure from surface tension pressure will have a higher bubble pressure than a larger bubble with a smaller Laplace pressure from surface tension. For example if the ambient pressure is 2.0 bar and a large bubble has a surface tension of 0.5 bar then its internal bubble pressure will be 2.0 + 2.5 = 2.5 bar. A smaller bubble with a surface tension of 1.0 bar will have an internal bubble pressure of 2.0 +1.0 = 3.0 bar.

If the inert gas tension is between the two bubble pressures then inert gas will diffuse into the larger bubble causing it to grow but will diffuse out of the smaller bubble causing it to shrink. This is shown in Figure 79 where the surrounding tissues are supersaturated giving a tissue Nitrogen pressure of 2.6 bar. The larger bubble has a bubble pressure of 2.5 bar and so Nitrogen diffuses from the tissues into the bubble, causing it to grow. The smaller bubble has a bubble pressure of 3.0 bar and so Nitrogen diffuses out of the bubble into the surrounding tissues, causing the bubble to shrink.

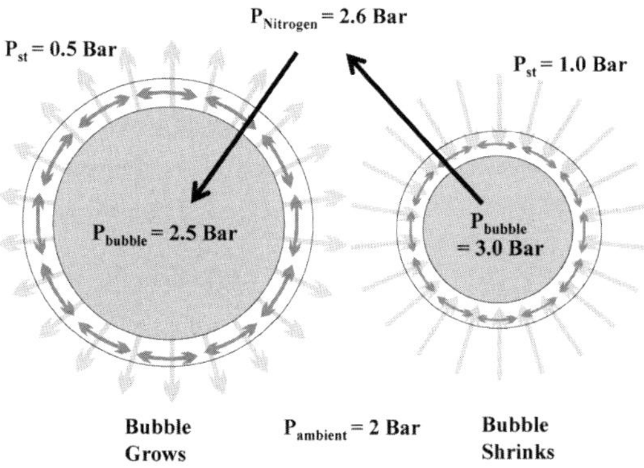

Figure 79: *Different size bubbles will be affected in different ways by a given ambient pressure*

The implication of this is that larger bubbles are more likely to grow and smaller bubbles are more likely to shrink at a given ambient pressure. At some point in the middle there will be a bubble whose size gives it a surface tension which, when added to the ambient pressure, gives a bubble pressure which is the same as the inert gas pressure in the surrounding tissues. This bubble is stable, neither growing nor shrinking. The size of this bubble is known as the critical radius.

Figure 80 shows a range of bubbles, those larger than the critical radius will grow and those smaller then the critical radius will shrink. Bubbles which are exactly at the critical radius will be stable.

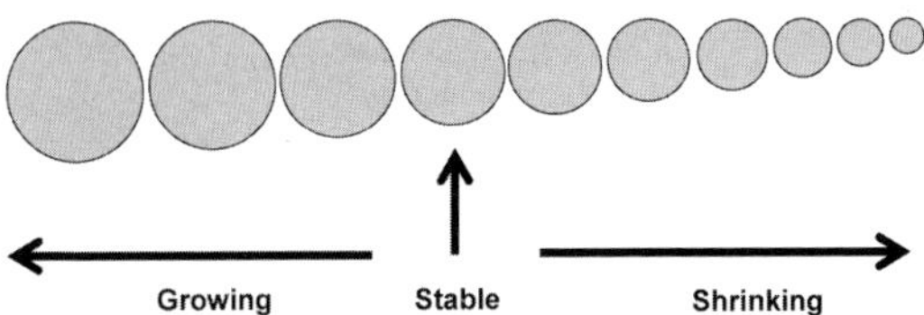

Figure 80: *Bubbles above a certain size will grow and those below it will shrink*

We could see these principles at work if we once again consider the standard visual aid for most decompression lectures: a bottle of soft drink. However, after Eric Maiken used bottles of beer to illustrate his Bubble Decompression Strategies presentation, it has become traditional to illustrate bubble model example using beer rather than soft drinks.

Initial bubble formation or, nucleation, in beer occurs at the point of imperfections in the glass rather than within the body of the liquid. Tiny scratches, marks and other minor faults in the surface of the glass allow bubble formation.

Shaking a bottle of beer before it is opened will also cause bubbles to form. This is due to the cavitation of the agitated liquid. If the bottle is then opened there is already a larger number of bubbles and gas will diffuse rapidly into these pre-existing bubbles causing the beer to froth out of the bottle. If the bottle is allowed to sit for a while after it has been shaken the bubbles will decompress back into solution. This occurs because the surface tension of the bubble compresses them back down increasing the bubble pressure and allowing the gas to diffuse out of the bubble into the surrounding beer. Despite these bubbles shrinking, they may not completely disappear. It is believed that microscopic nuclei exist in all aqueous liquids. This includes beer as well as the aqueous liquid that makes up the majority of human tissues.

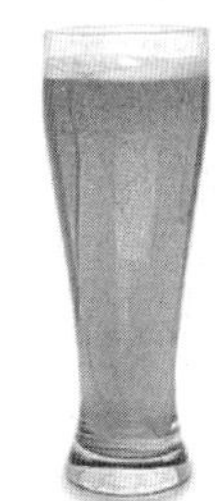

Figure 27: *Practical demonstration of bubble mechanics*

As bubbles rise up through the glass they grow larger. Depending on the height of the glass they may increase by a factor of two or three times. This increase is not due to Boyle's law. The reduction in pressure from the very bottom of the glass to the top is nowhere near enough to cause this amount of increase in volume. It would require a beer glass 10m / 33ft tall in order to have sufficient reduction in pressure to cause a bubble to double in size. The increase in size is caused by CO_2 diffusing from the liquid into the bubble. The pressure of the CO_2 dissolved in the beer is larger than the bubble pressure and so CO_2 diffuses into the bubble causing it to grow. As it grows, the surface tension will drop, reducing the bubble pressure and resulting in even more CO_2 diffusing into the bubble.

A bubble model will attempt to keep bubbles below this critical size so that they will shrink rather than grow. A traditional Haldane type ascent will bring the diver close to the surface and reduce ambient pressure. In reducing the ambient pressure and at the same time increasing the supersaturation we will encourage the bubbles to increase in size. In order to keep the bubbles from growing we need to keep the ambient pressure high and the supersaturation low and the only way to do that is to stay deeper. Thus bubble models lead to deep stops where we stop briefly at depth to allow the high ambient pressure and lower supersaturation to squeeze down the bubbles before they become too large, and the surface tension reduces allowing further growth. As a result of these stops, by the time we get to the shallower stops, we will have controlled the growth of these bubbles to the extent that there will be fewer larger bubbles than if we had made a direct ascent to the shallower stop depths.

Bubble models also include the concept of different tissue compartments that take up and release Nitrogen at different rates. In this context the fast tissues will have a higher Nitrogen loading then the slower tissues and on accent they will initially have a higher level of supersaturation. This will cause more bubbles to grow and these bubbles will grow faster than in a slower tissue with a lower level of supersaturation. This is balanced by the fact that faster tissues remove inert gas sooner than the slower tissues, which means that the supersaturation level drops very quickly in the fast tissues and so bubbles in these tissues don't have time to grow as big as they do in slow tissues.

Of course while we are doing the deep stops some of the medium and slow tissues, which were not saturated, will still be on-gassing. If we were to carry out very long deep stops or stop at very deep depths then this could cause a problem as the increased on-gassing in the slow tissues may result in longer decompression later on to allow these tissues to off-gas. Any bubble model must balance out the advantages of deeper stops in reducing bubble growth against the increased on-gassing in the mid to slow tissues.

Multiple Bubble Behaviour

The behaviour of multiple bubbles within the body and their impact on the onset of decompression sickness is the second key aspect of bubble models. Haldane and many subsequent researchers assumed that it was the formation of bubbles that caused decompression sickness but as we have seen a certain number of bubbles are formed on every dive. These do not trigger signs of decompression sickness. What then is the cause of decompression sickness if it is not bubble formation? Bubble models assume that there is a maximum number of bubbles that can be tolerated without causing decompression sickness. In other words the body can tolerate a certain number of bubbles without showing any signs of decompression sickness but if the number of bubbles formed exceeds a certain threshold then signs and symptoms of decompression sickness will occur. If this is true, then keeping the super-saturation level below that required to stimulate the critical number of nuclei should prevent decompression sickness.

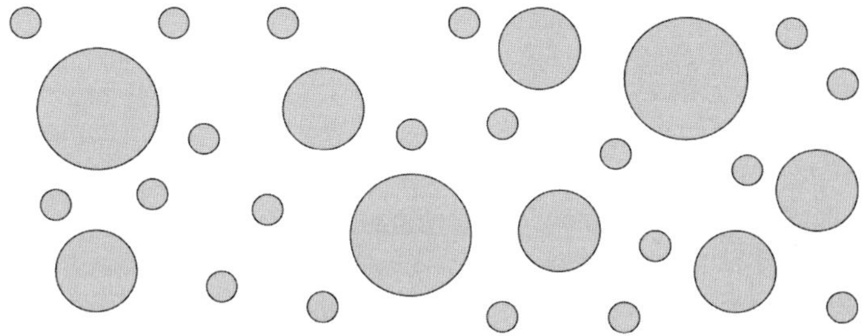

Figure 82: *Bubbles within the body will vary in size*

When bubbles form within in the body there will be a combination of bubbles of varying sizes and, as we have seen, at a given ambient pressure and supersaturation level, larger bubbles are more likely to grow then smaller ones.

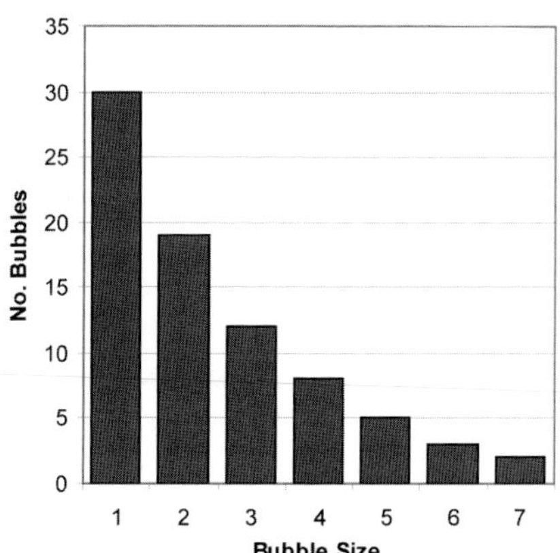

Figure 29: *Number of bubbles in each size category*

If we classified all of the bubbles that are formed according to their size and gathered all of the bubbles in each category together then we would find that there would be lots of smaller bubbles, a lower number of medium sized bubbles and even fewer large bubbles.

This is shown in Figure 29 where we can see that there are 30 bubbles of size 1, 19 bubbles of size 2 and so on up to 2 bubbles of size 7. The actual sizes of the bubbles are purely for illustration. However the pattern shown here with a large number of smaller bubbles and progressively fewer large bubbles is exactly the pattern we would expect to find. From this we can see that it is easy to tell how many bubbles are above or below a certain size. We can see that there are 5 + 3 +2 = 10 bubbles which are size 5 or greater.

We can easily re-draw Figure 29 to give us the cumulative total of bubbles of a given size or larger. If we add up all the bubbles of a given size or larger we get the graph shown in Figure 30. From this we can easily read off the number of bubbles which are of a certain size or bigger. We can directly read off that there are 10 bubbles which are of size 5 or bigger and slightly less than 50 bubbles which are size 2 or bigger.

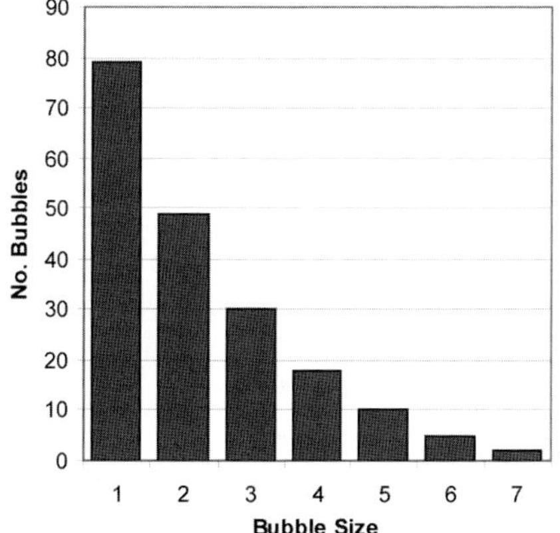

Figure 30: *Cumulative totals of bubbles of a certain size and greater*

The total number of bubbles that will be stimulated into growth is related to the minimum size stimulated into growth. The number of smaller bubbles is much higher than the number of larger bubbles so as the minimum size of bubble that is excited into growth is reduced so the total number of bubbles that will grow becomes much larger. Again we can see this in Figure 30. If bubbles of size 5 or above are excited into growth then a total of 10 bubbles will start to grow. However if bubbles of size 3 or above are excited into growth then a total of 30 bubbles will start to grow. So we can achieve our aim of preventing more than a critical number of bubbles from growing by ensuring that no bubbles smaller than a certain size are allowed to grow. If we wanted no more than 20 bubbles to grow then from Figure 30 we can see that we have to ensure that only bubbles of size 4 or above are allowed to grow. The certain size is known as the initial critical radius. In any bubble model there will be an initial critical radius for Nitrogen and another for Helium. In addition each compartment will have its own set of initial critical radii.

As we saw above for any given level of supersaturation we can calculate the critical radius which separates the bubbles that will grow from the bubbles that will shrink. We can also reverse this calculation to give us the supersaturation gradient that will cause only bubbles above a certain critical radius to grow.

By putting these steps together we can determine the supersaturation gradient which will ensure that only bubbles above our critical radius will grow which also means that the total number of bubbles that grow will be inside the limit required to avoid decompression sickness.

The dynamics of bubble growth will vary between fast and slow tissues. Fast tissues remove inert gas faster than slow tissues, meaning that bubbles don't have time to grow as big as they do in slow tissues.

Initially the bubbles grow faster because of the typically higher pressure difference, but this is greatly outweighed by the quick removal of source gas. There is competition between bubbles and blood for the gas in the tissues. Bubbles in fast tissues run out of gas for growth much sooner than bubbles in slow tissues. However most dive tables allow a higher gradient in the fast tissues, precisely because the bubbles can't grow as fast. However this higher gradient that normally is allowed means that bubbles in fast tissues initially grow faster than those in slow tissues (even though in the end the slow tissue bubbles usually grow bigger).

This means fast tissues can have lots of small bubbles, while slow tissues can have hardly any bubbles above the minimum number. Faster tissues have higher allowed gradients. These gradients stimulate many more bubbles into growth, but because the bubbles are small the maximum free gas limit is still maintained.

To summarise this section we can say simply that the primary job of a bubble model is to prevent excessive numbers of bubbles from growing. We can define "excessive" as "no bubble smaller than X". In order to achieve this goal, the model has to calculate for each compartment a supersaturation gradient such that only bubbles bigger than X will grow. The magical number X is known as the initial critical radius and is one of the fundamental parameters of any bubble model. The values for initial critical radius, one for Nitrogen and one for Helium, have been derived experimentally.

Gas Switches and Bubble Models

In Chapter 5 we introduced the idea of a gas switch from backgas to one or more decompression gasses. The advantages of accelerating our decompression by increasing the inert gas gradient and increasing the rate of off-gassing were described in terms of a traditional dissolved gas model. We now need to look at how a bubble model deals with gas switches and see if we still get the advantage off accelerated decompression in the context of a bubble model.

If we consider the alternative name for bubbles models, that is dual phase models, then it reminds us that these models deal with gas dissolved in solution as well as gas in a free phase (bubble) form. The effect of a gas switch on the dissolved gas part of the model is exactly the same as for a traditional dissolved gas model. By reducing the fraction of inert gas in the inspired gas the inert gas gradient is increased and this results in a faster rate of off-gassing from the tissues.

For bubble models there is a further consideration. As the inert gas gradient is increased and the rate of off-gassing is increased the dissolved gas pressure in the tissues will drop faster. For supersaturated tissues this increase in off-gassing will reduce the level of supersaturation. We have seen that bubble growth is related to ambient pressure and the level of tissue supersaturation. By reducing the level of tissue supersaturation we reduce the drive for the bubbles to grow.

Figure 85 shows the situation before a gas switch. The level of supersaturation means that the smaller bubble is shrinking but the larger bubble is growing. The critical radius can therefore be seen to be somewhere between the radii of the two bubbles shown.

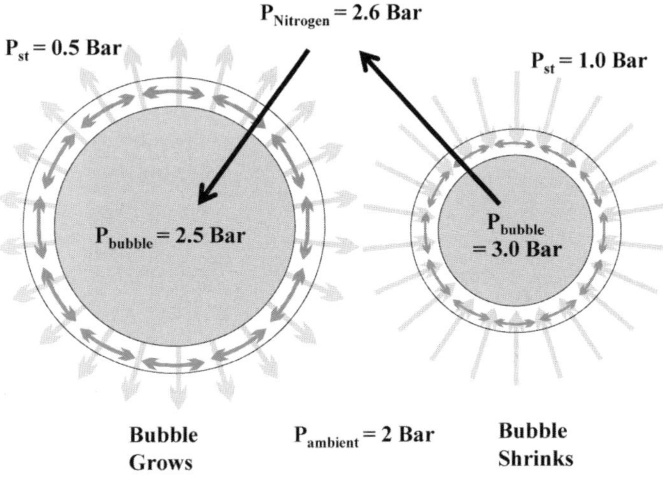

Figure 85: *Bubble dynamics before gas switch*

After the switch to the decompression gas the rate of off-gassing increases and the level of supersaturation drops. This is shown in Figure 86 where the inert gas tension is now lower than the bubble pressure in the larger bubble and so the inert gas in this bubble starts to diffuse out and it too starts to shrink. In this case the critical radius is now larger than the radius of the larger bubble. In other words bubbles which would have grown if we had continued to breathe back gas will start to shrink after the change to decompression gas. By changing the critical radius in this way we can afford to ascend earlier without allowing a sufficient number bubbles to grow so that in total the volume of free phase gas exceeds the critical volume.

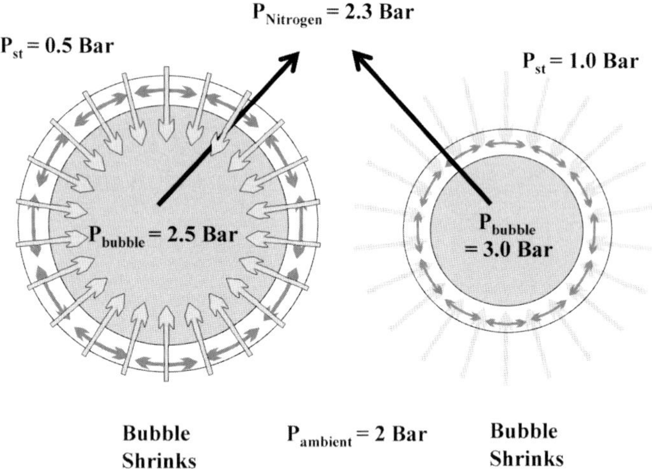

Figure 86: *Bubble dynamics after a gas switch*

From this we can see that switching to a decompression gas with a reduced level of inert gas can provide significant benefits in the context of a bubble model as well as in the context of a dissolved gas model.

In order to control bubble growth we have seen that we need to keep the ambient pressure relatively high whilst keeping the supersaturation low. In order to keep the ambient pressure high we have to remain at depths which are deeper than traditional decompression stops. If our decompression gas is chosen so that we can switch at shallow decompression stops then we will not get the benefit of reduced supersaturation in conjunction with increased ambient pressure. In order to get the benefit of both we need to perform a switch to decompression gas whilst still quite deep. This is one of the reasons for the increase in popularity of EAN50 as a decompression gas. By switching onto EAN50 at 21m the ambient pressure is still high and the benefits of the decompression gas will reduce the level of supersaturation.

Specific Bubble Models

Thermodynamic Model

The thermodynamic model was the pre-cursor of subsequent bubble model approaches. It was developed by Brian Hills in the late 1960 and early 1970's and later developed by other researchers. The model is more complicated than earlier models as it takes into account a number of factors that drive decompression rather than focusing on just one factor. The model takes into account gas dissolved in tissues as well as gas in the form of bubbles. It also takes into account gas uptake by diffusion and perfusion. Unlike many earlier models that assumed gas uptake was either perfusion limited or diffusion limited Hills' model combines both processes. Inert gas tension in the blood and tissues are obviously interrelated and Hills modeled this using a complicated feedback loop between the two areas.

The model assumes that a safe ascent can be calculated by balancing the constraints of allowing dissolved gas to come out of the tissues as fast as possible while at the same time preventing bubble growth. This is the key task of any bubble model and leads to the common dilemma that decreasing pressure (depth) is required to speed off-gassing of dissolved gas while increased pressure (or depth) is required to control bubble formation.

Hill's theories were based partly on research he carried out while studying Okinawan pearl divers operating in the Torres Straits of Northern Australia. This research was historically significant as well as being scientifically significant. The Australian pearl diving industry, which had begun in the 1850's, was being undermined by synthetic pearls and the whole industry was dying out. The study by Le Messurier and Hills captured a vast body of experience that would otherwise have been lost. The pearl divers regularly dived to depths of 90m 300 fsw for as long as one hour. They would carry out these dives twice a day, six days a week, and for ten months out of the year. Between 1850 and 1950 there were about 4,000 deaths and many more cases of residual decompression injury. To reduce this accident rate they began using decompression schedules that were developed by trial and error rather than being based on any underlying decompression theory. They would begin their decompression stops much deeper then required by traditional theory but ended up with less overall decompression times. The tables were developed empirically, but they worked. The results cannot be dismissed as a few unverified examples as the number of dives carried out is more than enough to show a statistically significant result. Over a million dives were carried out which means that these empirical tables were based on more test dives than any 'official' tables.

Similar results were reported by Farm and Hayashi amongst fishermen in Hawaii. These divers would make between 8 and 12 dives a day to depths beyond 106m/350 fsw. A typical dive series might start with a dive to 220 fsw, followed by two dives to 120 fsw and end with three or four more dives to less than 60 fsw–with little or no surface interval between dives. These dive profiles were way outside conventional theory and tables, but again they worked. Despite contradicting traditional theory when these dives are analyzed using bubble models it is clear that these empirical approaches are adopting the same strategy as have been adopted by modern bubble models.

Although called the Thermodynamic Model, Hills has said that it could have been more appropriately named the 'Zero supersaturation' model as, unlike traditional models which encouraged high levels of supersaturation, the thermodynamic model advocates an approach where there is a much lower level of supersaturation. Indeed when inherent unsaturation is taken into account the ascent can be considered to be zero supersaturated.

The thermodynamic model is based on a number of assumptions.

1. Only one critical tissue type is considered. This is due to the observation that it is typically a single type of tissue that first presents symptoms of DCS. In the case of caisson workers it is usually the lower limbs where DCS is first detected but for divers it is usually the upper limbs. The assumption is that if we can avoid DCS in these critical or marginal tissues then we will also avoid DCS in all other tissues.
2. The formation of gas nuclei or gas seeds occurs randomly throughout the various parts of the tissue as well as at various stages of supersaturation.
3. The formation of gas nuclei through cavitation, or any other method, occurring in a supersaturated tissue will result in 'dumping' gas into the gas nucleus. As a gas nuclei is formed the dissolved gas remaining in the adjacent tissues will quickly diffuse into the bubble causing the pressure in the tissue to drop and the corresponding pressure in the bubble to rise until equilibration is reached.
4. Phase equilibration: The growth of the gas phase until it is in equilibrium with the surrounding tissue , occurs quickly and is completed within a few minutes.
5. Once bubbles have formed they tend to coalesce causing physical pressure on tissues or nerves and triggering pain when this pressure reaches a certain threshold.
6. Once bubbles have formed they are only eliminated by inherent unsaturation.

Just like any other decompression model the thermodynamic model attempts to select the pressure (or depth) where the driving force for inert gas elimination is at its maximum. However this model assumes that the optimum point will vary depending on whether a gas phase exists or not. If no gas phase exists, that is no bubbles have been formed, then the optimum point is the lowest pressure (and hence shallowest depth) before bubbles will form. In this case it is better to ascend to shallower depth, as prescribed by a dissolved gas model, in order to obtain a greater inert gas gradient and increase inert gas elimination. However, if a gas phase exists, that is bubbles have already been formed, then the optimum point is the highest pressure (and deepest depth) where the gas phase still exists. Ascending any shallower than this point is the worst possible action since more gas will be formed which will reduce the rate of off-gassing In addition supersaturated gas dissolved in the tissues will diffuse into the bubbles, reducing the inert gas tissue tension which then reduces the inert gas gradient and further slows the rate of off-gassing.

These two points coincide with each other at the position of thermodynamic equilibrium.

The need to maintain a higher level of pressure in order to control bubble growth leads to a much deeper first stop. The chart in Figure 87 shows the difference in the decompression profile for the thermodynamic model when compared to the US Navy and Royal Navy Models. This clearly shows the differences in decompression schedule between the thermodynamic model and traditional models.

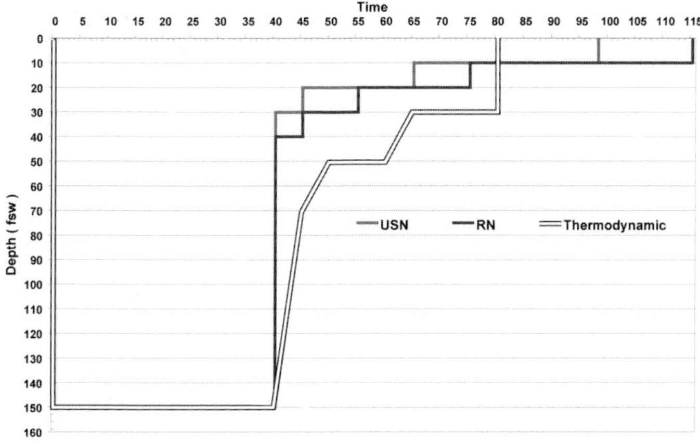

Figure 87: *Thermodynamic model compared to US Navy and Royal Navy models*

This graph also shows why Hills' model was considered such a radical departure. For researchers used to a dissolved gas frame of mind this was almost as revolutionary as when Copernicus first suggested that the Earth orbited the Sun rather then the other way around. The traditional model predicts that the deeper stops will slow the rate of off-gassing due to a lower inert gas gradient and that the mid range and slower tissues will still be on-gassing. In addition, the considerably shorter shallow stops would mean that there was insufficient time to off-gas enough to ascend to the surface without exceeding critical supersaturation and risking decompression sickness.

The thermodynamic model was such a radical departure from traditional models that Hills encountered significant skepticism. Despite years of advocating two-phase models he finally gave up and switched his attention to other areas of research. He says that "Haldanian methods were simply too deeply ingrained in the psyche of diving medical officers for any alternative to be considered". It would be another 20 years before the work of other researchers would make enough of an impact for bubble models to gain any level of widespread acceptance. It was only when these bubble models became more widely accepted that the value of Hills research came to be recognized.

Varying Permeability Model

The Varying Permeability Model (VPM) is a bubble model that considers both dissolved gas and free phase gas (bubbles). VPM, like many of the other bubble models, uses a multi tissue dissolved gas model to track the uptake and release of dissolved gas. It uses a 32 compartment model with 16 compartments tracking the Nitrogen loading and 16 compartments tracking Helium loading. Unlike a traditional dissolved gas model VPM only uses the 16 paired compartments to track gas loading. It doesn't monitor M-Values and instead the ascent limitations are introduced by bubble considerations rather than a critical supersaturation limit.

VPM assumes that gas seeds, or micronuclei, are present in the body at all times. These gas seeds are small enough to remain in solution but do not get completely crushed.

VPM was a natural development of the work of Brian Hills. During the 1980's a number of researchers at the University of Hawaii developed Hills' ideas and performed a number of experiments to determine the mechanics of bubble formation and growth. Their work was based on a series of laboratory studies on the formation and growth of bubbles in gel.

The group became known as the 'tiny bubble model group'. Although a number of researchers were involved, it was Dr David E Yount who led the project and he is the person most closely associated with the development of the model.

The VPM assumes that micronuclei exist in water at atmospheric pressure. These micronuclei will therefore also be present in tissues before the start of a dive as the tissues largely consist of water. Any nuclei larger than a specific 'critical' size will grow during decompression. The critical size is largely related to the dive depth. VPM aims to minimise the total volume of these growing bubbles by keeping the ambient pressure high, and the inspired inert gas partial pressures low during decompression. Several experiments have shown that the probability of bubble formation can be reduced if a high initial level of pressure is applied. Since solid or liquid nuclei would not be affected Dr Yount concluded that the nuclei must be primarily gas and so micro nuclei are also referred to as "gas seeds".

The assumption that gas seeds exist before the start of every dive is surprising. In theory, all bubbles should eventually dissolve as surface tension makes the bubble pressure higher than the surrounding dissolved gas pressure. This means that the gas in the bubble will diffuse out into the surrounding tissues. This causes the bubble to shrink which results in an increase in the surface tension and a corresponding increase in the bubble pressure. The increased bubble pressure will cause even more gas to diffuse out. This situation should mean that as the bubble shrinks the gas diffuses out even faster, causing it to shrink even further. Eventually the bubble should shrink completely and all the gas returns to a dissolved state.

Despite the explanation above, in reality, bubbles don't always dissolve. A number of explanations have been suggested as to why this doesn't always occur. The explanation proposed by the VPM model is that the tiny bubbles become 'stabilised' at a certain size by an elastic skin or membrane composed of "surface active molecules", known as surfactants.

These surfactants act like the skin of a soap bubble and form a layer around the gas bubble. The molecules can be thought of as having two ends. One end repels water (it is hydrophobic) while the other end attracts water (it is hydrophilic). Molecules with both ends will go to the gas-water interface, with the hydrophobic end inside the gas and the hydrophilic end in the water.

Just as each water molecule "pulls" towards each-other to create surface tension, each surfactant molecule "pushes" against the others. Surfactant molecules can be thought of as tiny springs pushing against each-other in the skin of the bubble. When a bubble is compressed by descending, the area available for each spring is reduced. Each spring pushes back more as it is squeezed against its neighbours. But just like real springs, eventually they can't push back any more. At this point, springs will start to be squeezed out of the bubble surface.

This skin formed by the surface active molecules counteracts the effect of surface tension. As the bubble is squeezed down and the effects of surface tension are reduced, the pressure inside the bubble will be equal to the ambient pressure. If the tissue pressure is equal to the ambient pressure, there is no pressure gradient for gas to diffuse out of the bubble. No diffusion means the bubble will not shrink and so it stabilises at its new smaller radius. This can be used to explain why smaller bubbles are only squeezed down to a certain size, rather than being completely crushed.

For slightly larger bubbles the effect of the surfactant molecules is reduced as the springs loose contact with each other and cannot push against each other to counteract the effects of surface tension. This means that the effects of surface tension once again start to play a part in the dynamics of bubble growth or shrinkage.

As the surfactants push together they can form a diffusion barrier. This just means that the concentration of surfactant molecules in the bubble's skin slows down the rate at which gas molecules diffuse out of the bubble and into the surrounding tissues.

We can once again use our beer analogy to illustrate the idea of surfactants. Traditional beers use ingredients which form a surface active layer around each bubble. This means that these beers have a naturally foamy consistency as the surfactant stop the bubbles from shrinking away to nothing. Many industrially produced beers and lagers do not have these natural ingredients and so the brewers must add chemicals to provide bubble skins in order to keep the beer from appearing flat.

A number of models to describe the exact behaviour of surfaced active models have been proposed. The two main models are those proposed by Tomas Kunkle and David Yount. Kunkle's model assumes that when surfactants leave the bubble they become part of the main body of the surrounding liquid and don't return or interact in any way with the bubble they left. His model also proposes that the strength of the diffusion barrier is related to how closely the surfactant molecules are squeezed together. As they are squeezed closer and closer together the resistance to diffusion increases.

Yount's model, on the other hand, assumes that the surfactants stay close to the bubble they have just left and so there is a reservoir of surfactants in the vicinity of the bubble skin. His model also plays down the 'springiness' of the surfactant molecules; the molecules do not push back against one another until they reach a certain threshold. At this point they push back fully and start to leave the surfactant layer. A better analogy for the behaviour of Yount's surfactants might be billiard balls rather then springs. The implication of this approach is that surfactants either don't block diffusion at all or block it completely causing the diffusion barrier to become completely impermeable at a certain pressure. This impermeability is reached at approximately 90m (300 ft) and so is not a concern for the majority of divers but does become of interest to deeper technical divers. The implication of this theory is that during descents past 90m (300ft) an impermeable bubble won't be crushed as much as a permeable bubble would have been as gas doesn't diffuse out as it shrinks.

Critical Volume Algorithm

The original VPM model used a bubble number limit where the ascent was limited to ensure that no more than a certain number of bubbles are formed. This works well for saturation diving but results in a decompression schedule that is far too conservative for 'bounce' dives, i.e. non-saturation dives. The solution adopted by Yount and Hoffman was to include the critical volume model that had been proposed by Hennessey and Hempleman. This model assumes that there is a critical total volume of gas in bubbles that triggers DCI. If we keep the total gas volume below this critical volume then we can avoid DCI.

The dynamic critical volume algorithm assumes that the body can eliminate or tolerate a certain number of bubbles and the associated volume of released gas for an indefinite period of time. It also assumes that the body can eliminate or tolerate an even greater "critical volume" of released gas for a limited period of time.

During the ascent gas is entering and leaving the free (bubble) phase and so the additional gas volume is dynamic. The rate at which the free phase gas inflates is assumed to be proportional to three factors; the gradient, time and number of bubbles.

As the number of bubbles increases then the volume of gas in those bubbles will also increase. Bubbles continue to grow over time and so a longer timeframe allows more growth and hence more volume than a shorter time frame. Finally the supersaturation gradient also drives the growth of bubbles and so a higher gradient means a faster rate of growth and a corresponding increase in total bubble volume

Therefore we can see that the volume of gas present can be found by calculating the product of these three factors

Total volume = Gradient x Time x Number of bubbles

The total volume of released gas in the body at any time should never be allowed to exceed the critical volume. If this volume is exceeded the volume of bubbles is likely to trigger decompression illness. However if the total volume is greater then the amount that can be tolerated indefinitely, but less than the critical volume, we have a more effective decompression profile without risking triggering DCI. The critical volume algorithm attempts to find the most efficient decompression profile that does not exceed the critical volume threshold.

The total volume of released gas in the body at any time should never be allowed to exceed the critical volume. If this volume is exceeded the volume of bubbles is likely to trigger decompression illness.

These ideas are shown in Figure 94. The top section of the diagram shows the dive profile with bottom time, ascent and surface interval sections. In the bottom section the red line shows the maximum gradient allowed. The actual gradient is in pink and we can see that it varies during the stops. At the start of the stop we are at the maximum gradient but during the stops we will off-gas and so the gradient will reduce. At the end of the stop we ascend up to the next stop where we once again reach the maximum gradient. The blue line represents the total free phase gas within the body. This increases as we ascend and can continue to increase well into the surface interval. It is essential that this never exceeds the critical volume which is represented by the dashed red line.

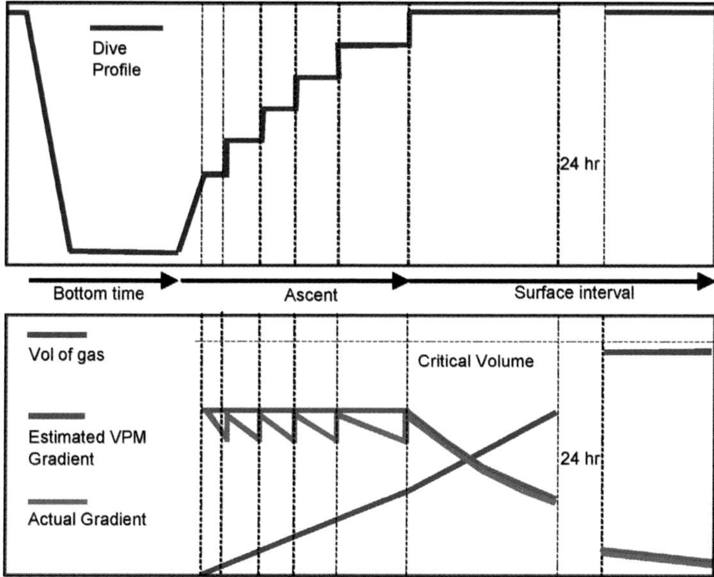

Figure 94: *Total gas volume is related to the maximum gradient*

For bounce dives the original VPM model resulted in conservative profiles. The critical volume algorithm attempts to find the most efficient decompression profile that does not exceed the critical volume threshold. This is achieved because if the total volume is greater then the amount that can be tolerated indefinitely, but less than the critical volume, we have a more effective decompression profile without risking triggering DCI.

The supersaturation gradient is really the only variable parameter and the only one that can be changed. This means that the task of the critical volume algorithm is to find out which supersaturation gradient gives us a volume of gas which is closest to our maximum value.

In order to achieve this task, the algorithm gradually increases the allowed tissue gradient until the total permitted gas volume is reached in each compartment. Starting with the initial gradient allowed by the original VPM model, the maximum allowed supersaturation gradient is increased and the total gas volume is recalculated. If it is less than allowed, the gradient is increased again and again, until the compartment maximum is reached. If the volume of gas is too large then it is recalculated with a smaller gradient until the volume of gas is less then our critical volume.

An example of this process is shown in Figure 95. In this example the orange lines represent the details of the initial ascent profile. The initial gradient generated an ascent which resulted in a total volume of gas that id considerably less then the critical volume. This means that we may be able to allow a higher gradient. In the second case, shown in blue, a higher gradient is allowed which in turn results in a more aggressive ascent profile. This generates a higher total volume of gas but still less than the critical volume. The next iteration, shown in purple, uses a slightly higher gradient which results in a shorter decompression profile and as a result a higher total volume of gas. This total level of gas is now just short of the critical volume and if we were to re-calculate the ascent based on a higher gradient we can see that the resulting gas volume would exceed the critical volume.

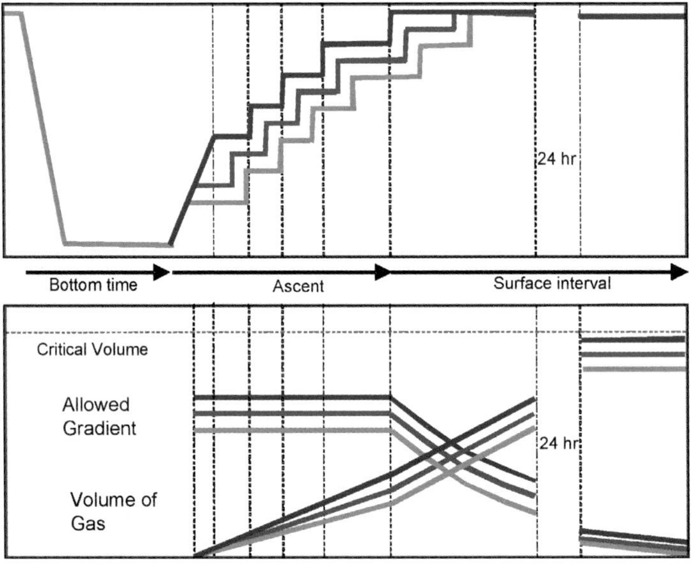

Figure 95: *Changing the allowed gradient until the critical volume is reached.*

Development of VPM

VPM and its subsequent revisions has become popular amongst the technical diving community. One of the reasons for this is that the intellectual content of the model has been made freely available which has allowed it to be incorporated into a number of PC planning programs. Between 1999 and 2001 David Yount, Erik Baker and Eric Maiken collaborated on a version of the algorithm that went beyond the original algorithm and incorporated multiple inert gases, repetitive dives and gas switches. This revised model was subsequently implemented in the V-Planner PC planning program. Sadly Dr Yount did not see the results of this collaboration as he died in April 2000 whilst playing tennis. As well as carrying out groundbreaking research into decompression theory he was professor of Physics and served as Chair of the department of physics and astronomy at the University of Hawaii and was vice president for research and graduate education. Dr. Yount wrote more than 150 research papers on high-energy physics, diving medicine, acoustics, and surface chemistry. He received the prestigious Stover-Link Award of the Undersea and Hyperbaric Medical Society in 1987 for his work on bubble formation.

Although very popular amongst technical divers it is now recognized that the original VPM model, now sometimes referred to as "VPM-A", had a flaw in the model. This flaw, however, only manifested itself in certain depth ranges. Most of the testing of the model took place in what was then the typical technical diving range of 50-80m. The results for dives in these depths were adequate. However as the use of the model moved out of this range, in either direction, the results started to become less reliable. As the depth increased the decompression predicted by the model became much too short whereas for shallower depths the decompression was far too long.

The reason for this flaw is that at the beginning of the ascent the model calculates an allowable gradient. This is the maximum allowable supersaturation gradient. Staying within this gradient ensures that bubble growth is not allowed to exceed the critical volume. This allowable gradient is calculated at around the first stop depth and is then used throughout the rest of the ascent. However the allowable gradient is only relevant at the depth at which it is calculated, as the diver ascends and the bubble dimensions change the allowable gradient is no longer valid.

In 2003, Erik Baker introduced a revision to the algorithm, which was designed to address the flaw in the original model. The new version accounts for the expansion of the bubbles in accordance with Boyle's Law and then recalculates the allowable gradient at each stop. The impact of this change at each stop is relatively small but when combined together over multiple stops can produce a significant change to the decompression profile. This change served to remove the problems that had been observed in the original model. For deeper dives the increase in bubble size forces the VPM model to reduce the allowable gradient allowed in the subsequent parts of the ascent and has the effect of increasing the length of the shallower decompression stops. However, it is not accurate to just say that this revision extends the decompression or makes it more conservative as for shallower dives it has the effect of reducing the overall decompression. This revision to the original model is usually called "VPM-B."

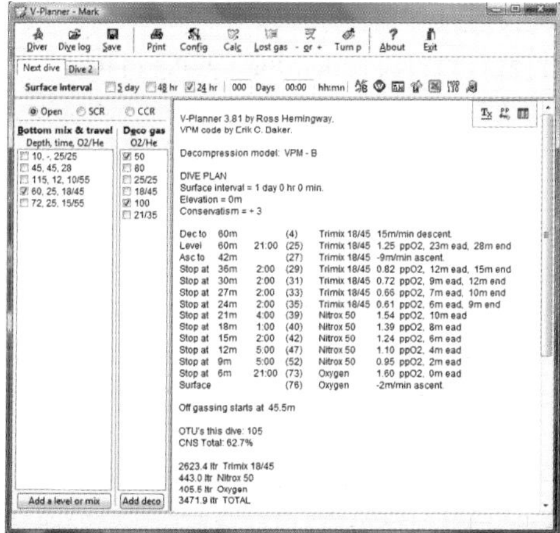

Figure 96: *A screen shot of the V-Planner decompression planning program*

In 2005 Ross Hemingway, the developer of the V-Planner program, introduced another revision to VPM, which further reduces the allowed gradients for shallow stops. The VPM-

B/E model variation is for exceptional, extreme, or extra long dives and exposures. This aspect of the model becomes active on dives with longer decompression stops, typically decompression times of over an hour in length. This results in a longer shallow section, more like that required by a traditional Haldane model. The output is similar to a combined VPM-B and Haldane plan.

Reduced Gradient Bubble Model

The Reduced Gradient Bubble Model (RGBM) grew out of the same approach as VPM. Its developer Bruce Wienke was a contributor to the overall bubble model theories which are embodied by VPM and was an advocate of VPM until he developed his own bubble model. Despite the fact that VPM and RGBM are now two distinct models it is still clear that RGBM shares at least a common development path and RGBM and VPM produce very similar decompression schedules, especially for single dives.

RGBM is a proprietary model and so its full parameters and implementation are not freely available. However, Weinke has published a number of papers and books which lay out the principles of RGBM.

RGBM is also a bubble or dual phase model that combines a weighted split between free-blood and dissolved-blood gradients, with the weighting fraction proportional to the amount of separated gas.

Managing bubble growth and limiting total bubble volume controls the initial, deep stops in an RGBM ascent. A traditional perfusion limited dissolved gas calculation then provides the controlling factor for shallow stops. In addition, because body tissues and blood are normally undersaturated with respect to ambient pressures at equilibrium, RGBM considers the "Oxygen Window" in its calculations.

In line with other bubble models RGBM features reduced no-stop time limits when compared to dissolved gas models. The other areas in which Weinke has extended the application of bubble models is in dealing with various 'real world' problems. This includes dealing with repetitive dives, reverse profile dives, multi day diving and diving at altitude.

The details of the individual dive, together with the implications of the 'real world' issues listed above can result in a situation where the volume of free gas in the body is higher than expected. Therefore in order to keep the total volume constant at the end of the dive RGBM enforces a reduction in the allowed gradient, hence the name reduced gradient bubble model. This is achieved by a set of bubble factors that are applied to the allowed gradient.

The first bubble factor is used to account for repetitive dives over the period of a few hours and is introduced to deal with the situation where bubbles created during pervious dives have not yet fully been eliminated. This factor will vary for each tissue compartment and with the length of the surface interval. Faster tissue compartment will be impacted more than slower tissue compartments. This bubble factor will introduce a significant reduction in the allowed gradient in the period immediately after a previous dive but the effect of the fact will drop off until it is negligible after 2-3 hours.

The second bubble factor accounts for the fact that deeper than previous dives (reverse profile dives) can excite previously crushed nuclei into growth. It is this feature that led Weinke and a number of other bubble modellers to speak out against the relaxation of limits on reverse profile dives at the 1999 Undersea Hyperbaric Medical Society (UHMS) conference to discuss this topic.

The third bubble factor accounts for repetitive diving over a period of several days and is used to compensate for the creation of new stabilised micronuclei in the days after the previous dive. The RGBM model assumes that a dive will crush a number of the micronuclei present in the body to the point where they are less likely to cause problems. This accounts for the phenomena of adaptability where divers who dive regularly appear to be less prone to DCS. Over the course of a few days the micronuclei regenerate and the adaptation is gradually reduced.

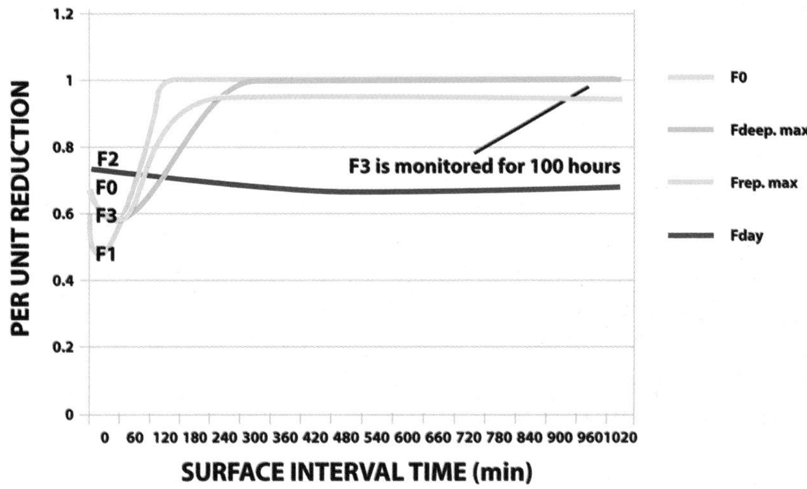

Figure 88: *Bubble factors applied to a baseline gradient*

Each bubble factor is applied to the base level gradient to produce a reduced gradient for subsequent dives. This is shown in Figure 88 where factors F1 (repetitive), F2 (multiday) and F3 (reverse) are combined to give an overall bubble factor F0. F0 is then multiplied by the allowable gradient to give the modified gradient for use on a subsequent dive. We can see from the graph that the effects of F1 and F3 are particularly significant for surface intervals of a few hours but then drop off for longer surface intervals.

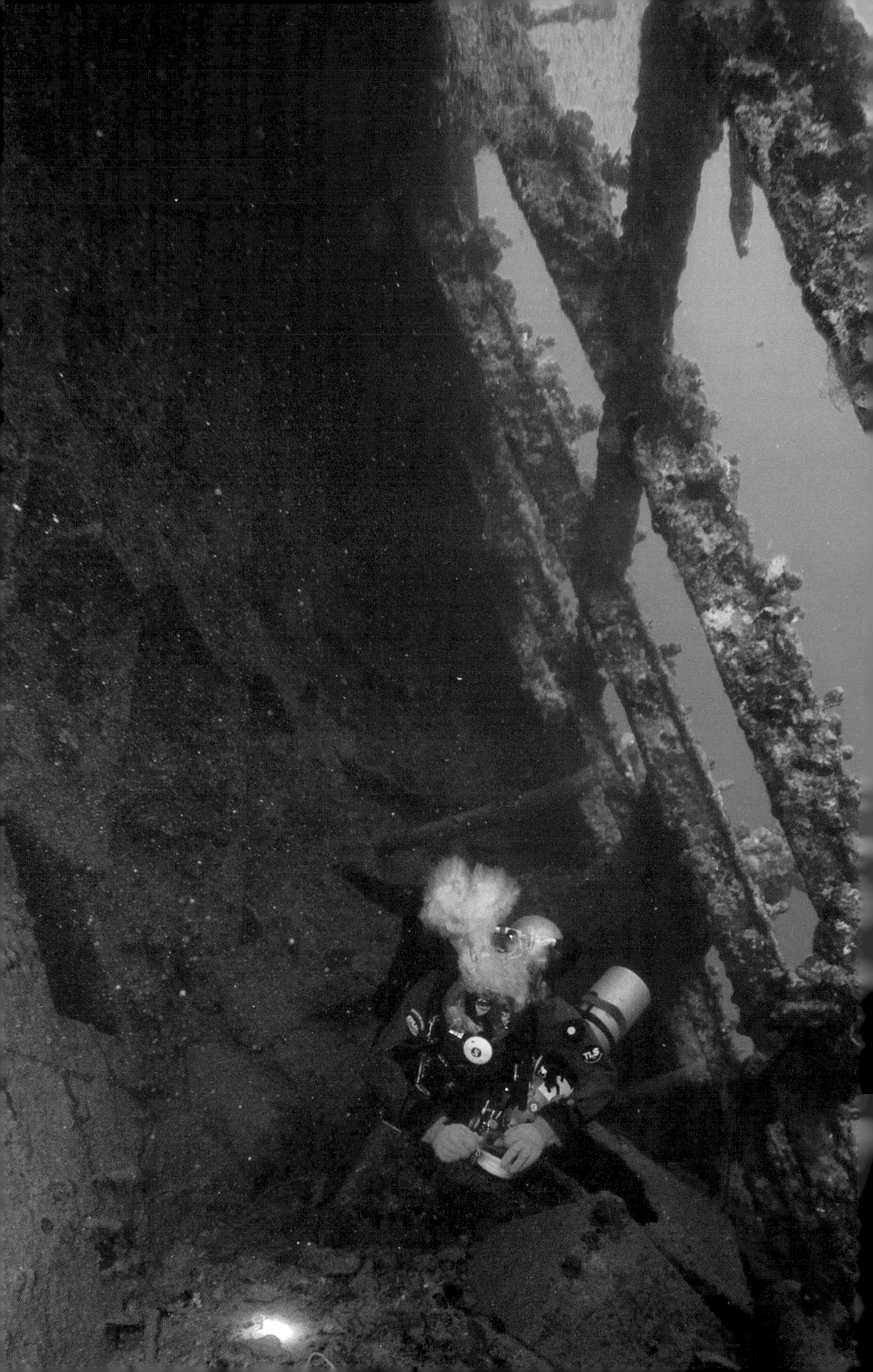
TLS

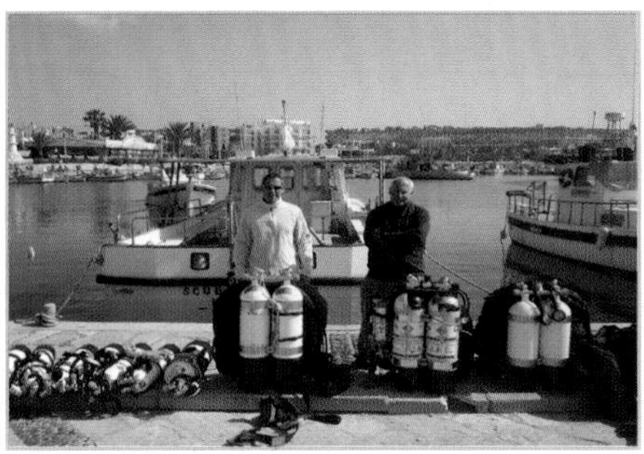

Mixed gas diving involves the use of multiple gas mixes

7 Mixed Gas

When breathing Air or Nitrox, our breathing gas is primarily made up of Oxygen and Nitrogen. We know that Oxygen is a metabolic gas and so is ignored from a decompression calculation point of view. This means that whether we are breathing air or Nitrox the only inert gas we are concerned about is Nitrogen. With Nitrox there is a lower percentage of Nitrogen than in air and so at any given depth the partial pressure of nitrogen will be lower than if we were breathing air. Other than the change in the partial pressure of nitrogen the decompression principles for air and Nitrox are identical.

Air and Nitrox have limits when used for deeper diving. The Nitrogen in air becomes increasingly narcotic below 30m and the narcosis increases in severity as the depth increases. Motor skills, memory, problem solving, logic and other higher cognitive functions all become impaired as narcosis increases. Different agencies impose different limits on the maximum depth we can dive on air as a result of the increased level of narcosis. This varies from 30m to 73m.

The oxygen in air also causes a problem for deeper diving. Oxygen toxicity becomes a risk as we go deeper and the partial pressure of oxygen increases. 1.6 bar is considered the maximum partial pressure for oxygen and on air this is reached at 66m. Many agencies specify a lower ppO_2 of 1.4 which results in a maximum depth on air of 55m. With nitrox we have a higher percentage of oxygen in the breathing mix and so the ppO_2 is higher at a given depth than for air. For example on EAN32 we reach 1.4 ppO_2 at just below 33m. This means that Nitrox is not suitable as a deep diving gas.

In order to safely plan deep dives we need a breathing mix with less nitrogen in order to reduce nitrogen narcosis and less oxygen to reduce the risk of oxygen toxicity. We could potentially replace all of the inert nitrogen with another gas although we must always leave

Left: A diver begins to enter a wreck

a certain fraction of oxygen in order to maintain the body's metabolism. To achieve this we replace part of the Nitrogen and Oxygen with a third gas which has lower narcotic potential and is not toxic at depth.

Choice of Gas

Various other gases have been considered as a replacement for Nitrogen and at least part of the Oxygen in our breathing mix. Most of the gases suitable for use in a breathing mixture belong to the family of Noble gases, so called because of their reluctance to combine with any other elements. As such the Noble gases are chemically inert. Despite the fact that these gases are chemically inert they are not biologically inert and can have a variety of effects on the body.

Argon

Argon was the first of the noble gases to be discovered and its name derives from the Greek word 'argos' or 'lazy' because of its chemical inertness. Argon is the most common of the noble gases found on earth. It is regularly used by divers for suit inflation as it is denser than air and so acts as a better insulator. However Argon is twice as narcotic as Nitrogen and so gives us no advantage over Nitrogen in the breathing mixture. In addition the density of Argon makes it difficult to breath at depth.

Neon

Neon has been used in conjunction with Oxygen (Neox) as a breathing gas as it is much less narcotic then Nitrogen. In experiments Neon has been shown to produce no symptoms of narcosis at depths of up to 1200fsw. Breathing mixtures using Neon produce less voice distortion then using Helium or Hydrogen. Neon also has lower thermal conductivity then Helium which means that it is not such a cold gas to breath or use as suit inflation. However, Neon is extremely expensive which has limited the experiments on its use. Most of the research into using Neon as a breathing gas has focused on its use in conjunction with Helium.

In addition Neon is a very dense gas and as such its rate of diffusion into tissue is very slow. This means that for very short deep dives the decompression obligation is low as very little Neon has been absorbed by the tissues. As the dive time increases and more gas is dissolved in the tissues the decompression times become extremely long as a result of the time it will take for the Neon to come out of solution.

Hydrogen

Hydrogen suffers from a major disadvantage as a breathing gas in that when mixed with Oxygen percentages over 4% it becomes explosive. A gas mixture with less than 4% Oxygen will not support life on the surface and in fact only becomes breathable below 35m. This means that a higher Oxygen content mix must be breathed down to at least 35m. This is followed by a second mix which contains 4% oxygen and some combination of Nitrogen and/or Helium. This second mix acts as a buffer, reducing the Oxygen content in the presence of an inert gas to the point where the diver can switch to a mixture of 4% oxygen and 96% Hydrogen. Despite the logistical problems involved with using Hydrogen there is a long history of experiments in using hydrogen in a breathing mix. This is because Hydrogen is the lightest element and as such is the least dense gas at depth which makes it very easy to breathe even at extreme depths.

The first recorded attempt to use hydrogen as a breathing mix was in 1789. French scientist Antoinne Lavoisier, widely regarded as the Father of Modern Chemistry, and his colleague Sequin exposed guinea pigs to mixtures of hydrogen and oxygen (Hydrox).

Swedish Engineer Arne Zetterstrom is most closely associated with research into hydrogen as a breathing gas. It was Zetterstrom developed the buffering approach to deal with the transition from air to Hydrox without risking an explosion. In 1944 he used this technique to dive to 110m/363 feet on Hydrox. In 1946 he was attempting to dive to 160m/528 feet but died when his surface crew raised him to the surface without completing his required decompression. Although his death was not related to his use of Hydrox as a breathing gas it cast a shadow over further research into this controversial breathing mix and served to stifle further research for many years.

The US Navy carried out a number of experimental dives during the 1960's and 70's. Research was carried out to try to develop realistic tissue saturation times for the development of Hydrox decompression tables.

Bill Fife at Texas A & M University successfully conducted simulated hydrox dives in a decompression chamber to a depth of 300m/1,000ft. In the ultimate show of faith in his work, Fife subjected himself to deep dives using hydrox and at one point he held the world's record for a hydrox dive at 129m/425ft. In 1976, Fife began developing the first hydrox diving tables in a project funded by the Texas Sea Grant College Program. Fife's initial tables were good for dives up to 30 minutes at 100m/300ft.

Further experimental Hydrox dives were carried out by Comex in the 1980's. They found a further problem with Hydrogen in that the narcotic effects below 150m were much more pronounced than the narcotic effects of Nitrogen. The narcotic symptoms were more like the symptoms of a hallucinogenic drug such as LSD than the symptoms of alcohol. This work suggested that Hydrox had an effective limit of 150m/500 ft for useful work.

French commercial diving company Comex carried out an extensive research programme into the use of Hydrogen based breathing mixtures during the 1980's and 90's. They carried out a series of record breaking dives achieving depths of 534 m in 1988 and then 701m in 1992. In the mid 90's they demonstrated the feasibility of combining hydrogen and helium breathing mixtures. The Hydra 12 project demonstrated the feasibility of what is known as the helium in/hydrogen out technique. Within the saturation diving chambers the divers breath standard helium based mixtures but while working on the seabed they are supplied with a helium/hydrogen breathing mixture (Hydreliox). During the Hydra 12 project the divers spent 12 days in saturation and carried out 8 dives of between 2 and 6 hours. After carrying out the hydreliox dives the divers were tested with Doppler ultrasound equipment which showed no detectable bubbles. Comex continued research into the decompression rate from Hydrogen based dives compared to Helium based dives. Initial animal testing seemed to indicate that decompression with Hydrogen was faster then decompression with Helium for the same decompression risk.

Krypton and Xenon are significantly more narcotic than Nitrogen and so are unsuitable as candidates for use in diving breathing mixes.

Helium

The idea that nitrogen narcosis could be reduced if the breathing mix was diluted with a gas other than nitrogen was first suggested as early as 1919. Professor Elihu Thompson, an electronics engineer and inventor, proposed Helium for the purpose. The problem with this suggestion was that in 1919 the price of helium was over $2500 per cubic foot and so this solution was not economically viable. When Helium was discovered in four Texas natural gas wells this completely changed the economic situation. The United States now had an exclusive monopoly on the world's supply of helium and the volume available meant that the price dropped from $2500 per cubic foot to a few cents per cubic foot. Helium was now a viable option for use in breathing mixtures.

In 1925 Thompson, in conjunction with the US Bureau of Mines and thc US Navy, began practical experiments in the use of Helium as a diving gas. Initially experiments were carried out on animals in laboratory experiments in Pittsburgh. These dives involved the use of Heliox (Helium and Oxygen). Initial experiments showed that while breathing heliox animals could be decompressed faster than if they were breathing air. With a 20% Oxygen and 80% Helium mix it was established that ⅙ of the decompression time compared with an air breathing mix was required. These experiments were repeated on human subjects and the same results were found when decompressing for ¼ of the time required for air.

During these experiments divers confirmed Prof Thompson's theory that using Helium would remove some of the symptoms of nitrogen narcosis. Divers were able to function normally at depths that would have resulted in incapacitation from narcosis had they been breathing air. Divers also reported that helium based mixes were easy to breathe due to the light nature of the gas. However they also reported problems with becoming chilled while breathing Helium. The characteristic changes to the voice, resulting in very high pitched speech, also made communication difficult between divers and support staff.

Prof Thompson also suggested that, as the helium was not consumed, it could be recycled and used again. All that was required was an effective way of removing or 'scrubbing' the carbon dioxide produced by the diver. As we have seen previously significant developments in diving are often made not by the Navies of the major powers or by commercial organisations but by enthusiastic independent amateurs or entrepreneurs. This was the case with Max Nohl who, working with Edgar End and John Craig, had developed a new type of diving helmet which also included a Helium/Oxygen system complete with a device to remove the carbon dioxide. This early mixed gas rebreather had been designed with the intention of photographing the wreck of the Lusitania. When this project was abandoned the team decided to test their device by attempting a new world depth record. In December 1937 Max Nohl set a new world depth record by diving to 127m/420ft in the cold waters of Lake Michigan.

The US Navy had also resumed serious research into the use of helium. At about the same time that Max Nohl was making his 127m/420ft dive the Navy was carrying out a chamber dive to 150m/500ft using heliox. During this dive the Navy diver was not told his depth. When asked what he thought his depth was, the diver replied, "It feels like a hundred feet." During his decompression, the diver was then told that his actual maximum depth had been 180m/500ft.

Spurred on by their success the US navy proceeded with further research into helium diving. This was put to practical use when in 1939 the submarine *USS Squalus* sank off the Isles of Shoals in 74m/243 feet. Divers were working under incredible time pressure in order to save the men trapped inside. When diving on air they were unable to reattach a cable for a rescue bell due to the incapacitating effects of narcosis. Heliox was used and the diver was able to reattach a cable for a rescue bell. 33 men were saved during this operation and the submarine was later salvaged. The rescue of the 33 men and the successful salvage was a very high profile success. This success, coupled with the growing spectre of war, prompted the US Government to increase funding for deep diving research and training.

The outbreak of World War II resulted in the US Government prohibiting the export of helium for strategic reasons. This meant that research into the use of helium for diving, or indeed any other application, was almost entirely restricted to the US for 20 years. The British Navy was allowed a restricted supply of helium for research but only after permission was granted by the US Secretary of Interior, the Secretary of Defence and the President himself. The British research was carried out on a vertical wall in Loch Fyne. This Scottish Loch was ideal for deep diving experiments as it was over 150m/500ft deep. Diver First Class Wilfred Bollard set a new record of 164m/540ft. He took 7 ½ minutes to descend, spent 5 minutes on the bottom and then spent 8 hours 26 minutes decompressing. The dive was not a complete success as the ascent time was increased by three hours to allow for treatment for a bend. Bollard had suffered elbow pain when transferring from the Davis submersible decompression chamber (which he had entered at 57m/190 feet) to the main decompression chamber at 9m/30 feet.

Helium was first used for recreational diving in the 1970's. Like many other technical diving innovations this was driven by the cave diving community. In 1970 two divers died while exploring Mystery Sink in Florida. Hal Watts, one of the pioneers of technical diving and for many years the holder of the depth record on compressed air, was asked to retrieve the body. Despite being considered one of the leading proponents of deep air diving Watts thought that using Heliox would give him a safety advantage given the depth and the effort involved in a double body recovery. Despite successfully recovering the bodies Watts suffered decompression sickness while completing his decompression stops. The incident coloured Watts' view of Heliox and he returned to using air.

In 1975 Experienced cave divers Lewis Holtzin and Court Smith used Heliox for deep cave diving. On their first dive, to 80m/265 feet, Holtzin died when he suffered oxygen toxicity during decompression. Although not related to the use of Heliox on the dive the death of Holtzin nevertheless cast a shadow of the use of Heliox. In 1980 Dale Sweet used heliox to reach 109m/360 feet in the cave Die Polder Sink #2. Although six months later, cave diving legend Sheck Exeley made the same dive on compressed air, the era of helium based mixes for deep exploration, both for cave diving and deep wreck exploration, had started. In 1981, German cave diver, Jochen Hasenmayer, descended into the French Vaucluse cave system to reach a depth of 144m/476 feet using Heliox. This was a new world record for a surface-to-surface scuba dive. In 1983, Hasenmayer made another Heliox dive. This dive was to 207m/685 feet and another world record

Most of the early research into the use of Helium used Heliox, a mixture of Helium and

Oxygen. Heliox as a breathing gas has two disadvantages. At depths in excess of 120m divers on Heliox start to experience muscle spasms and tremors. These tremors are known as High Pressure Nervous Syndrome (HPNS). Research by Peter Bennett at Duke University showed that by adding a small percentage of Nitrogen into the breathing mixture prevented the onset of HPNS.

The other disadvantage of Heliox is that Helium is an expensive gas and the high Helium percentages required for Heliox make this an expensive breathing mixture. This is not a major problem for commercial or military use but as recreational divers began to dive deeper the cost of using Heliox was a significant factor. Adding Nitrogen into the mixture reduces the risk of HPNS and also reduces the cost of the mixture. This mixture of Helium, Nitrogen and Oxygen is termed Trimix.

For all of the reasons above Trimix (Oxygen, Helium and Nitrogen) has become the gas of choice for deep technical dives in the recreational area whereas Heliox is still the first choice for commercial divers..

A summary of the various physical properties of the gases discussed is shown in Table 22 below.

Gas	Helium	Neon	Hydrogen	Nitrogen	Argon	Krypton	Xenon
Symbol	He	Ne	H	N	Ar	Kr	Xe
Narcotic level	4.26	3.8	1.83	1.0	0.43	0.14	0.039
Density	Low	Medium	Low	Medium	High		
Tissue Solubility	Low	Low	High	Medium	High		
Cost	Medium	High	Low	Low	Medium		

Table 22: *Physical Properties of Gases*

Trimix

Trimix is any combination of Helium, Nitrogen and Oxygen. A variant where Helium is topped up with Air (containing Nitrogen and Oxygen) is known as Heliair or "poor mans mix". Trimix mixes can be normoxic, hypoxic or hyperoxic.

Normoxic mixes contain a level of Oxygen which is at or near the level found in normal air. Generally a mix with between 18-21% Oxygen is considered Normoxic. The balance will be made up of Nitrogen and Helium. Normoxic mixes are generally used for depths down to 60m. At this depth the amount of Oxygen in the mixture will start to approach a partial pressure of 1.4 Bar which most training agencies recommend as the maximum partial pressure for back gas.

Hypoxic mixes are those with less then 18% Oxygen. Mixtures such as this where the Oxygen is reduced are used for greater depths as the reduction in Oxygen percentage allows the diver to descend to a greater depth before reaching the maximum partial pressure of Oxygen. However a mix with less than 18% Oxygen is considered to low a percentage to breathe at the surface. As a result an additional gas, known as a travel gas, must be breathed during the initial part of the descent until the depth is such that the partial pressure of Oxygen is sufficient to support life.

The third type of Trimix, a hyperoxic mix, is one in which the percentage of Oxygen is higher than normal air, that is higher than 21%. Hyperoxic mixes are sometimes used in the 30-55m range where divers want to reduce the effect of narcosis whilst still benefiting from the decompression advantages of reduced overall inert gas content in the gas.

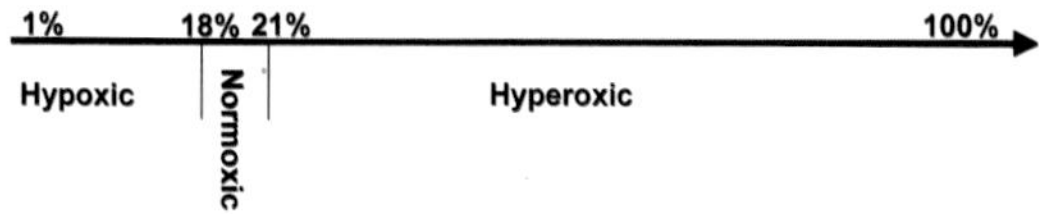

Figure 89: *Hypoxic, Normoxic and Hyperoxic Oxygen levels*

From a decompression point of view Trimix adds a number of considerations. Rather than a single inert gas we now have two different inert gases to deal with. If Helium and Nitrogen had exactly the same properties then this wouldn't be too much of a problem but in fact Helium and Nitrogen, as can be seen from Table 22 above, have quite different physical properties. It is dealing with these properties that makes trimix decompression theory more complicated than air or nitrox decompression.

Helium molecules are much smaller than Nitrogen molecules and so will diffuse into and out of tissues much faster then Nitrogen. This has led to Helium being referred to as a 'fast gas'. Helium uptake and elimination in the body has traditionally been tracked by using the same approach as for Nitrogen, i.e. assuming a half time for each tissue. However due to the fact that Helium is a 'fast' gas the halftimes for helium are usually taken to be 2.7 times faster than Nitrogen for the same tissue. This is shown in Table 23 where the half times for Nitrogen and Helium for each of the compartments in Bühlmann's ZHL-16A model are shown.

Compartment	Half-time Nitrogen	Half-time Helium
1	4	1.5
2	8	3.0
3	12.5	4.7
4	18.5	7.0
5	27	10.2
6	38.3	14.5
7	54.3	20.5
8	77	29.1
9	109	41.1
10	146	55.1
11	187	70.6
12	239	90.2
13	305	115.1
14	390	147.2
15	498	187.9
16	635	239.6

Table 23: *Nitrogen and Helium half times for ZHL-16A*

The result of the faster half time is that a given compartment will saturate with Helium much faster then it will saturate with Nitrogen. For any given dive at the end of the bottom time more compartments will be saturated with Helium than with Nitrogen and most compartments will have a higher level of saturation of Helium than Nitrogen.

This is shown in Figure 90 which represents tissue loadings for Helium and Nitrogen. These loadings are for a 60m dive for 40 minutes using 20/40. 20/40 was chosen for this example as it means that the inert gas portion of the breathing mix is 40% Helium and 40% Nitrogen. The equal percentages of Helium and Nitrogen make it easier to compare the behaviour of the two gases.

We can see that compartments one to three are saturated with Helium and compartment four is very close. In contrast only compartment 1 is saturated with Nitrogen and all the others are at a lower level of saturation. We can also see that in most of the compartments the level of Helium loading is higher then the level of Nitrogen loading.

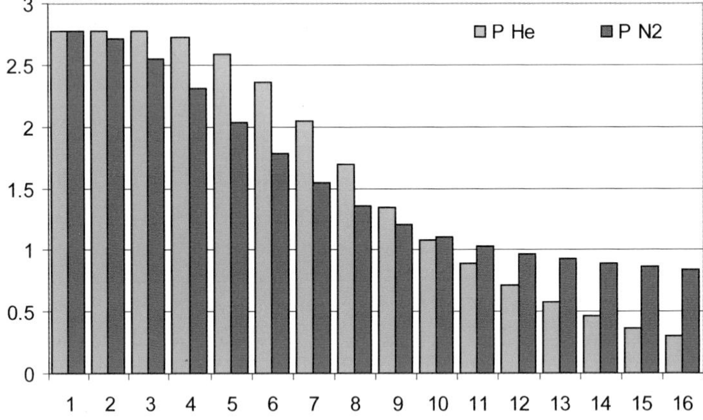

Figure 90: *Tissue loadings at the end of the bottom time*

The exception to this is the slower compartments eleven to sixteen. The reason for this is that all compartments already have a Nitrogen loading from being saturated with Nitrogen at the surface, but do not have any Helium loading. The existing Nitrogen loading is quickly overtaken by the Helium loading in the faster compartments but in the slower compartments it will take a long time for the Helium to on-gas enough to overtake the Nitrogen loading already present.

During the initial part of the ascent the higher level of helium in the faster tissues means that the diver will reach supersaturation and potentially critical supersaturation earlier then if they had been breathing Nitrogen. As a result the first decompression stop may be deeper than an equivalent Nitrogen dive.

The faster half time for Helium means that it on-gasses faster and has a higher initial level of saturation but the other side of the coin is that Helium also off-gasses faster. This means that the Helium is eliminated faster then Nitrogen and during the later part of the dive Helium levels may be lower than Nitrogen levels. This is clearly shown in Figure 91. This shows the tissue loading at the 24m stop for the same dive used above. As we can see the Helium loading in the faster tissues has dropped significantly. It is now considerably lower than the

Nitrogen loading for compartments one through four. In the mid range compartments five to ten the Helium level is still higher then the Nitrogen level as these compartments haven't has sufficient time to off-gas enough for the Helium to drop back below the Nitrogen. The slowest compartments, eleven to sixteen, still have a higher level of Nitrogen due to the initial loading from saturation at the surface.

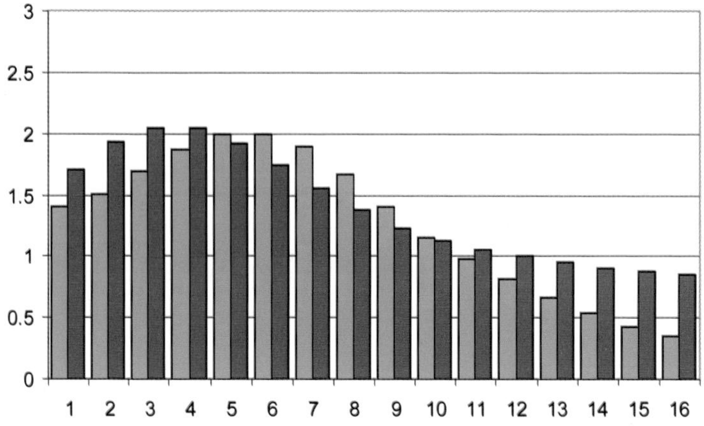

Figure 91: *Tissue loadings during ascent*

Another difference between Helium and Nitrogen is the Helium is less soluble then Nitrogen. The solubility of Helium in blood is 0.0087 atm^{-1} whereas the solubility of Nitrogen in blood is 0.0122 atm^{-1}. The size of bubbles formed by various inert gases is related to the amount of gas dissolved in the tissue, which in turn is related to the solubility of that gas in the tissue. A gas which has a high solubility will allow a greater amount of gas to be dissolved and so larger bubbles can form. On the other hand a gas which has a lower solubility will allow a lesser amount of gas to be dissolved and so smaller bubbles will form. As Nitrogen is 1.4 times more soluble in blood than Helium, more Nitrogen can dissolve in the blood than Helium, which in turn means that Nitrogen will form larger bubbles than Helium.

Breathing Trimix we will have two inert gasses diffusing into and out of the tissues. Although diffusion is a result of a partial pressure gradient, gasses are not pushed into the tissues by the force of the pressure. When we pump air into a cylinder, the pressure is used to push air into the cylinder. However, diffusion works in a different way as it is the movement of individual gas atoms or molecules due to random atomic or molecular movement that cause the gas transfer. This means that diffusion of an individual gas into or out of a tissue is dependent only on the partial pressure gradient of that particular gas, and not on other gases present in the tissue. In other words the diffusion of Nitrogen is unaffected by the partial pressure gradient of Helium or of Oxygen in the tissues. Equally the diffusion of Helium is unaffected by the partial pressure gradient of Nitrogen or Oxygen. As a result the diffusion of Helium in and out of the tissues is driven purely by the partial pressure gradient of Helium and the diffusion of Nitrogen is driven purely by the partial pressure gradient of Nitrogen.

It is a common misconception that gases present in tissue are exerting a "pressure" that "holds" other gases out of the tissue. As we have just seen, this is not true. A tissue can become saturated with a particular gas but if another gas is introduced it will also start to diffuse into the tissue. This is shown in Figure 102 below. The tissue is saturated with Nitrogen as the tissue partial pressure and the blood partial pressure are the same. If Helium is introduced then it will start to diffuse into the tissue as the partial pressure in the blood is higher than in the tissue and so a partial pressure gradient is introduced.

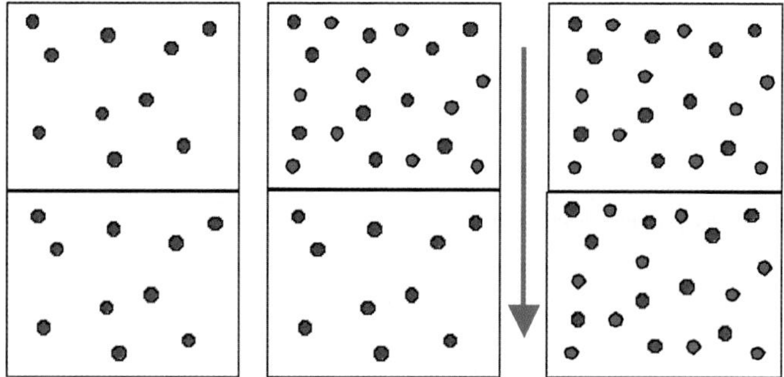

Figure 102: *A gas can diffuse into a tissue even if it is currently saturated with another gas*

Equally it is possible to have one gas diffusing into a tissue while another gas is diffusing out of the tissue. This is shown in Figure 103. The tissues are saturated with Helium and Nitrogen as the blood and tissue partial pressures are the same for both Helium and Nitrogen. If the breathing mixture is changed so that there is more Nitrogen and less Helium then Nitrogen will start to diffuse into the tissues while Helium diffuses out of the tissues.

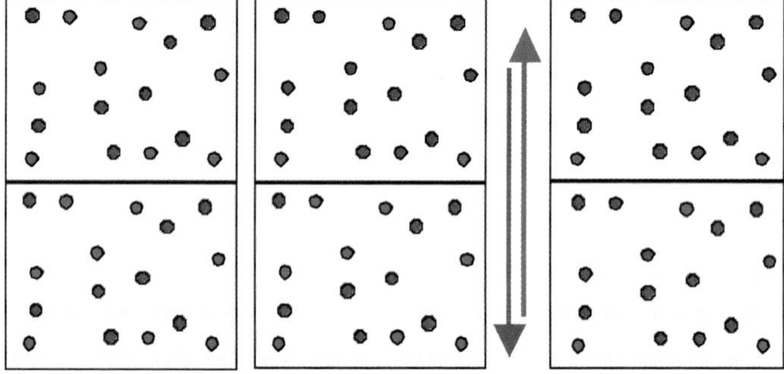

Figure 103: *One gas can diffuse into a tissue while another gas is diffusing out*

The reason why this is possible is that a gas in saturation in a liquid only constitutes a very small percentage of the liquid. There is still plenty more "room" for other gases. For example, if water is saturated with Nitrogen on the surface (1 bar) at 37°C, the Nitrogen molecules are only 0.01% of the total molecules (water and Nitrogen). If the amount of Nitrogen is doubled (2 bar), then Nitrogen molecules increase to only 0.02% of the total number of molecules. There is still plenty of scope for additional inert gas molecules to be absorbed into the liquid even if it is saturated with Nitrogen. As we can see, the concept that gas atoms or molecules dissolved in tissue can "push" other gas molecules out of the tissue is not correct.

Trimix Decompression

We have seen that Helium is a faster gas than Nitrogen and so will be absorbed into the tissues faster. If we were breathing a Trimix with equal fractions of Helium and Nitrogen then at the end of a dive more tissues will be saturated with Helium than would be saturated with Nitrogen. Even those tissues that are not yet saturated will have a higher loading of Helium than Nitrogen. This was shown earlier and is repeated again in Figure 92

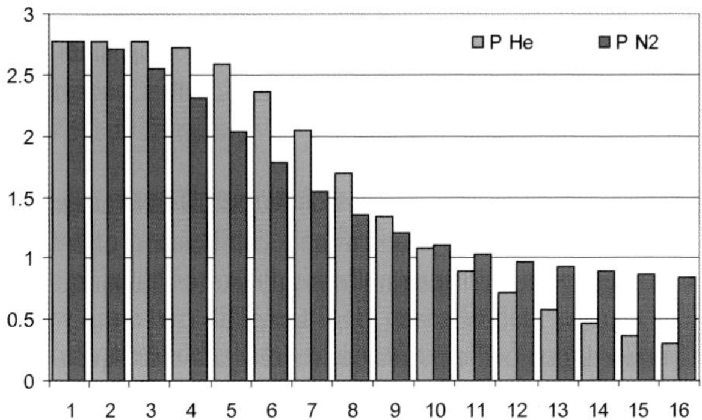

Figure 92: *Tissue loadings at the end of the bottom time*

More dissolved helium and a higher level of saturation means that saturation and critical supersaturation will be reached sooner on a Trimix dive than on an equivalent Air or Nitrox dive. However during the ascent Helium will be off-gassing at a faster rate than Nitrogen. This means that a stop may be required sooner and so the first stop may be deeper for a Trimix or Heliox dive to the same depth than one using air or nitrox. That is unless the Helium has off-gassed enough during the ascent to keep the supersaturation level below critical supersaturation. It is often stated as a fact that Trimix always requires deeper stops but this is not always the case.

As the diver ascends the helium will off-gas faster then the nitrogen. This means that towards the end of the dive a larger amount of Helium will have been off-gassed.

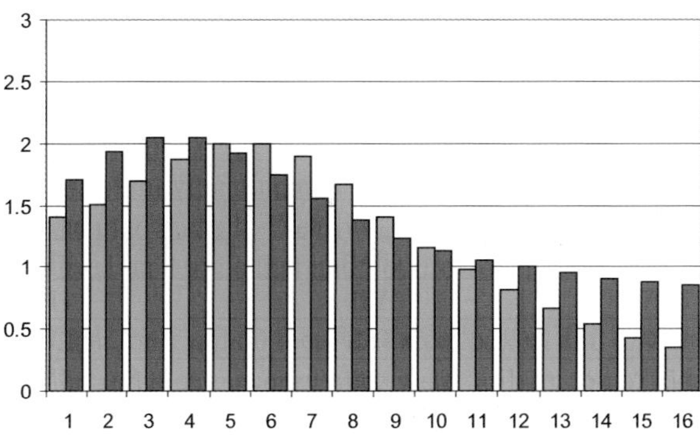

Figure 93: *Tissue loadings during ascent*

This complex interaction of on and off gassing for Helium and Nitrogen means that it is very difficult to say that one gas is better or worse from a decompression point of view. It is also difficult to say whether the decompression for a Trimix based dive will be longer or shorter than for an Air dive. However, as a general rule of thumb, for dives with a bottom time of less than 2 hours Traditional deco models have produced longer decompression schedules for helium based mixtures than for air. For dives with a bottom time of less than 2 hours the progression is;

Nitrox ➛ Air -➛Trimix ➛ Heliox

This shows that a Nitrox based bottom gas will produce the shortest decompression profile, followed by Air and Trimix with Heliox producing the longest decompression schedule. Traditional decompression approach generates these results because the Helium on-gasses faster and so more compartments will have reached saturation than with Nitrogen and so there is more gas to be off-gassed.

As the bottom time reaches 2 hours the overall decompression time converges and then for dives of over 2 hour bottom time the order is reversed with helium based mixtures giving shorter overall decompression times

Heliox ➛ Trimix ➛ Air ➛ Nitrox

The longer bottom time has allowed more compartments to become saturated with Nitrogen, catching up with the number of saturated compartments on the Helium based dive. The compartments saturated with Helium will not absorb any more Helium, as they are saturated, but will off-gas faster then the compartments saturated with Nitrogen. Two hours is roughly the point where the slower off-gassing of Nitrogen starts to overtake the faster on-gassing of Helium as the determining factor.

Modern approaches to decompression are much more sympathetic of Helium. Although Helium on-gasses faster it also off-gasses faster. When combined with gas switching to accelerate the rate of off-gassing of the Helium it is possible to generate decompression schedules which are shorter for Helium based mixes, even when the bottom time is less than 2 hours.

If Trimix back gas is breathed throughout the ascent and decompression then the partial pressure of each gas in the breathing mixture decreases as the ambient pressure is decreased. This is shown in Figure 94.

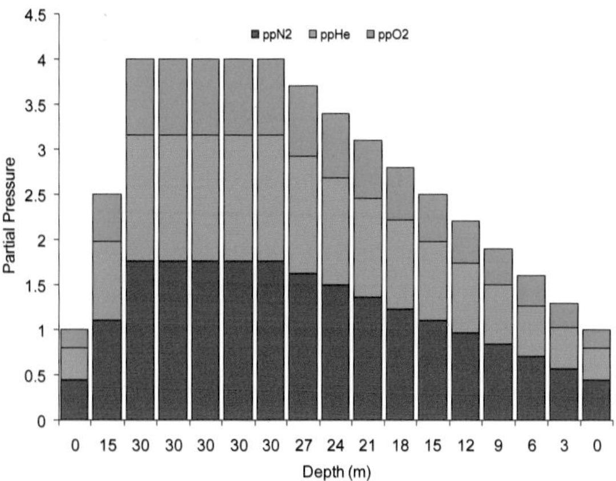

Figure 94: *Partial pressure of constituent gasses when decompressing using Trimix 21/35 back gas*

However, as we have already seen, it is possible to switch to a different mix, usually a rich nitrox mix, on the decompression stops. If we are breathing air or nitrox then switching to a rich nitrox mix simply reduces part of the nitrogen in the breathing mixture with oxygen. In the case of trimix it is more complicated as we are replacing a mixture with three gases (Oxygen, Helium and Nitrogen) with a mixture of two gases (Oxygen and Nitrogen). In this case the fraction of helium in the mix drops to zero as the mix now contains no Helium. However there will still be nitrogen in the new mixture and we need to consider the implications of this.

With Nitrox diving the increase in the fraction of oxygen replaced part of the nitrogen, but for Trimix diving the increase in the oxygen fraction is primarily reducing the helium. This is shown in Figure 95. In this example the diver is breathing 21/35, that is a trimix with 21% Oxygen, 35% Helium and 44% Nitrogen. When the diver reaches his 21m stop he switches from his 21/35 mixture to a decompression gas of 50% Nitrox. This deco gas contains 50% Oxygen and 50% Nitrogen. This means that the Oxygen content has gone from 21% to 50%, the helium has gone from 35% to zero but the Nitrogen has gone from 44% up to 50%. So the diver is now getting slightly more nitrogen then when he was breathing his back gas.

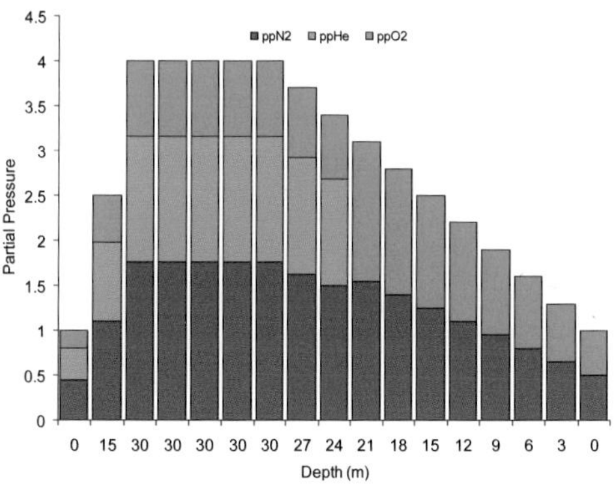

Figure 95: *Partial pressures when switching to EAN50 for decompression*

The result of this gas switch is that there is now a large inert gas gradient for Helium and so the Helium will come out of the tissues even faster. However the inert gas gradient has actually increased for Nitrogen and so the Nitrogen will not come out any faster and some tissues may even briefly start on gassing nitrogen again.

We can see that in this case the switch to the deco gas has accelerated the off-gassing of helium but has done nothing to accelerate the off gassing of nitrogen. Helium is a fast gas and so we are accelerating the off-gassing of what is already a fast gas. This means that by the later stages of the decompression schedule there may be little or no Helium present and the last few decompression stops will largely be driven by the Nitrogen in the tissues.

This is illustrated in the following sequence of graphs. In Figure 96 we can see the tissue loadings at the 24m stop.

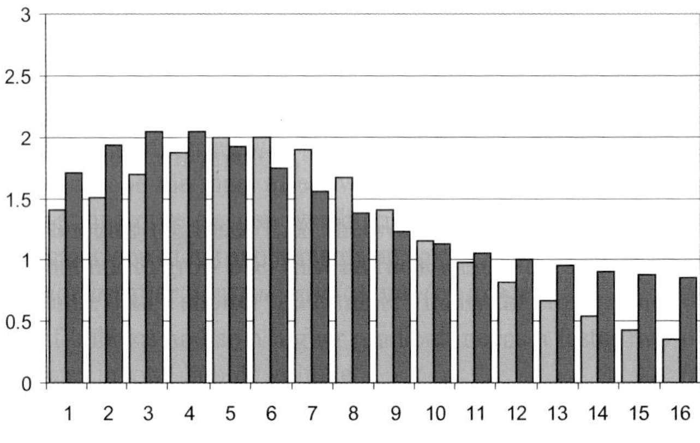

Figure 96: *Tissue loadings at 24m stop*

Compare this with Figure 97 which shows the tissue loadings at the 18m stop, after the switch to 50% deco gas at 21m. The rate of Helium off-gassing has clearly been accelerated as shown by the significant drop in tissue loading in the fast tissues. The Nitrogen loadings on the other hand are virtually unchanged.

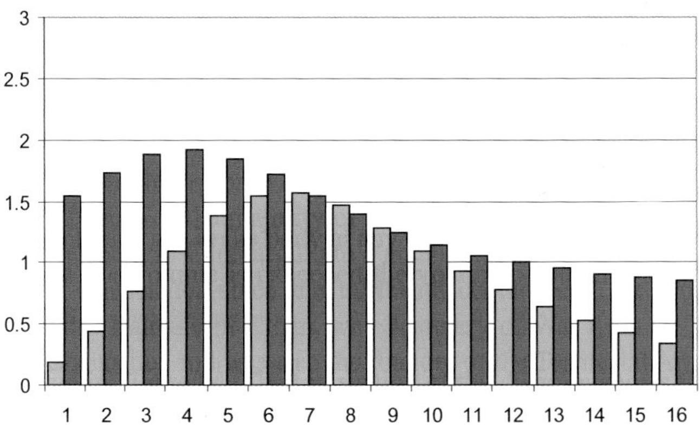

Figure 97: *Tissue loadings at 18m stop – after switch to deco gas*

By the time we reach the 9m stop, as shown in Figure 98, the Helium loadings in compartments 1 and 2 have dropped to zero and the loadings in the other tissues are all now well below the level of Nitrogen loading.

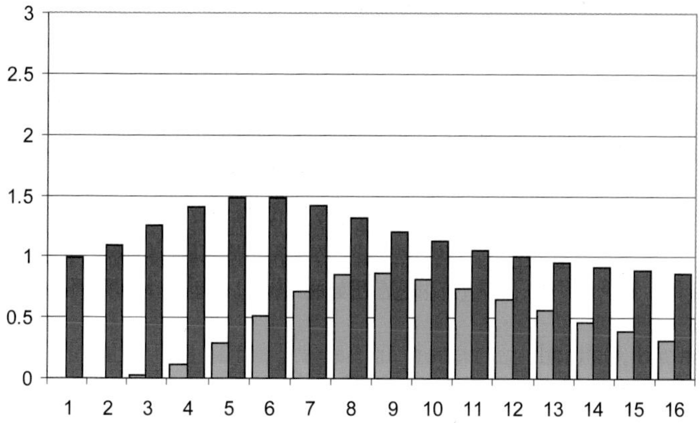

Figure 98: *Tissue loadings at 9m stop*

Finally on ascending to the surface after clearing the 6m stop we can see in Figure 99 that the tissue loadings for Helium are zero for a number of the fast compartments and are well below the level of Nitrogen loading in all the others

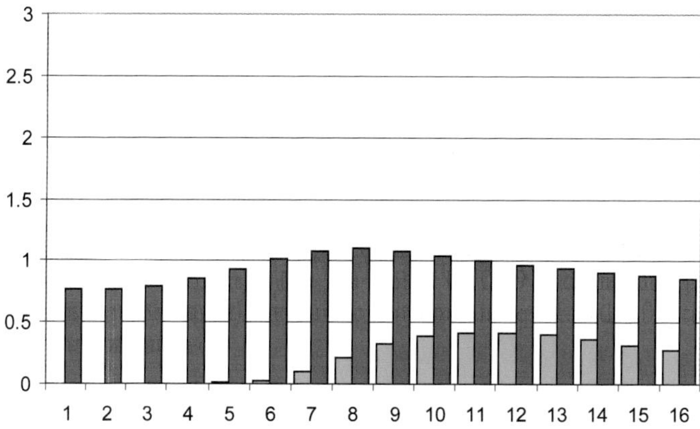

Figure 99: *Tissue loadings at surface*

A different choice of decompression gas will give a different pattern to the off-gassing. If the diver is using EAN80 as a decompression gas, as shown in Figure 100, then the situation is changed. The higher percentage of Oxygen (80%) means that in addition to removing all of the helium we have also removed a large portion of the Nitrogen. When switching to the decompression gas the oxygen changes from 21% to 80%, Helium still goes from 35% to zero and now the nitrogen drops from 44% to 20%. This means that most of the inert gas has been removed or at least reduced. As a result the off gassing of both helium and nitrogen is accelerated. The disadvantage of this approach however is that due to the risk of CNS toxicity we cannot switch to EAN80 until 9m (compared to 21m for EAN50). So although the inert gas gradient is greater for EAN80 than it is for EAN50 we cannot start to use it until much later.

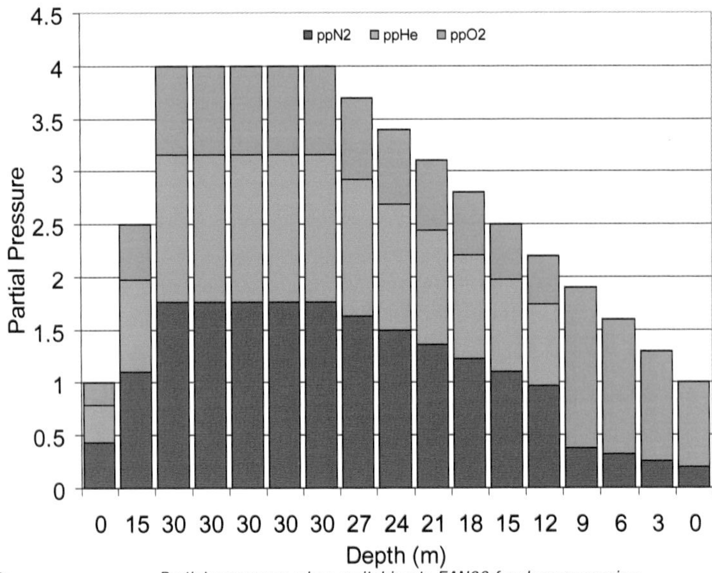

Figure 100: *Partial pressures when switching to EAN80 for decompression*

The same is true of using 100% Oxygen for decompression. This is shown in Figure 101. In switching to pure Oxygen we remove all of the helium and nitrogen and so the inert gas gradient is at its maximum, but we cannot do this until our 6m stop, forcing us to carry out all of the decompression stops prior to 6m on our trimix back gas.

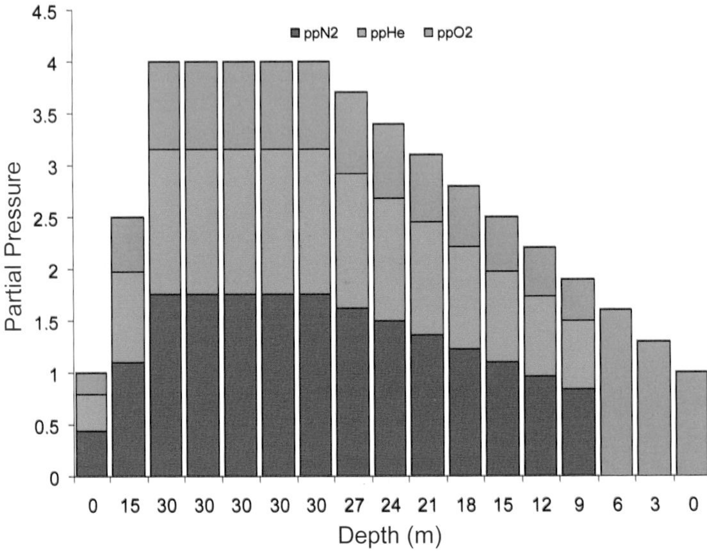

Figure 101: *Partial pressures when switching to 100% Oxygen for decompression*

The balance between the pros and cons of the various deco gases can be offset by using multiple deco gases. A weaker nitrox mix is used at depth. This allows us to initially remove the helium but does little to replace the nitrogen, a richer mix is then used later to remove the nitrogen. Combinations of EAN50 and Oxygen or EAN40 and EAN80 are common.

Helium in Decompression Gases

When using a rich nitrox mix for decompression after a dive using Air or Nitrox as a back gas the increased amount of Oxygen results in a decreased amount of Nitrogen. This in turn increases the inert gas gradient and allows accelerated off-gassing. The partial pressures of Oxygen and Nitrogen immediately before and after a switch from EAN32 to EAN50 are shown in Table 24.

	Oxygen	Nitrogen
EAN32	1.0	2.1
EAN50	1.55	1.55

Table 24: *Partial pressure before and after gas switch from EAN32*

The partial pressure of Nitrogen drops from 2.1 to 1.55 after the gas switch resulting in an increased inert gas gradient and an increased rate of off-gassing. Compare this to the situation in Table 25 where the partial pressures before and after a switch from Trimix 18/35 to EAN50 are shown in Table 25

	Oxygen	Helium	Nitrogen
TX 18/35	0.56	1.08	1.46
EAN50	1.55	0	1.55

Table 25: *Partial pressure before and after gas switch from Trimix 18/35*

In this case the partial pressure of Helium drops to zero, resulting in the maximum possible inert gas gradient. This gives the maximum rate of off-gassing for Helium at that depth. However the partial pressure of Nitrogen increases from 1.46 to 1.55. This decreases the inert gas gradient and so slows down off-gassing for Nitrogen. So, unlike the Air or Nitrox example, this same choice of decompression gas has now slowed Nitrogen off-gassing rather than accelerated it. In this example switching to EAN50 is accelerating our Helium off-gassing but is slowing down our Nitrogen off-gassing.

Of course by using Trimix rather than Nitrox we had already reduced the amount of Nitrogen in the back gas. This reduction meant a lower partial pressure of nitrogen on the bottom and so a lower level of Nitrogen tissue loading. So you could say that the inclusion of Helium had already accelerated our Nitrogen off-gassing by replacing it in the first place.

Switching to EAN50 also provides two further advantages. The point at which we reach critical supersaturation or exceed our M-Value is related to the point where the total dissolved gas tension exceeds ambient pressure by a certain amount. This means that the sum of all inert gas tensions must be considered. Even though the Nitrogen tension may be dropping slowly the more rapid reduction of Helium inert gas tension means that the total inert gas tension is also rapidly reduced. Secondly, by switching onto a gas with 50% Oxygen at 21m we are increasing the partial pressure of Oxygen to 1.55 Bar. As we saw earlier there is an argument that by increasing the partial pressure of Oxygen, opening the Oxygen window as it is sometimes called, we can reduce the likelihood of bubbles forming or help to reduce the size of any existing bubbles.

We know that Helium is a faster gas then Nitrogen and will off-gas at a faster rate than Nitrogen. This means that by switching to a Nitrogen based decompression gas we are accelerating the off-gassing of an already fast gas without accelerating the off-gassing of the slower gas. Including a percentage of Helium in the deco gas is sometimes used in order to adjust the balance between the off-gassing of the two inert gasses.

In switching to a deco mix of 50/25 (50% Oxygen and 25% Helium) we can increase the off-gassing gradient for Nitrogen as well as the gradient for Helium. Table 26 shows that when switching from 18/35 to 50/25 the partial pressure of Helium drops from 1.08 to 0.775 and the partial pressure of Nitrogen drops from 1.46 to 0.775.

	Oxygen	Helium	Nitrogen
TX 18/35	0.56	1.08	1.46
TX50/25	1.55	0.775	0.775

Table 26: *Partial pressure before and after gas switch from Trimix 18/35 to 50/25*

Of course in this example the drop in Helium partial pressure and the corresponding increase in the off-gassing gradient is not as great as if we had removed all of the Helium but the increase in Nitrogen off-gassing is the benefit we get in this trade off.

The benefits of using a Helium based decompression gas will depend on a number of factors. One of the most important is the length of the dive. For shorter dives using Trimix we will build up a relatively low Nitrogen loading in the middle and slower compartments due to the initial displacement of Nitrogen by Helium and the fact that the short bottom time means that there is less time for the slower gas to on-gas. In this case using EAN50 will allow the Helium to off-gas rapidly and the relatively low levels of Nitrogen will off-gas in a reasonable time.

For a longer dive there is more time for Nitrogen to on-gas into the tissues. The higher Nitrogen loading will require a longer decompression. On switching to EAN50 the Helium will rapidly off-gas but the high levels of Nitrogen will take much longer to off-gas. In this case switching to 50/25 will be beneficial as it will still allow a certain level of accelerated off-gassing of the Helium but will also allow accelerated off-gassing of the Nitrogen.

In some cases it may even be advantageous to use 50/50, that is 50% Oxygen and 50% Helium. In this case the off-gassing gradient for Nitrogen is increased to the maximum amount but the gradient for Helium is kept the same or even increased slightly.

Decompression gases including Helium are typically used in conjunction with very high Nitrox mixes or 100% Oxygen on the shallower stops. This final switch to 100% Oxygen will remove all remaining traces of inert gas from the breathing mix and so will maximize the gradient for both Helium and Nitrogen.

Rebreather divers using Trimix will get a similar effect. During ascent the partial pressure of Oxygen is kept constant. In order to achieve this as the diver moves shallower the percentage of Oxygen introduced into the breathing loop is gradually increased. This has the corresponding effect of decreasing the percentage of both Helium and Nitrogen. In this way the gas gradient for both of the inert gases is increased and off-gassing is accelerated. Many rebreather divers will then flush their units with 100% Oxygen at the final stop to remove all the inert gas from the breathing loop and help 'clean up' any remaining inert gas by ensuring the gradient for both Helium and Nitrogen is at a maximum. Flushing the unit will also remove the inert gas that has been off-gassed into the breathing loop.

Isobaric Counter Diffusion

Isobaric Counter Diffusion is a term that is used to describe the situation where one inert gas enters a tissue faster than another can leave it. The inert gas entering the tissue can cause the tissue tensions to rise above the critical supersaturation point causing bubbles to form. This bubble formation can occur with no change in depth, hence the name Isobaric, meaning "same pressure". Commercial divers and the early technical diving pioneers have been aware of Isobaric Counter Diffusion (ICD) for many years but ICD was first observed in the Laboratory by Kunkle and Straus in 1974. The term Isobaric Counter Gas Transport has also been used to refer to the same situation.

As ICD depends on the presence of more than one inert gas it is not relevant to the air or nitrox diver. Even if the diver is using Air or a weak nitrox as back gas and one or more rich nitrox mixtures for decompression gas there is still no risk of ICD as we are still only dealing with a single inert gas: Nitrogen. ICD only becomes a problem if there is more than one inert gas present and so this means it is only a concern if we are using a set of gases that contain helium in addition to Nitrogen. The metabolic gases such as Oxygen and Carbon Dioxide are not relevant for ICD.

ICD is also only a problem under certain conditions and for recreational divers it is never an issue. Even for recreational technical dives it does not become a major issue until we start to look at dives in excess of around 80m. In fact ICD as long been disregarded by some areas of the technical diving community as irrelevant or even a myth.

The fact that ICD is not a single phenomenon but rather a group of several, related phenomena has made it easy for this aspect of decompression to be shrouded in myth and uncertainty. However, as technical divers are descending deeper and staying longer than ever before, ICD is becoming more of a risk. During the late 1990's and early 2000's a number of incidents occurred which raised the profile of ICD and made consideration of ICD a mainstream concern. Although still primarily a concern for those at the very edge of technical diving it is still a condition that should be considered during deeper dive planning

There are at least three situations during which ICD can occur. The first is more of a theoretical risk than a real risk but the second two situations are much more relevant.

The first of the instances of ICD occurs when the subject is immersed in a lighter gas than the one he is breathing. This was a phenomenon studied by Idicula and Lambertsen in 1975. The test subjects, in this case pigs, were surrounded by helium and were breathing a neon based gas. The experiment was intended to study the effects of a dense gas on breathing mechanics. Neon was used in order to duplicate the density of helium at a much deeper depth. What Idicula and Lambertson found was that the pigs developed red patches on their skin. Despite being well inside what should have been a safe decompression schedule they had suffered extensive skin bends.

The scientists were intrigued by this unexpected result and reasoned that the red patches on the skin had been caused by the rapid ingress of helium through the skin. Helium had diffused through the skin and the partial pressure of the Helium, when added to the partial pressure of the neon in the tissues (from the lungs through the blood stream) had been enough to exceed the M-value for the tissue. The sum of the partial pressures was such that bubble growth could occur. This would only occur if the test subjects were immersed in a very rapidly diffusing gas and breathing a slowly diffusing one. The phenomena has variously been termed 'steady state', 'subcutaneous' or 'superficial' counter diffusion.

Interesting though this experiment may have been, it wasn't very relevant for real divers. We tend not to be surrounded by Helium while breathing Neon based mixtures. When using rich Helium mixes together with Nitrogen based nitrox mixes we tend to use the heavier and slower diffusing Nitrogen based nitrox for suit inflation rather than the lighter and faster diffusing Helium based gas. This is one of the reasons why Helium rich Trimix should not be used for suit inflation. The other reason of course being that a Helium based gas will conduct heat away from the body faster than a Nitrogen based gas, resulting in faster cooling of the body which, in itself, can have decompression implications. If Argon is used for suit inflation then again we are surrounded by a much slower diffusing gas than the one we are breathing and so ICD is not a risk.

The fact that this experiment was so far from a real situation caused many people to discount the ICD phenomenon completely. George Irvine, Former Project Director for the WKPP, was famously quoted as describing ICD as something that only occurs when Santa Claus performs a lewd sex act on the Easter Bunny. Despite these comments there are other situations where ICD is a real concern with regard to the risk of decompression sickness.

The second instance where ICD can occur is when switching from breathing a nitrox (heavy) mix back to a helium (light) mix, for example if switching to back gas during an air break. In this case the Helium in the back gas starts to re-enter the tissues faster then the Nitrogen is leaving it. The overall tissue gas supersaturation increases and can exceed the critical supersaturation limit. This is known as Deep Tissue ICD.

The greater the nitrogen in the deco gas, and the greater the concentration of helium in the bottom mix, the greater the risk when switching back to bottom gas. The risk increases as the ingradient for He increases, and the outgradient for N_2 decreases. This can happen late in the decompression schedule when a diver switches to back gas before switching to a new deco gas; for an air break in order to manage the CNS clock or in the unfortunate situation when he discovers his deco gas is running out and switches to back gas. The risk also increases with the length of the switch back to the lighter gas. Luckily this means that for dives in the 60-90m range short air break switches from Nitrox to Trimix are not a high risk provided that the total air break duration is less than 30 minutes. This is consistent with accepted practice which has seen air breaks used as a matter of course for dives which would have otherwise have pushed the CNS limits. For dives beyond 100m and dives where the total air break time exceeds 30 minutes then an alternative strategy is required.

There are a number of fairly straightforward strategies for avoiding these situations. For the first instance simply avoid switching back to back gas before switching to your next deco gas, instead switch directly from deco gas 1 to deco gas 2. As switching to back gas between deco gases is an unnecessary step all we are doing here is removing an extra step which introduces problems. In other words simplifying the process and increasing the safety.

Air breaks are a different matter, when using high PO_2 for deco then CNS toxicity limits may be approached and traditionally an air break has been introduced to reduce the loading and reduce the risk of a CNS oxygen toxicity hit. Adopting an air break strategy without risking ICD means that we have to find a way of switching from our high FO_2 mix without going back to a high FHe mix. This can be achieved by switching to your travel gas or a weaker O_2 deco gas. So for example if we are using 10/50 as back gas, 30/30 as travel, 50% as first deco and 100% as final deco gas then on our final deco stop on 100% O_2 at 6m we can switch to the 50% during our air break and reduce the PO_2 from 1.6 to 0.8. The alternative is to use a lower PO_2 for decompression and so reduce the CNS loading. This will increase the overall decompression time but with the advantage of reducing the risk of CNS oxygen toxicity and reducing the need for air breaks.

The third instance of ICD is the most controversial although it appears to have been the first to be recorded. During the early days of commercial diving in the North Sea saturation diving was less common and it was far more common for divers to perform bounce dives using heliox (Helium and Oxygen) mixtures. Some of the tables devised for this procedure called for a switch from heliox to air at 24m. At this switch divers would occasionally show signs of loss of balance, extreme vertigo and vomiting. The symptoms were identical to those of someone suffering from an infection in the inner ear, specifically the semi-circular canals which are involved in control of balance. For many years it was thought that the bubbles causing the damage occurred in the vestibule part of the ear, hence "vestibular bends" was the name given to that specific type of decompression sickness.

With deeper Trimix dives, using higher percentages of Helium, similar effects have been noticed if divers switch to a Nitrogen rich decompression gas. Nitrogen, with its high solubility, can cause problems with ICD if introduced to a tissue that is already saturated with Helium which has low solubility. The nitrogen dissolves into the tissues quicker than the helium can come out, creating a super saturation situation, hence bubbles of helium and/or nitrogen are formed in the tissues. Mark Ellyat describes the effect using the following analogy. A bath tub is filled with small polystyrene balls (Helium) until it is completely filled. Water (Nitrogen) is added to the bath and quickly the Polystyrene Balls are displaced, causing them to spill over the side. This spillage would be seen as damage, as the baths capacity (body tissue) has been exceeded.

The pioneers of technical diving started to experience these problems when they started to dive deeper and introduced Helium into the mix to reduce the effects of narcosis and oxygen toxicity. German cave diver Joachen Hasenmeyer reported symptoms of vestibular DCS during his exploratory dives in Vacluse in Southern France. In 1981, when planning his record breaking 881ft dive in Nacimiento del Rio Mante in Mexico, US cave diver

Sheck Exley was aware of the problems encountered by Hasenmeyer and a similar problem reported by Gene Melton. The approach he adopted to try and avoid the situation was to gradually switch onto his shallow mix, taking a single breath from the stage cylinder before switching back to his deep mix for two breaths followed by a switch to the shallow mix for two breaths before switching back to the deep mix for one breath "Finally I switched over to air completely, bracing myself for the severe narcosis and dreaded vestibular hit, all the while doing my best to count off the seconds required for the stop. Nothing happened, no narcosis, no sudden lapse into unconsciousness."

An example of the sort of gas switches which may cause problems such as this is a dive to 100m using 10/50 helium trimix (i.e. 10% oxygen, 50% Helium and 40% Nitrogen) followed by a switch to Air at 60m in order to get of the Helium followed by the use of EAN50 for decompression. The diagram below shows that when the switch to Air is made at 60m the partial pressure of Nitrogen in the gas being breathed spikes up from 2,8 bar to 5.53 as the Helium is removed and replaced with Nitrogen.

If we consider a more detailed example of a diver decompressing on air at 20 metres, i.e. 3 bar ambient pressure, after a Trimix dive. Supposing he arrived at the stop with tissue partial pressures of 2.5 bar helium and 0.5 bar nitrogen. On arriving at the 20 metre stop he switches to air. There is now no helium in the decompression gas and so the helium starts to offgas, however the Nitrogen partial pressure has been increased and so the tissues start to on-gas Nitrogen. After decompressing on air for 10 minutes the tissue partial pressures have changed due to isobaric counter diffusion, to 2.3 bar helium and 1.0 bar nitrogen. Our diver has not exceeded the critical supersaturation levels for either gas individually (i.e. neither exceeds 3 bar). However, the partial pressures are additive when it comes to the tendency to form a bubble. Thus bubble formation will now occur, although it will be difficult to tell if this is for helium, nitrogen or a possibly mixture of both.

So how do we avoid this type of ICD problem? Ideally the best solution would be for our decompression algorithms to take into account the inert gas tensions in the relevant tissues of the body and to generate decompression profiles that avoided the situation occurring or at least highlight that there is a risk of ICD with the gas mixes chosen. This would require a model of the causes of ICD to be built into the decompression algorithm. Researchers Doolette and Mitchell have published a mathematical model which simulates the processes involved in ICD and specifically the situation in the inner ear with respect to gas tensions. However, to date, no decompression program or tables embodies this algorithm. See below for further details of this model.

In the absence of a model which predicts or avoids the root causes of ICD there are a number of 'rules of thumb' which can easily be used to try and avoid ICD situations

The most straightforward rule of thumb is that during decompression we never let our partial pressure of nitrogen rise significantly. This can be achieved by increasing the fraction of Oxygen as we decrease the fraction of Helium in order to keep the fraction of Nitrogen almost constant. By using trimix we have an advantage over heliox as the tissues will already have an inherent partial pressure of nitrogen, thereby decreasing the nitrogen gradient after the gas switch. For the North Sea divers breathing heliox, the only way to avoid increasing the nitrogen partial pressures would have been to carry out all decompression on pure oxygen, as any nitrogen in any of the decompression mixes would have increased the nitrogen partial pressure.

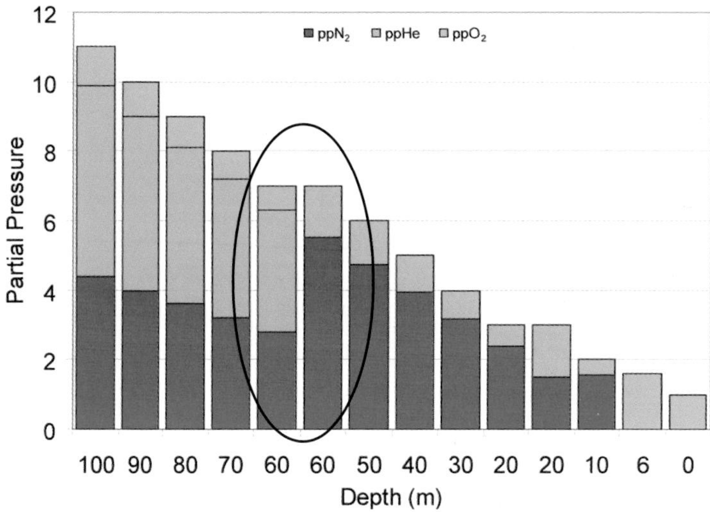

'never let the partial pressure of nitrogen rise significantly'

A key question when using the rule is the meaning of the word significantly. The most conservative interpretation is to never let the partial pressure of nitrogen rise at all. This ensures that there is never an increased in-gassing gradient for nitrogen but can be very restrictive in the choice of gasses we can use for decompression.

For a diver using a 10/50 helium trimix (i.e. 10% oxygen, 50% Helium and 40% Nitrogen) in order to maintain an equal nitrogen partial pressure during decompression he would have to switch to a nitrox deco gas with 40% Nitrogen and hence 60% oxygen. In order to avoid CNS oxygen toxicity we always plan to keep the PPO_2 below 1.6 Bar. So for a 60% Nitrox mix we wouldn't be able to switch to until we reach 17m. Our diver therefore would not be able to switch from his bottom mix until this depth was reached. Using one of the older decompression models this would have resulted in a significant time increase on the deeper stops, however newer decompression models result in shorter decompression schedules for this kind of dive. The following diagram shows the switches for this combination combined with pure O_2 from 6m

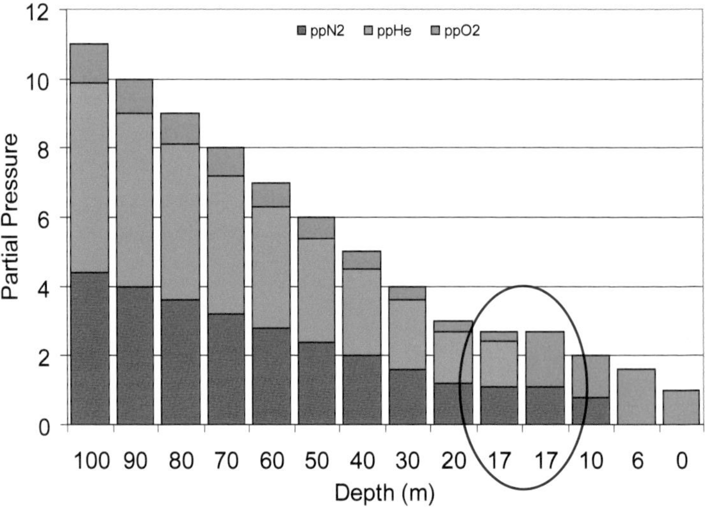

The other option is to switch to a travel gas which still contains some helium. This means that the partial pressure of Nitrogen is controlled by reducing the fraction of helium while at the same time increasing the fraction of Oxygen in coordination in order to keep the fraction of Nitrogen constant. So in the case of our 10/50 Trimix we could switch to a travel mix of 40/20 (40% Oxygen, 20% Helium and still 40% Nitrogen) at a depth of 30m. This maintains the Nitrogen pressure by replacing some but not all of the Helium with Oxygen. The diagram below shows this switch combined with a switch to 80% at 10m.

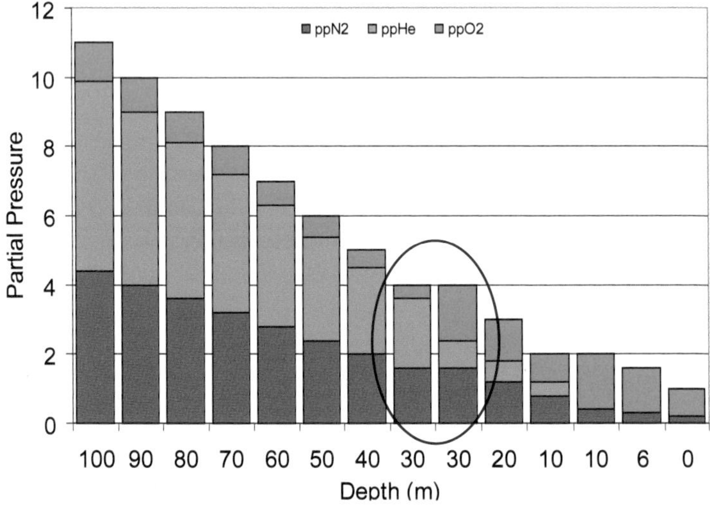

Other, less conservative, rules have been proposed to allow a certain increase in nitrogen partial pressure while trying to include some upper limit on the increase. This is an attractive approach as historically a great deal of decompression dives have been carried out with increases in the partial pressure of nitrogen and no resulting ICD problems. This implies that under many circumstances the partial pressure of nitrogen can be increased a certain amount without subsequent problems. The simplest such rule is not letting the partial pressure of nitrogen by a given amount, e.g. 0.5 bar. However, this is a purely arbitrary limit and is not based on any biophysical basis. In some circumstances it may be a safe limit but in others it may be far too high an increase.

A more recent approach suggested by Steven Burton attempts to put a limit on the relative changes in gas composition. The allowable changes are based on the physical properties of nitrogen and helium. As we have seen Helium is a fast gas and will diffuse in and out of a tissue approximately 2.65 faster than nitrogen, however nitrogen is approximately 4.5 times more soluble in lipid tissues than helium.

Burton's approach is based on the fact that the quantity of a dissolved gas in a fixed volume of a saturated tissue is equal to the current saturation pressure multiplied by the solubility factor in the medium. Obviously the total quantity of dissolved gas is the sum of the quantity of each of the inert gasses present. When switching from a high helium mix to a high nitrogen mix the higher solubility factor of Nitrogen offsets the decrease in pressure of the Helium. This results in an increase in the total quantity of dissolved gas. As nitrogen is approximately 4.5 times more soluble than Helium Burton proposes that by increasing the nitrogen percentage by no more than $1/5^{th}$ of the reduction in the helium percentage then the total quantity of dissolved gas will not increase and hence an ICD event can be avoided. The permissible percentage increase in nitrogen for a given percentage helium reduction is given in the table below.

% Helium Gas reduction	Permissible % Nitrogen Increase
10	2
20	4
30	6
40	8
50	10
60	12
70	14
80	16
90	18

Using these limits a switch from Trimix 20/25 to Nitrox 32 would not be allowed since Nitrogen jumps from 55 to 68% (a 13% jump), where the rule of 5ths would give a maximum allowable increase in %Nitrogen for a 25% drop in Helium of only 5%. However, a switch from Trimix 20/25/55 to Trimix 32/8/60 would be allowed.

The rule of 5ths approach has not been extensively tested however it was used to plan the gas mixes used on Mark Ellyatt's record breaking 313 meter open circuit Trimix dive.

The use of constant ppO_2 rebreathers can help to reduce the risk of this type of ICD. As the diver ascends the rebreather will maintain a constant ppO_2 by increasing the fraction of oxygen in the loop which will correspond to a reduction of both Nitrogen and Helium in the loop. This will optimize the decompression profile without introducing any risk of ICD. Problems can still occur however if the diver switches the diluent gas from a Helium rich to a Nitrogen rich gas or if they have to bailout to an open circuit bailout cylinder containing a high Nitrogen content.

The uncertainty over ICD is reflected in the fact that there is still no agreement on the site of the decompression bubbles that cause this form of DCS. Initially it was assumed that bubbles were forming in the inner ear, hence the term vestibular bends. However subsequent theories have suggested that the bubbles do not form in this region but in the cerebellum of the brain. This part of the brain controls muscles and receives the impulses from the semi-circular canals of the ear; hence the symptoms displayed would be very similar to an injury in the semi-circular canals. This theory has a significant weakness in that there is no reason to believe that the cerebellum is more prone to DCS than any other part of the brain and so it is reasonable to assume that bubbles in the cerebellum would also result in bubbles in other parts of the brain and yet the symptoms of ICD are very specific to the inner ear.

In 2003, in response to a number of specific incidents and a growing focus on this area, Doolette and Mitchell published a paper which provided a biophysical basis for inner ear DCS which once again focused on the inner ear as the site of the bubbles. This paper also suggested that inner ear decompression sickness was possible even without gas switches causing counter diffusion. Gas pressures in the inner ear were modeled and showed that for deep and/or long dives followed by a relatively rapid ascent significant supersaturation could occur during the early stages of decompression, prior to any gas switch. This supersaturation alone was enough to potentially result in bubble formation. However the authors did not deny the existence of ICD and their model showed that ICD can make an existing inner ear supersaturation situation even worse and could be the 'straw that breaks the camels back'.

Doolette and Mitchell described the inner ear as three compartments: a well perfused, (i.e. well supplied with blood) vascular compartment that contains many of the critical functional structures of the inner ear; and the endolymph and perilymph compartments which are two poorly perfused "water" filled chambers separated from the well perfused vascular compartment by a membrane. Gas uptake in the Endolymph and Perilymph is by diffusion of gas from the Vascular compartment. Figure 102 shows the various compartments of the inner ear and their gas uptake characteristics.

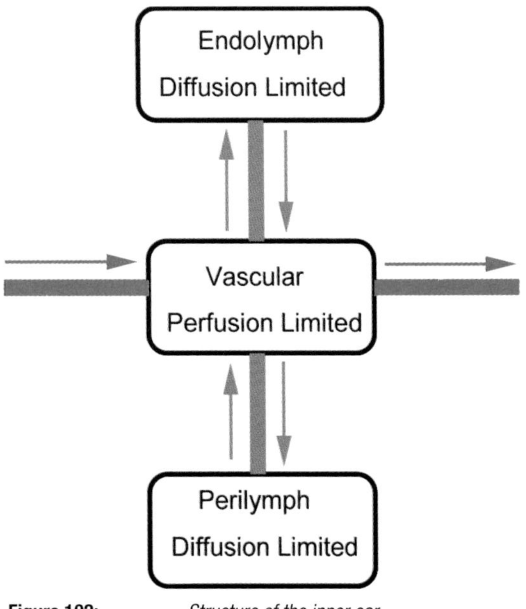

Figure 102: *Structure of the inner ear*

Gas enters and leaves all 3 compartments of the inner ear via the blood flow into the well perfused vascular compartment. Under increased ambient pressure the watery endolymp and perilymph compartments on-gas helium quickly by diffusion from the vascular compartment. During decompression, helium will be trying to leave all the compartments as the ambient pressure falls. However, the helium in the endolymph and perilymph compartments must diffuse into the vascular compartment before it will be carried away by the blood. Consequently the vascular tissues lag behind the rest of the tissues in off-gassing the helium. At a gas switch, the diver then changes from breathing a high helium mix to a high nitrogen mix. The blood quickly carries this nitrogen to the perfused vascular compartment of the inner ear. Here the rapid diffusion of helium from the endolymph and perilymph compartments into the perfused vascular compartment exceeds the transfer of nitrogen in the opposite direction and the washout of helium from the vascular compartment by the blood flow away from the tissue. For a short period, this process will further raise the inert gas tensions in the already supersaturated vascular compartment. A bottleneck can occur as Helium diffuses into the vascular at the same time as nitrogen arrives by perfusion. This increase in inert gas tension can be enough to exceed critical supersaturation resulting in bubble formation in the vascular compartment. As mentioned earlier, the vascular compartment contains many of the critical functional structures of the inner ear and bubbles forming in this area will result in the symptoms of inner ear or vestibular DCS.

Wherever the bubbles occur the result is the same; severe disability which can leave survivors with permanent balance problems or, in the worst case, completely unable to walk. For commercial diver decompressing in a dry chamber the symptoms are distressing but for SCUBA divers decompressing in mid water they are much worse. Vertigo causes the diver to feel like they are spinning and any movement to try and counteract this feeling only makes the situation worse. Clearly maintaining buoyancy and following the remainder of the decompression profile becomes extremely difficult in this situation.

It is clear that ICD is on the leading edge of decompression theory and practice. There is no complete scientific theory of the processes involved and empirical evidence is very much leading the way. This is an area where the technical divers who are pushing our knowledge of deeper diving are also acting as guinea pigs in our research of this phenomenon.

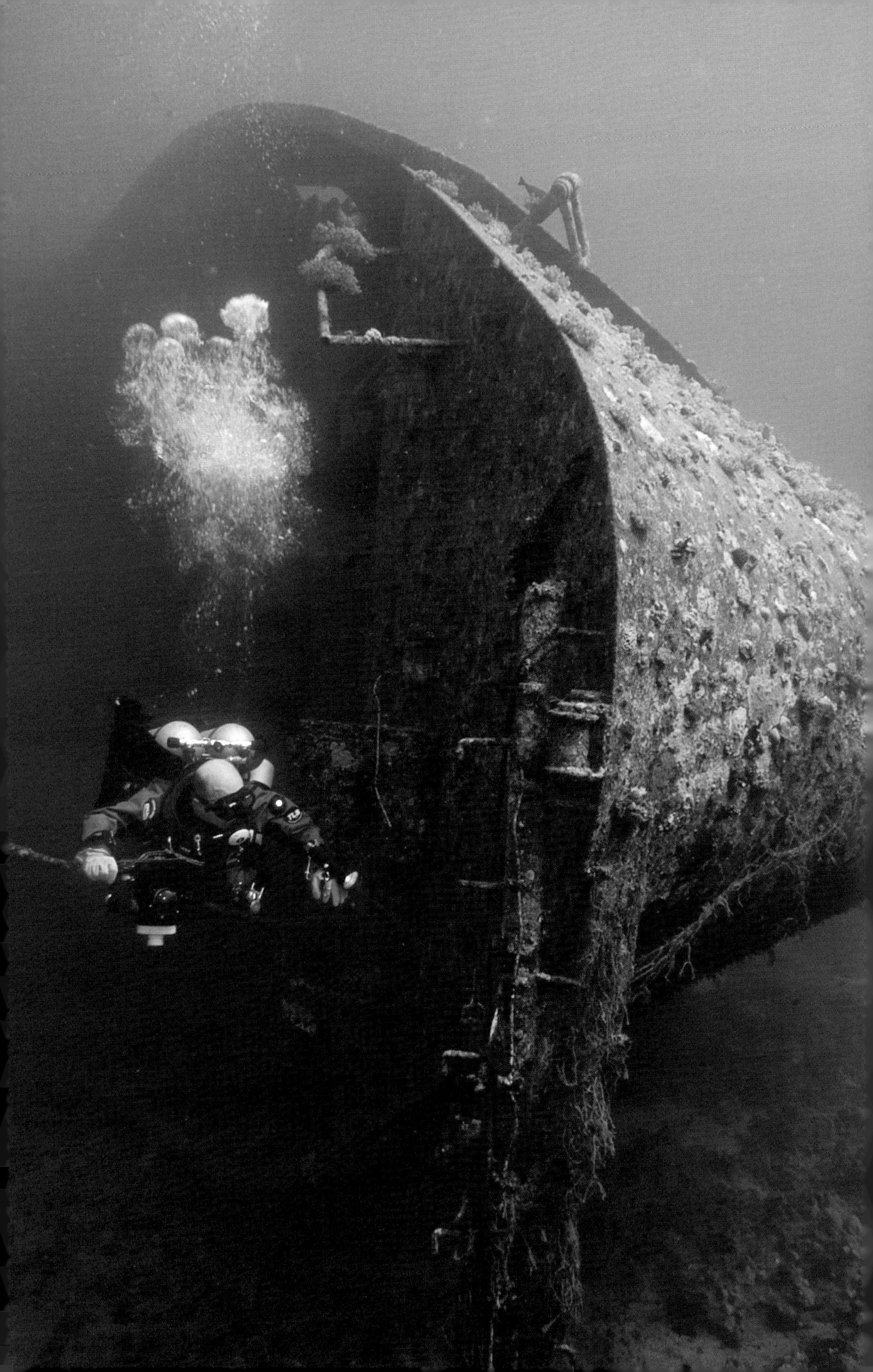

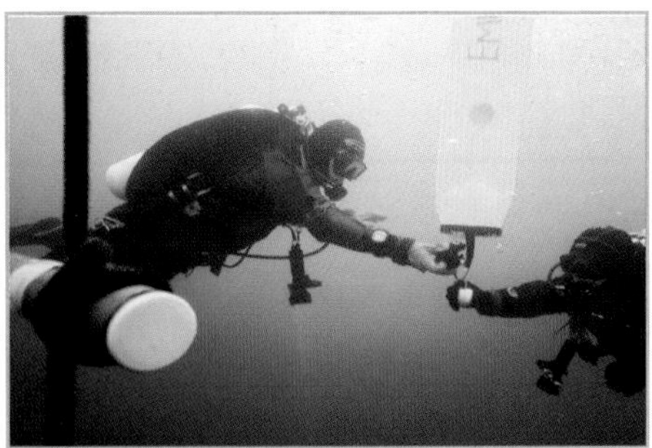

8 Other Decompression Models

John Scott Haldane's influential paper on the prevention of compressed air illness was published in the Journal of Hygiene in 1908, almost exactly 100 years before this book was published. His paper has had a significant effect on all subsequent research in the field of decompression theory. For almost 50 years his approach was adopted as the standard for studying decompression. Workman, Bühlmann and others added further refinements to his work but they were using his ideas as a framework. It wasn't until the 1950's that significant alternatives were proposed.

We have already looked at one of the major alternatives to the Haldanian approach, that of bubble models. Yet even in these modern bubble models we still find multiple tissue compartments with varying half times, exactly the concepts introduced by Haldane.

In addition to the two approaches of Haldanian versus bubble models there are a number of other decompression models that have been developed. In some cases these attempt to look again at the physiological processes going on in the body and provide a mathematical model which simulates these physiological processes. In other cases the models make no attempt to describe what is going on inside the body and instead simply try to come up with a mathematical model that allows divers to ascend without unacceptable levels of decompression illness.

In this chapter we will look at some of the more popular alternatives to Haldanian or bubble models. Despite sponsoring the original research by JS Haldane, the British Royal Navy developed an alternative method of calculating decompression schedules. These tables were developed by the Royal Naval Physiological Laboratory and are known that RNPL tables. These tables adopt a quite different approach to decompression modeling to the traditional approach inspired by Haldane. The British Sub Aqua Club (BSAC) has also developed a set

Left: Buoyancy control is important for all dives

of tables based on an alternative model. The BSAC has never published the details of their model but by investigating the research of the scientist who developed them, we can piece together some clues as to how they work. The US Navy has also looked at alternative models based on different assumptions as to how our body takes in and eliminates nitrogen. They have also put extensive effort into calculating decompression tables based on statistical or probability models.

RNPL – Slab Diffusion

The Royal Naval Physiological Laboratory (RNPL) was established in 1943, by the Royal Naval Scientific Service, to investigate physiological problems peculiar to the Navy, such as those connected with living conditions in submarines and the endurance of divers and swimmers.

The Royal Navy used the tables developed by John Scott Haldane in 1908 right up until the 1950's. Despite their widespread use there were known problems with the Haldane model for longer dives in excess of 36m/120ft. The US Navy progressed on the basis of making modifications to the basic Haldane theory to try to resolve the problems. The Royal Navy adopted a very different approach and went back to look at whether the fundamental assumptions underlying the Haldane model were correct. In the early 1950's Dr Henry Valance Hempleman (or Val as he was always known) and other researchers at the Royal Naval Physiological Laboratory (RNPL) developed an alternative model based on a completely different approach to Haldane's.

The RNPL tables are based on a "slab diffusion" model. Unlike the Haldane model, which assumes that uptake of inert gas is controlled by the rate of perfusion to the tissues, the slab model assumes that uptake of inert gas is controlled by the rate of diffusion of the inert gas from the capillaries through the tissue. The reasoning for this is that a perfusion limited model assumes that the blood and tissues are both 'well stirred' tissues; that is, that gas will diffuse quickly throughout the tissue. However Hempleman argued that whilst blood is a well stirred the bodies tissues cannot be considered in this way and that inert gas will take time to diffuse throughout the tissues. As a result of this the tissue cannot be thought to have a single partial pressure of nitrogen, except at saturation, as the areas of tissues closer to the capillaries will have a higher concentration of nitrogen than the tissues further away from the capillaries.

This is shown in Figure 103 where the capillary is shown in red passing through the centre of a section of tissue. Nitrogen is shown as diffusing outwards from the capillary into the tissue. Near the capillary there is a higher concentration of nitrogen, shown by the red shading. Further away from the capillary the concentration is lower.

Figure 103: *Diffusion of inert gas through the tissues*

With a large number of capillaries feeding an area of tissue then the structure of the tissues can be thought of as a number of parallel capillaries as shown in Figure 104.

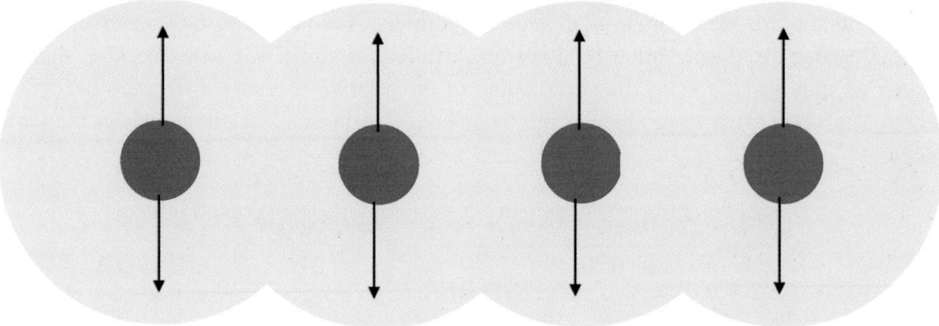

Figure 104: *Parallel capillaries*

This model goes one step further and assumes a single tissue compartment or slab, one end of the slab is exposed to the ambient pressure. As ambient pressure increases the inert gas pressure in contact with one end of the slab also increases and the inert gas starts to diffuse along the slab.

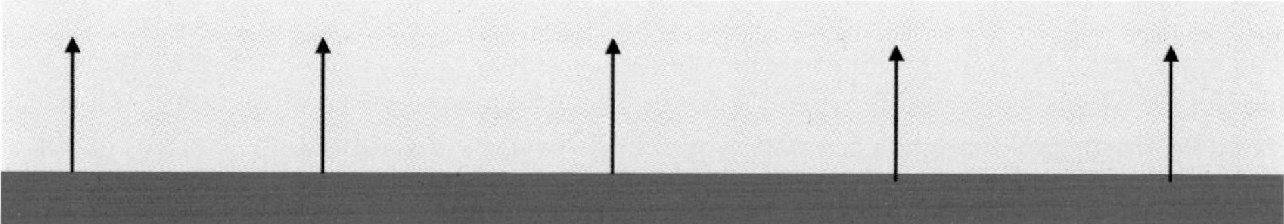

Figure 105: *Slab Diffusion Model*

The amount of gas in the tissue can be calculated using a diffusion equation. The amount of gas is proportional to the pressure of the gas in contact with the tissue and the square root of the time over which diffusion takes place. This equation introduces a non-linear relationship in the model. One side effect of this is that it prevents one from calculating equivalent air depths (EAD), unlike Haldane based tables such as the Bühlmann tables.

A key aspect of the model is the maximum volume of inert gas that is allowed to be present within the tissue before a bend occurs. If this limit is reached during the ascent then a decompression stop is inserted into the ascent profile until the volume of inert gas drops enough to allow ascent to the surface or to the next decompression stop without exceeding this limit. This means that the total volume of nitrogen had to below a specific fixed point before the diver could ascend to the surface from the last decompression stop. Similarly the total volume of nitrogen had to below a specific fixed point before the diver could ascend to the last decompression stop from the previous stop. As there is just a single compartment in the RNPL table this makes calculation of decompression schedules quite easy as the volume required to ascend from the 6m/20ft stop to the 3m/10ft stop, or from the 3m/10ft stop to the surface will always be the same regardless of the dive carried out. The only exception is the first decompression stop where there would be slightly less gas to release. As the same volume of gas was being released on each stop the time taken to release the gas was also the same for a particular decompression stop level. As a result the stops at each decompression stops level were always the same irrespective of the depth and time of the dive, again with the exception of the first stop. Longer and deeper dives would result in decompression stops starting earlier, i.e. deeper but would not result in longer stops. The stops became slightly shorter as they get closer to the surface due to the relative pressure difference becoming larger. The standard stops at each depth from 18m/60ft to 3m/10ft are shown in the table below

Stop Depth (ft)	Stop Length (mins)
18m/60ft	25
15m/50ft	24
12m/40ft	24
9m/30ft	23
6m/20ft	22
3m/10ft	22

HEMPLEMAN 1952.

This meant that the 9m/30ft stop would always be 23 minutes long, unless it was the first stop; the 6m/20ft stop would always be 22 minutes, again unless it was the first stop and the 10 ft stop would always be 22 minutes unless it was the only stop.

The tables were revised in 1968 to incorporate a variable ratio of tissue off-gassing so that the uptake of gas is assumed to be 1.5 times faster than the rate of elimination. This was based on the theory that gas elimination will be slowed by the formation of silent bubbles, and as such the theory was a forerunner of modern bubble models. Bubbles will slow the off gassing rate as the formation of bubbles and the diffusion of gas from the tissue into the bubble will reduce the tissue inert gas pressure. This means that the rate of diffusion from the gas in the bubble back into the tissues and into the circulation is much slower than if the gas remained in solution and diffused directly into the circulation. This model was published as the Royal Navy 1968 tables.

They were again modified in 1972 to address problems with longer and deeper dives. In addition Hempleman acknowledged that "the no-stop curve calculated for the 1968 table was somewhat over-conservative". The 1972 table was less conservative for no-stop times, although they were still very conservative for repetitive dives. At this point the tables were also converted to metric. These tables covered dives down to 75m and decompression times of over 3 hours.

One side effect of the 1968 and 1972 revisions was that the length of each decompression stop at a particular depth was no longer constant. Longer and deeper dives would now result in longer decompression times at each stop depth.

The British Sub Aqua Club (BSAC) adopted a version of the RNPL tables and these were subsequently published in BSAC qualification books up until 1987.The version adopted by BSAC was based on the RNPL 1972 Air Diving Tables but covered dives down to 50m, in increments of 2m and did not include dives requiring more than 30 minutes of decompression. The resulting table was simpler, more compact and was more suited to the type of diving being undertaken by sports divers at the time. The table became known as the RNPL/BSAC Decompression Table. The popularity of BSAC training in the UK and the simplicity of the tables meant that during the 1970's and 80's the majority of British divers used the RNPL/BSAC tables.

BSAC-88

The BSAC (1988) Tables, published in 1988 by the British Sub Aqua Club were intended to replace the old RNPL/BSAC tables. As sport diving, and in particular repetitive diving, became more popular, the manner of calculating repetitive dives was considered overly conservative. A new approach to recreational dive tables was devised for BSAC's use and included in the BSAC-88 tables. This was the first time that a standard set of decompression tables had been developed purely for a sports diving organization, previously sports divers had adopted military or commercial tables which had naturally been designed for military or commercial use rather than sports diving use.

The BSAC-88 tables are not, despite popular belief, a slab model. This misconception was not helped by Lippman in his book *Deeper into Diving* (page 325) who assumed, that Dr Tom Hennessey, the developer of the BSAC-88 Table, had used a slab model. Lippman may have made this assumption because Hennessey worked closely with Hempleman from 1976-1981 and co-authored a number of papers. The fact that Hennessey has never published a full description of the model has made it easy for this misconception to be repeated. In fact the BSAC-88 tables are based on quite a different approach to decompression modeling. While it is impossible to give a definitive description of the decompression model underlying the BSAC-88 tables it is possible to look at the research that Dr Hennessy published in the years leading up to the publication of the BSAC-88 tables in order to make some assumptions about the way his approach to decompression modeling was progressing.

Haldane's model assumed uptake was perfusion limited while Hempleman's slab model assumes that uptake is diffusion limited. Hennessy published a number of papers showing that a purely perfusion limited or a purely diffusion limited model was inadequate and that a combined perfusion/diffusion model gave a much more accurate representation over a range of conditions.

In 1987 Hennessy published a paper which described a model which combined the perfusion and diffusion aspects of gas uptake into a single model. This model combines both in the form of a single tissue complex which includes some tissues compartments which are perfusion limited and some which are diffusion limited. Each of the tissue compartments in the tissue complex interacts with each of the other compartments.

The diagram below shows a tissue complex with 4 compartments. Compartment 1 represents a fatty tissue and compartment 2 represents an aqueous tissue and both compartments are well perfused. This means that blood saturated with nitrogen at ambient partial pressure enters and leaves compartments 1 and 2 rapidly. As such we can say that these compartments are perfusion limited. Compartment 3 is a fatty tissue and compartment 4 is an aqueous tissue. There is no direct connection between the blood flow and compartments 3 and 4 so uptake in these compartments is limited by the diffusion from the other compartments in the tissue complex. As such we can say that these compartments are diffusion limited.

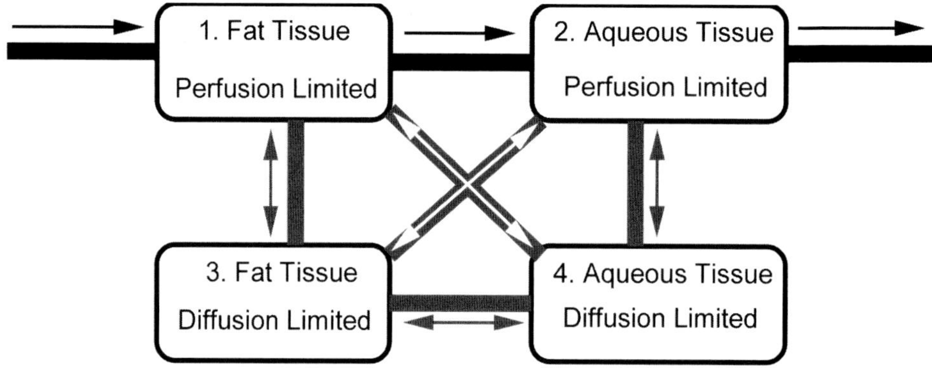

Figure 106: *Combined diffusion/perfusion limited tissue compartment*

Hennessy in conjunction with Hempleman had previously investigated the appearance of silent or asymptomatic bubbles during ascents which otherwise showed no signs or symptoms of decompression sickness. They proposed that DCS was not caused simply by the formation of bubbles but that it was caused by the formation of a critical volume of bubbles. This concept is known as the critical released gas volume concept. This concept was covered in Chapter 6 as it is a key part of modern bubble theories.

It is fair to assume that the BSAC-88 model incorporates some form of critical released gas concept which would predict that bubbles will form after every decompression. These bubbles will affect the gas uptake and release for subsequent dives. Hennessey's research has led him to believe that a diver may saturate more rapidly during a repetitive dive than during an initial dive of the same depth and duration, since any bubbles present will increase the uptake of nitrogen during the dive. Therefore the rates of gas uptake and elimination will vary from dive to dive, and it becomes necessary to treat the second and subsequent dives differently from the first when trying to predict safe decompression.

In contrast Haldane's decompression models assume that gas uptake and elimination occur at the same rate during any dive, and the models assume that this rate is the same on a repetitive dive as it is on a single dive. This may be true if significant bubbling has not occurred within the blood and tissues, but if bubbles are present, they will slow down off-gassing and may increase the rate of on-gassing.

As a result of the factors set out above, Hennessy designed a set of tables which become progressively more conservative as the number, depth and duration of dives increases. Rather than creating a single dive table to predict repetitive dives, he created a number of different tables to be used for different dives. These tables consist of a set of seven separate tables for use at sea level with additional tables for use at altitude.

Like the earlier RNPL model Hennessey's model also resulted in a non-linear relationship between time and tissue loading. As a result the EAD concept cannot be applied to the BSAC-88 tables. In order to deal with Nitrox Hennessy went on to calculate a specific set of Nitrox tables for use with EAN32 and EAN36.

In another difference to the majority of other tables the BSAC-88 tables define bottom time as the time from leaving the surface until reaching 6m during the ascent, or at 9m on dives requiring a 9m stop. For most other tables bottom time is defined as the time from leaving the surface to the time we leave the bottom. This consideration should be taken into account when comparing BSAC-88 tables with other tables.

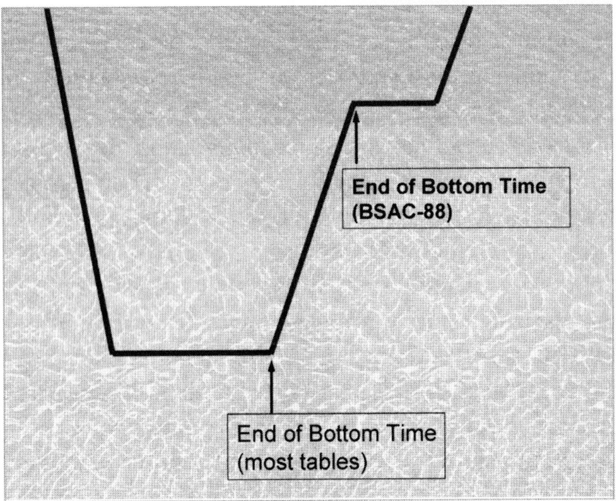

Figure 107: *BSAC-88 Definition of Bottom Time*

The BSAC-88 tables have been criticised for being overly aggressive for first dives, especially for deeper dives, and too conservative for repetitive dives. They have also been criticized for being 'old fashioned' or out of touch with modern decompression theory. Neither of these criticisms is entirely justified. When the difference in the definition of bottom time is taken into account the no-stop times for a first dive planned with BSAC-88 and Bühlmann tables for depths down to 50m are almost identical. However for decompression dives it is true that the decompression required for deeper and longer dives starts to become more aggressive than those given by other tables.

Hennessey's work on combining perfusion and diffusion is considerably more sophisticated then the solely perfusion limited assumptions that underlie the Haldane/Bühlmann models that have until very recently been the de-facto standard for other decompression tables. Furthermore the Hennessy/Hempleman critical released gas volume concept is a key part of modern bubble model approaches to decompression and when considered in this light the BSAC-88 tables can be viewed as much closer to 'modern' decompression theory than many people realise.

US Navy Exponential Linear Model

In 1977 the US Navy Seal community requested that the US Navy develop a decompression computer. Due to the kind of diving operations the SEAL teams were performing they would often perform long, multi-level dives and using standard air decompression tables resulted in excessively long decompression times. In 1978 the Navy Experimental Diving Unit (NEDU) began developing the Navy's decompression computer. The project was led by Captain Ed Thalmann, the Senior Medical Officer at NEDU.

Ed Thalmann is regarded as one of the leading authorities on decompression theory, but unlike Bühlmann, Workman and others his name is relatively unknown to most recreational divers. Most of Thalmann's research was carried out while serving in the US Navy. After serving as the medical officer aboard the nuclear Polaris submarine USS Thomas Jefferson, he was assigned to the Navy Experimental Diving Unit (NEDU). At NEDU, he was mainly involved in the development of new decompression tables as well as treatment of decompression sickness and in formulating 100 percent oxygen exposure limits. He spearheaded two major revisions to the Diving Medicine chapter of the U.S. Navy Diving Manual in 1985 and 1993.

The project to develop a US Navy decompression computer was originally going to use the US Navy standard decompression model as developed by Workman and others. Before confirming that they were going to adopt this model the project researchers retested the US Navy model in the context of real-time use for air and nitrox dives. The researchers found that the no stop limits were very safe and no incidences of DCS were detected, but for decompression dives in the 50-190 fsw (15-55m) range there was a 30-40% incidence of decompression sickness. Significant additional decompression time needed to be added to the calculated schedules in order for them to be safe. For some repetitive decompression dives with 60 minute surface intervals the decompression needed to be more than doubled (Thalmann 84).

Thalmann and his colleagues at NEDU began to develop a new model that could be incorporated into the decompression computer and would provide much safer decompression schedules for decompression dives as well as repetitive dives.

The model they developed assumed that inert gas such as nitrogen was absorbed into a number of parallel tissue compartments in the body at an exponential rate, just as Haldane and other researchers had assumed. Haldane's model also assumed that no bubbles are formed on ascent unless the supersaturation ration is exceeded. However as a result of Doppler ultrasound testing Thalmann knew that this is not true and that bubbles do indeed form on ascent, even if no overt signs or symptoms of decompression sickness are observed. The presence of these unanticipated bubbles will slow further off-gassing which in turn may cause more bubbles. This results in an overall rate of off-gassing which is slower than the exponential rate predicted by Haldane. Thalmann assumed that the off-gassing rate would be linear rather than exponential. Thus the model is termed an Exponential-Liner (EL) Model whereas the Haldane model is an Exponential-Exponential (EE) Model.

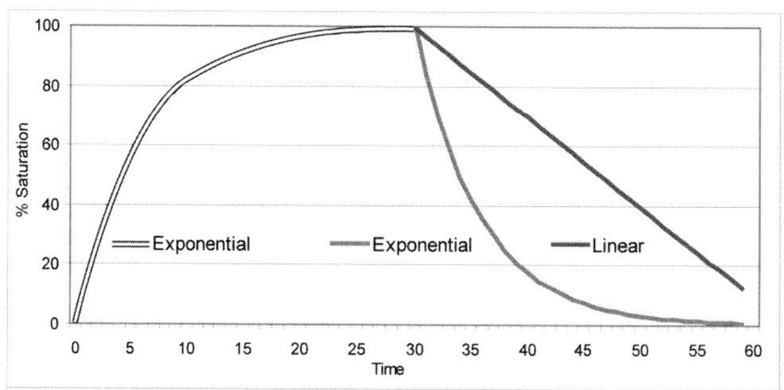

Figure 108: *Linear off gassing rate compared to exponential off gassing*

A linear off-gassing rate results in a slower ascent rate, longer decompression stops and a slower surface off-gassing rate. The slower ascent rate and longer decompression stops generated much more conservative decompression profiles which proved to be much safer for decompression dives than the previous US Navy tables. The slower surface off-gassing rate results in a higher nitrogen loading for subsequent repetitive dives which produces a much more conservative dive schedule for repetitive dives.

From 1985-87, Ed Thalmann worked as the U.S. Navy exchange officer with the Institute of Naval Medicine in England, where he continued his work on decompression table development. Dr. Thalmann finished his tour in the Navy at the Naval Medical Research Institute in Bethesda, Md. as its head of diving medicine and physiology research. There, he was principal investigator for the Navy's decompression research program. After leaving the Navy in 1993 Dr Thalmann joined DAN in 1995 as assistant medical Director, a post he held until his death in 2004.

The project to develop the US Navy's decompression computer was delayed due to a number of problems and changes of scope. First the SEALS decided that they needed the computer to be able to deal with gas switching, prototypes of the decompression computer suffered problems with continual flooding and a number of other problems. After Thalmann left NEDU, research and development of the dive computer project was continued by the Naval Medical Research Institute (NMRI) who developed a probabilistic method of determining decompression schedules. (See next section for details). However the probabilistic model developed by NMRI was judged too conservative and the Naval Special Warfare Biomedical Research Program, who were now leading the SEAL research progamme for the development of a decompression community made the decision to go with Thalmann's EL model (VVAL18). The model was incorporated into an existing commercial decompression computer known as the Cochran Commander, with the new version known as the Cochran Navy. The first version was delivered in 1996 and tested initially in the laboratory followed by field trials during 1998-99. At the end of 2000 all laboratory and field testing had been completed and all modifications completed and in January 2001 the computer, incorporating Thalmann's EL model, was approved for use by SEAL teams.

Probabablistic Models

Traditional decompression research had always proceeded from a physiological point of view. That is the researchers attempted to establish the mechanism in the body which controlled the on and off gassing of inert gasses. They would also attempt to identify the critical factor that resulted in decompression sickness. Haldane proposed that it was caused by bubble formation when a certain supersaturation ratio was reached. Hemplemann and Hennesy proposed that decompression sickness was caused only when a critical volume of gas in bubble form was present in the body. Once the researchers had produced what they considered a physiologically sound model of what was going on when the body was compressed and decompressed they would then attempt to create a mathematical model of this process. If the results of the mathematical model matched the real results from test dives then they assumed that the model was a good representation of what was happening within the body.

Clearly there is some uncertainty in this process and as we have seen there are clear theoretical problems with some of the physiological assumptions. As we have already seen there are known problems with some of the underlying models For example Haldane assumed that gas was held in solution until a certain supersaturation limit was reached, at this point bubbles would form and signs of decompression sickness would start to appear. We now know that this is not true and that silent bubbles occur on many dives where no signs of decompression sickness are observed. As a result one of the key physiological assumptions of Haldane's model has been shown to be false. Despite this flaw in the physiological underpinnings of the model the tables based on these models have been proven to result in many millions of incident free dives.

It is possible for a mathematical model to generate a set of tables which can produce incident free dives even if the underlying physiological model is flawed. This may sound surprising but remember that the models are often tested on a range of test dives and their parameters adjusted until they match the observed results. It is possible for a model to generate a wide range of results and so with enough parameters it is not so surprising that it can be tweaked to generate a set of results that match reality. In these cases the tweaking of the mathematical model is the important process, more so than the development of the underlying physiological model.

Taking this one step further, this means that it is possible to generate a set of tables which have no underlying physiological model but are still known to work. Statistical analysis can be used to analyse the safety level of a set of tables and predict an incidence level with a given level of certainty.

As we briefly mentioned, when discussing the US Navy's project to develop a decompression computer, a statistical approach to decompression modeling was developed by the US Naval Medical Research Institute (NMRI). This model is known as the Maximum Likelihood Statistical Method. This approach compares tables to diving data and adjusts the parameters of the tables until the tables match the desired level of probability of decompression sickness. In this way tables can be produced which generate a given DCS probability.

Probabilistic models are based on a binomial distribution. This just means that decompression sickness is considered a binary or yes/no situation. A dive is considered to result in either decompression sickness (yes) or no decompression sickness (no). Once a range of test dives have been carried out resulting in a set of binary yes/no results the distribution can be calculated and the incidence rate can be calculated with a given level of certainty.

The human body is an exceptionally complex biological system with many variables within each person let alone from one person to another. For this reason its behaviour is not easily predicted without a large number of test dives. As the number of test dives that are carried out is increased we can get a correspondingly increased level of confidence in the predictions. This is clearly a problem for decompression modeling as data on hundreds of repetitions of a dive profile is very rare and very few organizations have the facilities or funding to generate the number of test dives required. However, relatively simple statistical analysis tools can provide important information as to the number of trials needed to validate a given model, or the maximum risk associated with any number of incidences and tests. The table generated as a result may be described as having an incidence rate below 5%, with a 90% confidence level

Probabalistic analysis can also be applied to models based on physiological models in order to estimate the safety levels of these models. NMRI carried out significant work in this area during the late 80 and early 90's. They used probabilistic methods to analyse 4 models. The models were based on 3 or 4 tissue compartments and used either a traditional Haldane based exponential-exponential (EE) format or an exponential-liner (EL) format as proposed by Thalmann.

Starting in 1993 NMRI developed a new set of tables using exactly this statistical approach. Naval personnel made over 3,300 dives to test the validity of the model. The test dives were made in worst-case conditions, i.e. cold, hard, working dives. Extensive post-dive interviews conducted by medical personnel revealed even the most minor incidences of DCS. After extensive analysis, the navy chose a 2.3 % underlying incidence as an acceptable risk level. Although this seems high, with more than 1 predicted incident out of 50 dives, it should be noted that the 2.3 % incidence only applies when the model is pushed to its limits. Furthermore, the navy found that an incidence rate of less than 2.3 % significantly increased decompression times.

The new decompression tables generated by the NMRI probabilistic model were considerably more conservative than the existing Navy tables. They met with considerable resistance from Navy divers and the implementation of the tables was suspended.

DCIEM

The Defence and Civil Institute of Environmental Medicine is Canada's centre of expertise for defence research and development in human performance and protection, human-systems integration and operational medicine. The DCIEM Diving Tables and Diving Manuals are the result of more than 30 years of research and development and are considered to be one of the safest tables available for sports divers.
The DCIEM decompression theory is based on the work of D. J. Kidd and R.A. Stubbs. In the early 1960's Kidd and Stubbs were working for the Canadian Defence Research Medical Laboratory, one of the forerunners of the DCIEM. Their aim was to develop an instrument which would monitor a diver's depth and time history and provide instantaneous decompression information for oxygen-helium diving when complicated dive profiles and wide variations of gas mixtures would make the traditional tabular approach to decompression inadequate. In other words they were well ahead of their time in trying to develop a multi-gas, trimix compatible, dive computer.

The model was always intended to be used in a decompression instrument or decompression computer. The equations they developed describe the operation of a piece of hardware which is able to predict the safe decompression from a wide variety of dives rather than describing a physiological model for decompression. The initial versions of the computer were pneumatic-mechanical analogue instruments. Cavities, into which gas could enter at a controlled rate, were used to simulate the

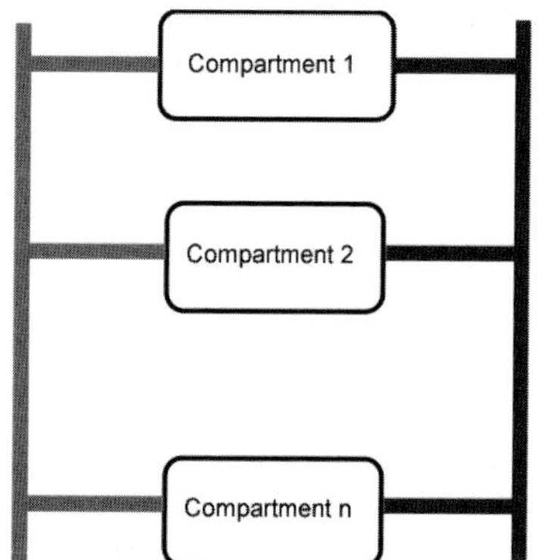

Figure 109: *Parallel Tissue Model*

different compartments. The instrument was known as a pneumatic analogue decompression computer (PADC). In 1965 the diver portable Mark VS PADC was developed followed by the surface based Mark VIS PADC a year later.

Early prototypes of the PADC were based on US Navy tables. Various changes were made to half-times, supersaturation ratios and the number of compartments in order to increase safety but ultimately they were dissatisfied with the US Navy tables and a purely Haldanean approach and decided to create a new model.

The Haldane model considers the various tissue compartments as a parallel sequence. Each compartment is considered separate to all of the others with no interaction or gas transfer between compartments and each compartment is considered to on-gas and off-gas directly into the blood stream and independently of each other. This is illustrated in Figure 109.

Kidd and Stubs concluded that in fact the tissues in our body do not act independently of each other and that there is indeed interaction between the compartments. They developed a serial model which was designed to model the interaction of the tissues. Serial decompression models assume that gas transfers from tissue to tissue during a dive, the compartments off-gas to each other even as they on-gas from other tissues of higher nitrogen tension. Only one tissue is assumed to be exposed to ambient pressure. The DCIEM tables are based on a four compartment serial model.

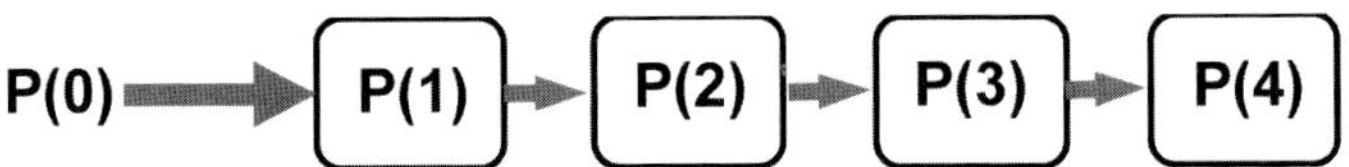

P(0): Ambient pressure (In initial dive, P(0) = Atmospheric pressure)
P(1) - P(4): Nitrogen pressure in compartments 1-4.

Figure 110: *Serial Tissue Model*

The approach taken by Kidd and Stubbs in testing their theory was to dive the model and, when symptoms of DCS occurred, to change the parameters of the model making it more conservative. They went through several variations of their air decompression model, improving the safety of the model after each iteration. By 1967, over 5,000 experimental dives had been conducted to validate the K-S (Kidd-Stubbs) model.

In 1970 it was discovered that for deeper dives hyperbaric chamber operators at DCIEM were not following the computed ascent profiles but were staying deeper by as much as 3m. This was due to an inherent distrust in the safety of the model for deeper dives. This distrust seemed to be justified as a series of dives, conducted in 1970-1971, where the ascent was carried out exactly as calculated resulted in a 20% incidence of DCI in the 60m to 92m depth range. The DCS incidence when the operators safety margin was applied was only 3.6%.

In 1971 Stubbs modified the model to take into account deeper dives. The modification he made was to make the supersaturation ratio depth dependent, with the ratio becoming more conservative with increasing depth. For deeper and longer dives this had the effect of introducing deeper decompression stops. In the same year the Defence Research Medical Laboratory and the Institute of Environmental Medicine merged to form the DCIEM and the K-S decompression model was approved in Canada as a safer alternative to the U.S. Navy tables.

In the late 1970's the PADC was replaced by the microprocessor controlled XDC-2 digital decompression monitor. The advantage of the digital computer was that the extensive calibration and maintenance procedures for each compartment of the PADC were no longer necessary. The only calibration necessary was for the depth sensor.
In 1979, DCIEM initiated a critical reevaluation of the K-S model using digital computers to control the dives and specially-designed Doppler ultrasonic bubble detectors to evaluate the severity of the dive profiles. Although thousands of dives had been conducted successfully there were three known problems with the model. Firstly, the no-decompression limits were extremely conservative. Some of the no decompression limits were less than half of those specified by other tables. This meant that there were a range of bottom times where decompression was required when using the computer but where no decompression was required with other tables.

The second problem was an excessively long decompression time when the third or fourth compartment became the controlling tissue. For example the decompression time required for a 70 minute bottom time at 36m was twice that required for a 60 minute bottom time at the same depth. This resulted in significantly longer decompression times than was seen with other tables.

Finally the third problem was that for a certain, small, range of bottom times the risk of DCS was higher than for other tables.

All three of these problems are clear if we examine a chart of total dive times for a range of bottom times.

Figure 111 shows the total dive times for a range of bottom times at 27m. The total times for the KS-1971 is plotted against times for Royal Navy Table 11 times and US Navy Standard Air times. As you can see for bottom times up to 60 minutes the KS model is more conservative than either of the other tables. Between 80 and 95 minutes it becomes the least conservative but then for bottom times over 100 minutes it is much more conservative by a large margin.

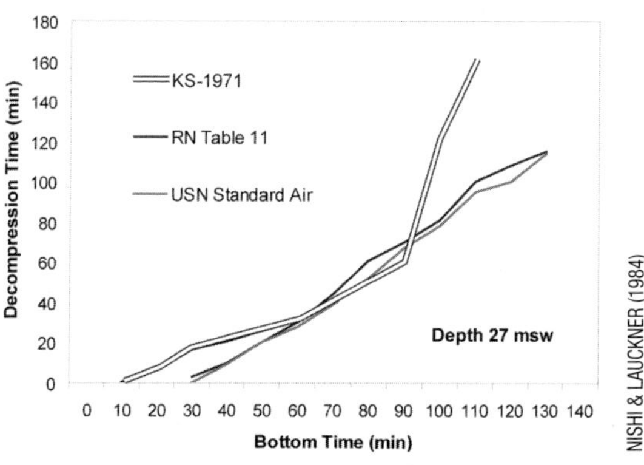

Figure 111: *Comparison of KS-1971 with Royal Navy and US Navy tables for a 27m dive.*

In order to deal with each of these known problems the two supersaturation constants "R" and "OFF" which control the supersaturation limits of the tissues were modified. In the 1971 model all four compartments used the same values for each of the two constants but in the 1983 revision each compartment was given its own value for the constants. This allowed more control over the behaviour of the model. For example, to increase the no decompression limits and reduce the decompression times for short exposures, the first compartment supersaturation ratio needed to be made less conservative. However the surfacing ratio was made more conservative for the second compartment in order to avoid the problem of aggressive decompression in the mid range. Of course in a serial model there is always a "downstream" effect with any changes to the first compartment affecting what happens to the second, third and fourth compartments and so this effect had to be considered when making any changes.

In order to reduce the problem of the long decompression times when the third and fourth compartments became the controlling compartments we must first of all understand the reason why this introduces such long decompression. This behaviour is a result of the model being limited to four compartments. For long bottom time dives, the fourth compartment saturates faster than in a model in which there are more compartments as it is the final compartment and hence the gas has no other compartments into which it can diffuse. This means that during the ascent there is more gas to be released which results in the correspondingly longer decompression times. With more compartments the gas would diffuse into the fifth, sixth, etc compartments and the "end compartment" effect would be reduced. One potential solution would obviously be to increase the number of compartments. It was calculated that 8 compartments would be required to accurately model the required behaviour. In fact the approach taken was to monitor the surfacing ratios for only the first two compartments (although all four compartments are still used for calculating the compartment pressure). By only monitoring the surfacing ratio for the first two compartments the model produces decompression times for long dives which are much shorter than those produced with the KS-1971 model. However they are still more conservative than the Royal Navy tables, US Navy tables or those generated with more 5 or more compartments.

Taken as a whole the changes resulted in a model where the no decompression limits are still conservative when compared to other models but considerably less conservative than the KS-1971 limits. Decompression times were also improved with overly conservative initial limits, aggressive mid range limits and very long decompression from long exposures being brought into line and resulting in a model which produced conservative, but not overly conservative dive schedules. Thousands of verification dives and many improvements of the theory have been performed and the dive table for air diving was released in 1992. The present theory is based on this dive table.

The DCIEM Manual published in 1992 contains decompression tables for air, enriched air (Nitrox) and Helium-Oxygen (HeO_2). Air decompression tables were developed in the 1980's for Canadian Forces operational use. These tables have also been adopted by foreign navies, commercial diving companies and other civilian organisations. The Sport Diving tables were a result of the original air diving tables adapted for use by recreational divers and have had a wide acceptance by the sport diving community. In addition to air tables, full Nitrox tables are also included as well as Helium-Oxygen decompression tables (HeO_2). HeO_2 tables were developed between 1986 and 1991 to replace the US Navy partial pressure tables for operational mixed gas diving to 100 metres.

The DCIEM tables are available commercially and are generally considered to be one of the safest and most conservative sports diving tables. NAUI adapted the 1995 DCIEM Sports Table for use in all NAUI courses and these were used until they were replaced by RGBM based tables in 2002. The DCIEM model has also been adopted by Citizen for use in its Cyber Aqualand range of dive watches.

In April 2002, DCIEM changed its name to Defence R&D Canada - Toronto. However, due to the close association of the name DCIEM with diving tables and manuals, these products continue to be marketed under the familiar and trademarked DCIEM name.

Ratio Deco

Ratio deco is a topic that has become popular, especially amongst internet discussion groups, in the last few years. The term has been popularised and is most closely associated with the GUE training agency but a number of other versions of the concept have been developed. Ratio deco can be defined as any set of rules that allow you to calculate the amount of mandatory deco and ascent rates based on the average depth of the dive and the length of the bottom time.

Ratio deco is based on patterns that can be found in decompression schedules. The basic concept is that by looking at a large number of decompression profiles it is possible to detect patterns in the profiles. These patterns can then be used as a shortcut to calculate the schedules required.

Ratio deco is not a decompression theory in itself. It is possible to identify patterns in the decompression scheduled generated by any of the various models discussed so far. However the two main versions of ratio deco approaches have both developed from modern decompression models that try to control the growth of bubbles during the ascent and as such they both produced ascents which are similar, but not identical, to a bubble model or gradient factor based decompression schedule. Given that ratio deco is not a separate theory in itself we will not spend too much time discussing it but will simply give an overview of the GUE version of ratio deco as well as another similar but subtly different version.

The key point of ratio deco is that there is a ratio which relates the bottom time of the dive to the amount of deco that needs to be done. This ratio will vary according to the depth with deeper depths requiring a higher ratio of decompression than shallow depths. For example one version of ratio deco may give a 1:1 ratio at 40m. This means that each minute of bottom time at 40m will give 1 minute of decompression. However at 60m the ratio would be 1:2 so that each minute of bottom time would give 2 minutes of decompression. These reference depths are often known as set points.

For depths that fall between the ratio points a calculation is made to take this into account. For every 3 metres (or part) shallower than the reference depth, we take 5 minutes off the deco. For every 3 metres (or part) deeper than the reference depth we add 5 minutes. So for example at 46m we are 6m deeper than the reference depth and so we would add 10 minutes onto the decompression. At 37m we are 3m shallower and so would subtract 5 minutes from the decompression.

The depth used for the calculation, depending on the particular version used, can either be the maximum depth of the dive or can be the average depth. Clearly using the maximum depth provides an additional level of conservatism as we are treating the dive as a square profile. However, there may be times when this is overly conservative and an average depth may be more suitable.

So for a 43m dive for 25 minutes we would take our decompression time to be 25 minutes plus an additional 5 minutes as we are 3m deeper than the 40m set point. This gives a total decompression time of 30 minutes.

Once the overall amount of decompression has been calculated it is then allocated between the various parts of the ascent. The ascent can be split into a number of phases. The initial part of the ascent, the first deep stop, the ascent from the first deep stop, the gas switch, ascent from gas switch and then shallow stops.

During the initial part of the ascent the focus is on getting up out of the on-gassing zone and as such the ascent rate should be brisk. Typically an ascent rate of 9 or 10 metres per minute it used. A slower ascent rate will allow additional on-gassing and will invalidate the subsequent profile. The depth of the first deep stop is determined slightly differently in the two versions. For the GUE version the first deep stop is calculated as 20% of the maximum depth in ATAs whereas the generic version places the first deep stop at 2 ATA (or 20m) above the average depth or at 21m for dives at a depth of 40m or shallower. So for a 43m dive, by using 80% of ATAs the first stop would be at 32m whereas by using 20m above maximum depth the first stop would be at 23m. In both cases we would probably round the stop depth to a multiple of 3m so the first stops would be at either 33m or 24m.

From the first stop up to the gas switch depth the ascent rate would be 3 metres a minute. The gas switch would then be at 21m for a switch to 50%. This gas switch would typically be at least 3 minutes.

The decompression time is then split evenly between the intermediate stops (21m-9m) and the shallow stops (6m) with half the decompression being carried out between 21m and 9m and the other half being carried out at 6m. In the example above, with 30m of decompression this would mean 15 minutes between 21m and 9m and 15 minutes at 6m.

The distribution of decompression over the intermediate stops can be achieved any one of three ways. The first is to simply distribute the time evenly over the stops. This is the method used in the GUE version of ratio deco. In our example there are 15 minutes of decompression to be distributed between 5 stops. This gives a straightforward 3 minutes at each stop as shown in the table below. This option has the benefit of being very easy to calculate but the justification for equal weighting for each decompression becomes weaker for shallower stops.

Stop Depth (m)	Time (minutes)
21	3
18	3
15	3
12	3
9	3

The second option is to use an 'S-curve' shape. This involves padding the deep and shallower parts stops at the expense of the middle stops. The justification for this is that at the deeper stops you are still getting a significant advantage from the decompression gas and so it makes sense to make the most of this advantage. At the end of the section the gas is coming out more slowly and so we need to slow up the ascent by extending the stops in order to avoid pushing the superaturation limits too hard. In the middle, when there is no major advantage from the deco gas but we have not yet started to push the supersaturation limits the stops can be brief.

Stop Depth (m)	Time (minutes)
21	4
18	3
15	2
12	2
9	4

The third option to use an exponential pattern where the stops get longer as you get shallower. In the example below the 15 minutes of stops is spread over the 5 stops in an exponential manner except that the full 3 minutes is spent at 21m as this is the gas switch stop. The remaining time is calculated by taking time from the deepest portion (18m) and adding it to the shallower portion (9m). Similarly time is taken from the 15m stop and assigned to the 12m stop.

Stop Depth (m)	Time (minutes)
21	3
18	1
15	2
12	4
9	5

In our example the 6m stop would be where we carry out the remaining 15 minutes of decompression, followed by a slow ascent to the surface.

For dives in the 40-50m range, with a single decompression gas the calculations are quite straightforward. For deeper dives, involving multiple decompression gasses, there are more steps involved. In these cases the idea of patterns is extended to the various phases of decompression stops.

For these dives the amount of decompression spent in each phase is related to the amount of decompression done in the other phases. For example, the table below shows that the 6m stop time is the same as the time from 21m-9m. However the stop time between 21m-9m is twice as long as the stop time between 36m-24m.

Stop Range (m)	Time
6	1 x 21-9
21-9	2 x 36-24
36-24	2 x 57-39
57-39	2 x 72-60

Ratio deco has a number of advantages. It allows the diver a great deal of flexibility in calculating their decompression schedule. If the exact depth is not known or if a wreck is large and you are not sure what part of the wreck you will end up on or if you end up spending time at different depths then this can be taken into account. Similarly if the bottom time of the dive varies from the plan then the decompression can be easily recalculated. It also allows the diver to carry out the dives without expensive wrist mounted Trimix dive computers.

Ratio deco also has a number of disadvantages or limitations. It will only work if the diver is using a consistent set of gasses. Clearly the decompression required will vary if the diver is using a different breathing mixture. Therefore in order to use any ratio deco scheme the diver must use consistent combinations of backgas and decompression gasses.

Ratio deco only works within a set range of parameters. For example as the bottom time increases the ratio concept breaks down. So at certain depths it may work for bottom times of between 10 and 40 minutes but will start to give inaccurate results beyond 40 minutes.

The level of conservatism, when compared to the base model, will very at different depths. Whilst ration deco might match very closely the decompression schedule generated by the base model at the set point depths it may become less conservative as you move deep from the set point depth.

One final disadvantage of ratio deco is that it requires the diver to carry out a certain level of mental arithmetic in order to calculate the decompression plan. None of the arithmetic is difficult but some divers struggle with mental arithmetic and for these the risks of making a mistake may be too great to justify the use of this method. For dives involving a 1:1 ratio with a single decompression gas then ratio deco calculations are quite straightforward. As the depth increases and the amount of decompression increases as well as the number of decompression gasses being carried the calculations become increasingly longer and more involved. In an emergency situation this situation may become even worse. In addition it is essential that any diver using this method uses it often enough to keep the process fresh in their mind. Many divers dive only infrequently and do not have enough opportunity to practice the method often enough for it to become something that they can rely on.

This section is not meant to teach you how to use ratio deco in practice. It is a purely theoretical discussion designed to illustrate some of the concepts behind ratio deco rather than teach you how to use it. A number of points of detail, which are essential to calculating a real profile, have been left out in order to focus on the concepts.

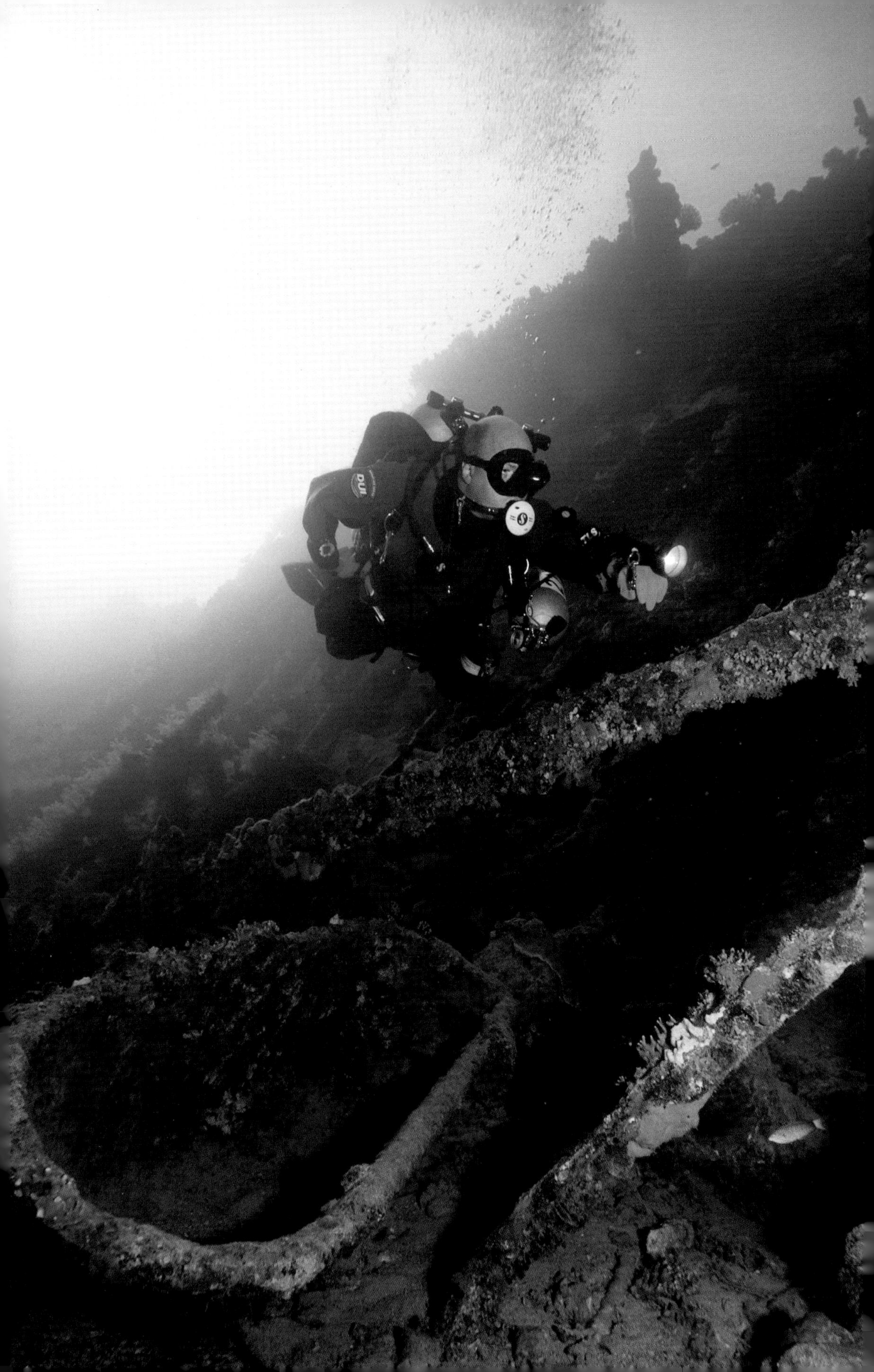
DUI

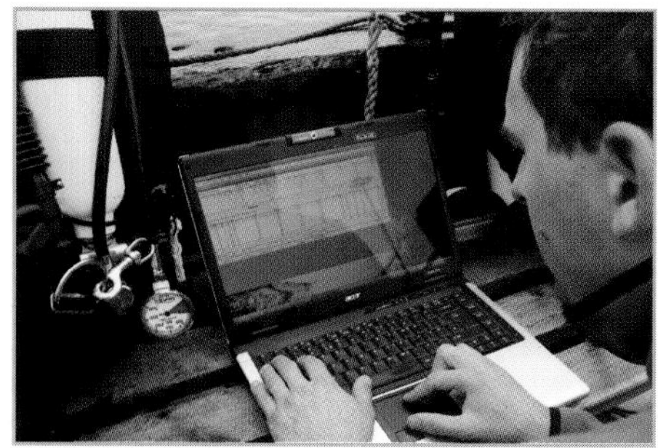

PC planning tools make decompression calculation much simpler

9 Decompression Calculations

Throughout the main body of this book I have tried to avoid formulas and a detailed mathematical treatment of the models we have discussed. This was primarily to focus on the concepts behind the models rather than the details of their implementations but was also to avoid putting off those who are less mathematically inclined. If you are one of those people who are not happy with maths then you should skip this chapter completely. However if you are interested in the calculations behind some of the decompression algorithms then this section is for you.

In this section I have gathered together many of the mathematical descriptions of the various models as well as several tables which provide the relevant 'parameters' to many of the models. Where a model has gone through a number of revisions I have tried to list out the formulas and parameters for each of the revisions so that it is possible to see how the model has developed.

Compartments, Half Times and Surfacing Ratios

Haldane (1908)

Compartment	Half time	Ratio
1	5	2:1
2	10	2:1
3	20	2:1
4	40	2:1
5	75	2:1

Left: A diver approaches the end of his bottom time on the wreck of the Ulysses

Hawkins (1935)

Compartment	Half time	Ratio
1	5	5.5:1
2	10	4.5:1
3	20	3.2:1
4	40	2.4:1
5	75	1.8:1 – 2.0:1

Yarbrough (1937)

Compartment	Half time	Ratio
1	20	2.45:1 – 2.8:1
2	40	1.75:1 – 2.0:1
3	75	1.75:1 – 2.0:1

Van Der Aue (1951)

Compartment	Half time	Ratio
1	5	3.8:1
2	10	3.4:1
3	20	2.27:1
4	40	2.06:1
5	75	2.00:1

Workman M-Values (1965)

Workman's presentation of M-values in the form of a linear equation was a significant step in the evolution of the dissolved gas decompression model. His M-values established the concept of a linear relationship between depth pressure [or ambient pressure] and the tolerated inert gas pressure in each "tissue" compartment.

$M = \Delta M \times D + M_0$

Where:

M	Tolerated inert gas pressure in hypothetical tissue compartment
ΔM	Slope of M-value line
D	Depth pressure (gauge pressure)
M_0	Intercept at zero depth; surfacing M-Value at sea level

No.	Half Time	M_0 (msw)	M
1	5	31.7	1.8
2	10	26.8	1.6
3	20	21.9	1.5
4	40	17	1.4
5	80	16.4	1.3
6	120	15.8	1.2
7	160	15.5	1.15
8	200	15.5	1.1
9	240	15.2	1.1

Bühlmann

Bühlmann published two sets of M-values; the ZH-L12 set from the 1983 book, and the ZH-L16 set(s) from the 1990 book (and later editions). The "ZH" in these designations stands for "Zurich" (named after his hometown), the "L" stands for "limits," and the "12" or "16" represents the number of pairs of coefficients (M-values) for the array of half-time compartments for helium and nitrogen. The ZH-L12 set has twelve pairs of coefficients for sixteen half-time compartments and these M-values were determined empirically (i.e. with actual decompression trials).

No.	Half time	M_0 (msw)	ΔM
1	2.65	34.2	1.2195
2	7.94	27.2	1.2195
3	12.2	22.9	1.2121
4	18.5	21.0	1.1976
5	26.5	19.3	1.1834
6	37	17.4	1.1628
7	53	16.2	1.1494
8	79	15.8	1.1236
9	114	15.8	1.1236
10	146	15.3	1.0707
11	185	15.3	1.0707
12	238	14.4	1.0593
13	304	12.9	1.0395
14	397	12.9	1.0395
15	503	12.9	1.0395
16	635	12.9	1.0395

The ZH-L16A set has sixteen pairs of coefficients for sixteen half-time compartments and these Mvalues were mathematically-derived from the half-times based on the tolerated surplus volumes and solubilities of the inert gases. The ZHL16A set of M-values for nitrogen is further divided into subsets B and C because the mathematically-derived set A was found empirically not to be conservative enough in the middle compartments. The modified set B (slightly more conservative) is suggested for table calculations and the modified set C (somewhat more conservative) is suggested for use with inwater decompression computers which calculate in real-time.

ZH-L16A Set of M-Values for Nitrogen (1990)

Compartment	Half time	M_0 A (msw)	M_0 B (msw)	M_0 C (msw)	ΔM
1	4.0	32.4	32.4	32.4	1.9802
1a	5.0	29.6	29.6	29.6	1.7928
2	8.0	25.4	25.4	25.4	1.5352
3	12.5	22.5	22.5	22.5	1.3847
4	18.5	20.3	20.3	20.3	1.2780
5	27.0	19.0	19.0	18.5	1.2306
6	38.3	17.8	17.5	16.9	1.1857
7	54.3	16.8	16.5	15.9	1.1504
8	77.0	15.9	15.7	15.2	1.1223
9	109	15.2	15.2	14.7	1.0999
10	146	14.6	14.6	14.3	1.0844
11	187	14.2	14.2	14.0	1.0731
12	239	13.9	13.9	13.7	1.0635
13	305	13.5	13.4	13.4	1.0552
14	390	13.2	13.2	13.1	1.0478
15	498	12.9	12.9	12.9	1.0414
16	635	12.7	12.7	12.7	1.0359

The individual a and b coefficients for each compartment can be calculated using the following formula:

$a = 2 \times t_{ht}^{-1/3}$
$b = 1.005 - t_{ht}^{-1/2}$

Where:

a	Bühlmann a coefficient
b	Bühlmann b coefficient
t_{ht}	Half time for the tissue compartmen

ZH-L16A Half-times, "a" and "b" values for Nitrogen and Helium

Compartment	Half-time N_2	N_2 a Value	N_2 b Value	Half-time He	He a Value	He b Value
1	4	1.2599	0.5050	1.5	1.7435	0.1911
2	8	1.0000	0.6514	3.0	1.3838	0.4295
3	12.5	0.8618	0.7222	4.7	1.1925	0.5446
4	18.5	0.7562	0.7725	7.0	1.0465	0.6265
5	27	0.6667	0.8125	10.2	0.9226	0.6917
6	38.3	0.5933	0.8434	14.5	0.8211	0.7420
7	54.3	0.5282	0.8693	20.5	0.7309	0.7841
8	77	0.4701	0.8910	29.1	0.6506	0.8195
9	109	0.4187	0.9092	41.1	0.5794	0.8491
10	146	0.3798	0.9222	55.1	0.5256	0.8703
11	187	0.3497	0.9319	70.6	0.4840	0.8860
12	239	0.3223	0.9403	90.2	0.4460	0.8997
13	305	0.2971	0.9477	115.1	0.4112	0.9118
14	390	0.2737	0.9544	147.2	0.3788	0.9226
15	498	0.2523	0.9602	187.9	0.3492	0.9321
16	635	0.2327	0.9653	239.6	0.3220	0.9404

Conversion from Workman M-Values to Bühlmann Coefficients

It is straightforward to convert between Workman style M-Values and Bühlmann style a and b values using the formulas below

Workman to Bühlmann
$a = M_0 - \Delta M\ P_{amb}$
$b = 1 / \Delta M$

Bühlmann to Workman
$M_0 = a + P_{amb} / b$
$\Delta M = 1 / b$

Where:

a	Bühlmann a coefficient
b	Bühlmann b coefficient
ΔM	Slope of M-value line
P_{amb}	Ambient pressure (absolute)
M_0	Intercept at zero depth; surfacing M-Value at sea level

The DCAP MM11F6 model (1988) for Nitrogen

The MM11F6 set of M-values are the values used by Hamilton Research's Decompression Computation and Analysis Program (DCAP). This set of M-values was developed by Dr. Bill Hamilton and colleagues during development of new air decompression tables for the Swedish Navy. In addition to air diving, the MM11F6 M-values have also been used for trimix diving and were the basis of many of the early custom decompression tables.

Compartment	Half Time	M_0 (msw)	M
1	5	31.90	1.30
2	10	24.65	1.05
3	25	19.04	1.08
4	55	14.78	1.06
5	95	13.92	1.04
6	145	13.66	1.02
7	200	13.53	1.01
8	285	13.50	1.00
9	385	13.50	1.00
10	520	13.40	1.00
11	670	13.30	1.00

The DSAT Recreational Dive Planner (PADI) model (1987)

The M-values used for the RDP were adopted from the Doppler bubble testing and tested by Dr Merrill Spencer and tested by Dr. Raymond E. Rogers, Dr. Michael R. Powell, and colleagues with Diving Science and Technology Corp. (DSAT), a corporate affiliate of PADI. The DSAT M-values were empirically verified with extensive hyperbaric chamber and in-water diver testing and Doppler monitoring.

Compartment	Half Time	M_0 (msw)
1	5	30.42
2	10	25.37
3	20	20.54
4	30	18.34
5	40	17.11
6	60	15.79
7	80	15.11
8	100	14.69
9	120	14.41
10	160	14.06
11	200	13.84
12	240	13.69
13	360	13.45
14	480	13.33

Variable Permeability Model (VPM)

In addition to tracking free phase gas VPM, like any other dual phase model, also tracks dissolved phase gas. As such it also incorporates a set of compartments and half times.

Compartment	Half Time
1	1
2	2
3	5
4	10
5	20
6	40
7	80
8	120
9	240
10	480
11	720

The rest of the mathematics for the VPM and other bubble models is beyond the scope of this book. The mathematics for these models is an order of magnitude more complicated than for the rest of the models discussed. For those readers wishing to find out more details then there are a number of references on page 241.

Alveolar Partial Pressure

When we breathe in, the mixture of gases that we inhale is diluted once it enters the lungs. This is largely due to the presence of water vapour and Carbon Dioxide in the lungs.

The air or breathing mix in a scuba cylinder is very dry. Compressors typically filter out much of the moisture content when filling a cylinder. When this dry air is breathed in it is humidified by the upper airways (nose, larynx, trachea). The water vapor is gaseous and so dilutes the breathing gas. A constant vapor pressure at 37 degrees Celsius of 0.0627 bar (47 mm Hg) has to be subtracted from the ambient pressure.

Carbon Dioxide is added to the breathing gas by gas exchange in the lungs. Since the partial pressure of Carbon Dioxide in dry air (and in common breathing mixtures) is negligible, the partial pressure of the Carbon Dioxide in the lungs is a result of the Carbon Dioxide produced by the body. This will be equal to the arterial partial pressure of 0.0534 bar (40 mm Hg).

Finally the partial pressure of Oxygen in the lungs is reduced as Oxygen is removed from the breathing gas by respiratory gas exchange in the lungs

The process of Oxygen consumption and Carbon Dioxide production is characterised by the *respiratory quotient* RQ, the volume ratio of Carbon Dioxide production to the Oxygen consumption. Under normal conditions the lungs take up about 250 ml of Oxygen, while producing about 200 ml of Carbon Dioxide per minute, resulting in an RQ value of about 200/250=0.8.

Depending on physical exertion and nutrition RQ values range from 0.7 to 1.0. The most commonly used values are those published by Schreiner, the US Navy and Bühlmann.

Source	RQ
Schreiner	0.8
US Navy	0.9
Bühlmann	1.0

The Schreiner RQ value is the most conservative of the three RQ values. Under equal circumstances using the Schreiner value results in the highest calculated partial alveolar pressure and hence the highest partial pressure in the tissue compartments. This leads to shorter no decompression times and hence to less risk for DCS.

The *alveolar ventilation equation* gives us the partial pressure of the inert gas with respect to the ambient pressure:

$$\mathbf{P_{alv}=[P_{amb} - P_{H2O} - P_{CO2} + \Delta P_{O2}]\ Q}$$

$$\mathbf{P_{alv}=[P_{amb} - P_{H2O} + (1 - RQ)/RQ\ P_{CO2}\ ]\ Q}$$

Where:

P_{alv}	Partial pressure of the gas in the alveoli (bar)
P_{amb}	Ambient pressure, i.e. the pressure of the breathing gas(bar)
P_{H2O}	Water vapor pressure, at 37 degrees Celsius 0.0627 bar (47 mm Hg)
P_{CO2}	Carbon Dioxide pressure, we can use 0.0534 bar (40 mm Hg)
ΔP_{O2}	Decrease in partial Oxygen pressure due to gas exchange in the lungs
RQ	Respiratory quotient: ratio of Carbon Dioxide production to Oxygen consumption
Q	Fraction of inert gas in the breathing gas. For example N_2 fraction in dry air is 0.78

No Decompression Limits (NDL)

The No Decompression Limit equation allows us to calculate the maximum time we can spend at any particular depth before exceeding the no decompression limit.

$$\mathbf{P_{no\_deco} = [M_0 - P_{alv0} - R\ (\ t\_asc - 1/k)\ ]\ e^{k\ t\_asc} + P_{alv0} - R/k}$$

Where:

M_0	Partial pressure limit (M-value) at sea level (bar)
t_asc	Time needed for ascending, t_asc=depth/v (min)
P_{no_deco}	Partial pressure at which ascending has to be started (bar)

Palvo	Alveolar partial pressure
d	Depth (m)
k	Logn(2)/Half time

Saturation level

Bühlmann

$$P_{comp} = P_{begin} + [\ P_{gas} - P_{begin}\ ] \times [\ 1 - 2^{-t_e/t_{ht}}\ ]$$

Where:

P_{begin}	Inert gas pressure in the compartment before the exposure time in bar
P_{comp}	Inert gas pressure in the compartment after the exposure time in bar
P_{gas}	Inert gas pressure in the mixture being breathed in bar
t_e	Length of the exposure time in minutes
t_{ht}	Half time of the compartment

Shreiner

$$P_t(t) = P_{alv0} + R\ [t - 1/k] - [P_{alv0} - P_{t0} - R/k]\ e^{-kt}$$

Where:

$P_t(t)$	Partial pressure of the gas in the tissue (bar)
P_{t0}	Initial partial pressure of the gas in the tissue at t=0 (bar)
P_{alv0}	Initial (alveolar) partial pressure of the gas in the breathing mix at t=0 (bar)
k	A constant depending on the type of tissue
R	Rate of change of the partial inert gas pressure in the breathing mix in the alveoli (bar/min) $R=Q\ R_{amb}$, in which Q is the fraction of the inert gas and R_{amb} is the rate of change of the ambient pressure.
t	Time (min)

Ascent ceiling

The ascent ceiling equation gives us the minimum depth to which we can adcend without exceeding our critical supersaturation limit. The ascent ceiling also represents the depth of the first decompressions stop (normally rounded down to 3m intervals). The calculation can also be used to show if the dive is a no-decompression dive (when the ascent ceiling is zero or negative).

The ascent ceiling is calculated by using the a/b coefficients. Other Haldanean models use M-values which represents the maximum tissue loading for a specific depth which will not produce DCI in that tissue. Each tissue has its own pair of a/b-values, nitrogen and helium. The following equation is used to calculate the ascent ceiling for each tissue:

$$P_{amb.tol} = (P_{comp} - a) \times b$$

Where:

P_{comp}	inert gas pressure in the compartment
$P_{amb.tol}$	pressure you could drop to
a and b	a and b values for that compartment and the gas in question

Each tissue will have a different ascent ceiling and the deepest ceiling is the one which should not be violated.

For Trimix dives the inert gas pressure in the compartment Pcomp is made up of the Nitrogen Pressure and the Helium pressure:

Pcomp = Pn -Ph

Where:

Pn	Current Nitrogen loading
Ph	Current Helium loading

There are a/b coefficients for both helium and nitrogen so for Trimix dives you must decide which to use. You can either use the nitrogen set which will give a more conservative schedule or you can interpolate the value based on the proportions of each gas load in each tissue.

For example, if a tissue has 2.65bar of nitrogen in it and 1.34bar of helium then the total gas loading is 3.99bar. Nitrogen makes up 66% of the total loading and helium makes up 34% of it. So you would take 66% of the nitrogen a or b value and 34% of the helium a/b value:

a = [a(n2) x Pn + a(he) x Ph] / (Pn + Ph)
b = [b(n2) x Pn + b(he) x Ph] / (Pn + Ph)

Where:

Pn	Current Nitrogen loading
Ph	Current Helium loading
a(n2)	Bühlmann a value for Nitrogen
a(he)	Bühlmann a value for Helium
b(n2)	Bühlmann b value for Nitrogen
b(he)	Bühlmann b value for Helium

For a Workman based approach the ascent ceiling is calculated from the M0 and _M values:

$$dmin = (Pt - M_0)/\Delta M$$

Where:

dmin	Ascent ceiling
Pt	Compartment Tissue tension at the end of the dive (bar)
M	Partial pressure limit for the tissue tension at depth d (bar)
M_0	The partial pressure limit at sea level (bar)
ΔM	Increase of M per meter depth (bar/m)

Decompression stops

The depth of the decompression stops are determined by the ascent ceiling. The decompression stop is usually rounded to the next deeper multiple of 3m. So if the ascent ceiling is 13m then the decompression stop is rounded to 15m.

To calculate the length of the decompression stops you simply calculate the ascent ceiling for each minute until the ascent ceiling is equal to or less then the next decompression stop depth.

Calculating a decompression profile

The steps above can be combined to give a step by step process for calculating a decompression schedule;

1. Calculate the partial pressure (tissue tension) in each tissue compartment at the end of the dive (just prior to the ascent).
2. For each compartment, calculate the minimum depth (dmin) to which the diver is allowed to ascend.
3. From all the values dmin obtained in step 2, choose the deepest depth.
4. Round the largest depth calculated in step 3 to the next deeper multimple of 3m. This will be the depth for the first decompression stop.
5. Let the diver ascend to the decompression stop. Calculate the gas loading during this ascent.
6. For each compartment, calculate the period the diver has to spend at this depth before proceeding to the next, shallower fixed decompression stop depth.
7. From all the values obtained in step 6, choose the largest period.
8. Round up this period to a whole minute.
9. Update the divers tissue tension in each tissue compartment for the stay at the decompression stop depth.
10. Repeat step 5-9 for each decompression stop depth until the surface is reached.

Gradient Factors

Gradient factor calculations involve determining how far each tissue compartment has travelled from ambient pressure towards its M-Value. This is known as the gradient factor and is calculated using the following formula:

$$\text{Gradient Factor} = \frac{\text{Tissue Compartment Pressure} - \text{Ambient Pressure}}{\text{M-Value} - \text{Ambient Pressure}}$$

In this case a gradient factor of 1.0 would indicate that the tissue is at its M-Value whereas a gradient factor of 0.0 would indicate that the tissue is at ambient pressure.

A gradient factor ascent involves keeping the gradient factor calculated above below a maximum gradient factor value which is determined by;

$$\text{Max GF} = \text{High GF} + \frac{\text{High GF} - \text{Low GF}}{\text{Hi GF Depth} - \text{Low GF Depth}} \times \text{Current Depth}$$

But as the high gradient factor is reached at the surface then Hi GF Depth is 0 and so this can be re-written as

$$\text{Max GF} = \text{High GF} + \frac{\text{High GF} - \text{Low GF}}{\text{Low GF Depth}} \times \text{Current Depth}$$

Saturation Diving

A simple model relating the rate of ascent from a saturation dive to the inspired oxygen partial pressure assumes that the ascent rate is a linear function of the Oxygen partial pressure.

$$\text{rate} = k.PO_2$$

Where:

rate	ascent rate
k	an empirically determined constant
PO_2	Oxygen partial pressure

To develop a saturation decompression procedure, the value of k (sometimes called 'Vann k') and the resulting ascent rate is adjusted in successive dives until the incidence of DCS becomes acceptably low.

DCIEM

The operation of the Kidd-Stubbs (KS) model is described by the following set of equations;

$$dP1/dt = A((B+P0+P1)(P0-P1) - (B+P1+P2)(P1-P2))$$
$$dP2/dt = A((B+P1+P2)(P1-P2) - (B+P2+P3)(P2-P3))$$
$$dP3/dt = A((B+P2+P3)(P2-P3) - (B+P3+P4)(P3-P4))$$
$$dP4/dt = A(B+P3+P4)(P3-P4)$$

Where:

Pi	the pressure in compartment i,
P0	the ambient pressure
A	0.0002596, gas flow constant (air, P in msw)
B	83.67, gas flow constant (air, P in msw)

And the safe ascent depth, i.e. the ascent ceiling, for the original model

SAD = Pt/1.8 – Psl

Where

Pt	the largest of the four compartments pressures
Psl	Pressure at sea level (10.06 msw)

And the safe ascent depth, i.e. the ascent ceiling, for the 1971 revision to the model

SAD = Pt/R – OFF – Psl

Where:

Pt	the largest of the four compartments pressures
Psl	Pressure at sea level (10.06 msw)
R	1.385
OFF	3.018

The supersaturation ratio can be obtained from the above as;

SR = Pt/(SAD)+Psl)
R/(1-(R x OFF)/Pt)

And the surfacing ratio (SAD = 0) as

SR0 = Pt/Psl

The DCIEM 1983 used the same basic model but rather than using the same constants R and OFF for all four compartments different constants were used.

First Compartment
R = 1.3 OFF = 4.8

Second Compartment
R = 1.385 OFF = 2.5

Third/Fourth Compartment
1/R = 0.0 OFF = 0.0

Ratio Deco

GUE Ratio Deco Calculations

Ratio Set Points

Depth (m)	Ratio
45	1:1
66	1:2
90	1:3
105	1:4.4
120	1:6

First Deep Stop

First Deep Stop = 80% of Max depth in ATA

Generic Ratio Deco Calculations

Ratio Set Points

Depth (m)	Ratio
30	1:0.5
40	1:1
50	1:1.5
60	1:2
70	1:2.5
80	1:3
90	1:3.5
100	1:4
110	1:5
120	1:6

First Deep Stop

First Deep Stop = Max depth – 2 ATA

First Deep Stop = Max depth – 20m

Acknowledgements

Many people have read various sections and early versions of the book. In particular Ross Hemingway, Dr Tom Hennessy, Dr Chris Powell, Crawford Foster, Mark Ellyatt, Steve Lewis and Janos Suto provided invaluable feedback on various aspects of early drafts. I am particularly grateful to Dr Mike Powell, formerly of NASA, and possibly better known as Dr Deco. Dr Powell provided a number of references and answers to various questions during the research of the book. Without his help the book would not have been as complete. Crawford Foster, Surgeon Commander Royal Navy and Head of Diving and Hyperbaric Medicine at the Institute of Naval Medicine also reviewed a draft copy of the book. He also helped to track down a number of the research reports detailing the development of the Royal Navy's work on decompression theory. Dr Peter Bennett, Founder of DAN and Executive Officer of the UHMS, also reviewed the final version and was very supportive of the idea. I am very grateful that he also agreed to write the foreword to the book.

Dr Richard Vann, Assistant Research Professor in Anesthesiology, Safety Officer and Director of Applied Research at the Duke Hyperbaric Center, and Vice President for Research at DAN, also provided a very detailed and useful review of the draft version of the book. Dr Vann picked up some details and errors that would otherwise have not have been spotted and helped with information on some of the more detailed points of various theories. He also provided a number of very useful references.

Gene Hobbs of the Centre for Hyperbaric Medicine and Environmental Physiology at Duke University Medical Centre was extremely helpful in the development of the book. Gene is the founder of the Rubicon Research Repository. The repository includes electronic versions of many of the most important and influential papers on decompression theory. When I started writing this book many of the papers I wanted to consult were not easily available. Now, many of the papers referenced are available online at the Rubicon Repository. This makes the task of anyone wanting to investigate further into the source material immeasurably easier. For more information on the Rubicon Repository visit www.rubicon-foundation.org

Many of the photographs in the book as well as the cover were provided by Gareth Lock. Gareth undertook a TDI Decompression Procedures course with me and so experienced first hand the course that prompted this book. Gareth is rapidly establishing a solid reputation as a deep wreck photographer by combining his passion for photography with that of wreck diving. Further examples of his work can be seen at www.imagesoflife.co.uk

I would also like to thank my parents for supporting me in everything I have done. Finally I have to thank Kate, my wife. As well as supporting me all the way through the writing of the book she proof read the whole book. She was largely responsible for shaping my enthusiastic outpourings into something more readable.

References and Further Reading

General

Bookspan J., 1997, *Diving Physiology In Plain English,* Bethesda: Undersea And Hyperbaric Medical Society.

Bennett PB, Elliott DH, eds. *The Physiology and Medicine of Diving.* 4th ed. London: W B Saunders, 1993

Bennett PB, Elliott DH, Brubakk AO, Neumann TS. eds. *The Physiology and Medicine of Diving.* 5th ed. Edinburgh: W B Saunders, 2003

Edmonds C, Lowry C, Pennefather J, *Diving and Subaquatic Medicine.* 3rd Edn, Butterworth Heineman, 1991.

Mount T and Gilliam B (Eds.) *Mixed Gas Diving: The Ultimate Challenge For Technical Diving.* Watersport Publishing, San Diego, CA

U.S. Navy Diving Manual, Revision 4, Supervisor of Diving, Naval Sea Systems Command United States Navy, 1999.

1 Historical Perspective

Boycott, A.E., Damant, G.C.C., & Haldane, J.S. *The Prevention of Compressed Air Illness,* Journal of Hygiene, Volume 8, (1908), pp. 342-443.

Boyle R. *New pneumatic experiments about respiration.* Phil. Trans. R. Soc. London 5: 2011-2031, 1670

Jackson, RW, 2001 *Rails across the Mississippis: A History of the St Louis Bridge.* University of Illinois Press

McCullough, D 1983. *The Great Bridge: The Epic Story of the Building of the Brooklyn Bridge.* Simon and Shuster

Mount T and Gilliam B (Eds.) *Mixed Gas Diving: The Ultimate Challenge For Technical Diving.* Watersport Publishing, San Diego, CA

Nobel Lectures, *Physiology of Medicine 1901-1921,* Elsevier Publishing Company, Amsterdam, 1967

Quintana, R. Prof Dr med *Albert A Bühlmann – In Memorial.* Nitrox Diver Vol 94-2 1986, p4

Stillson, GD. 1915. *Report on Deep Diving Tests.* US Navy Research Report. Bureau of Construction and Repair

Triger M. 1845 Letter to Monsieur Arago. *Compte Rendus de l'Academie des Sciences.* Paris. 20:445, 1845.

Workman, R.D. 1965. *Calculation of decompression schedules for nitrogen-oxygen and helium-oxygen dives.* Research Report 6-65. U.S. Navy Experimental Diving Unit, Washington, D.C.

2 Decompression Principles

Baker, E.C. 1998. *Understanding M-values.* Immersed. Vol. 3, No. 3, 23-27.

Bennett, P.B. 1996. *Rate of ascent revisited.* Alert Diver, January/February 1996: 2.

Boycott, A.E., Damant, G.C.C., & Haldane, J.S. *The Prevention of Compressed Air Illness,* Journal of Hygiene, Volume 8, (1908), pp. 342-443.

Marroni A, Bennett P.B, Cronje F.J, Cali-Corleo R, Germonpre P, Pieri M, Bonucelli C, Balestra C. "A deep stop during decompression from 82 fsw (25m) significantly reduces bubbles and fast tissue gas tension" Undersea and Hyperbaric Medicine Journal, Volume 31 No 2.(2004)

Pilmanis AA, 1976. *Intravenous gas emboli in man after compressed air ocean diving,* office of naval research contract report, N00014-67-A-0269-0026, Washington, DC.

Workman, R.D. 1965. *Calculation of decompression schedules for nitrogen-oxygen and helium-oxygen dives.* Research Report 6-65. U.S. Navy Experimental Diving Unit, Washington, D.C.

3 Decompression Illness

Bove, A. *Risk of decompression sickness with patent foramen ovale* Undersea Biomedical Research, Volume 25, Number 3, page 175-8, 1998

Conkin J, Powell MR. *Lower body adynamia as a factor to reduce the risk of hypobaric decompression sickness.* Aviat Space Environ Med. 2001 Mar;72(3):202-14.

Claybaugh JR and Lin YC, 2004. *Exercise and decompression: a matter of intensity and timing* J Physiol 555.3 (2004) 588

Dervay JP, Powell MR, Butler B, et al. *The effect of exercise and rest duration on the generation of venous gas bubbles at altitude.* Aviat Space Environ Med (United States), Jan 2002, 73(1) p22-7

Divers Alert Network. 1992. *Underwater Diving Accident & Oxygen First Aid Manual.* Divers Alert Network, Durham, North Carolina.

Doolette, D & Mitchell, S. 2003. *Biophysical basis for inner ear decompression sickness.* Journal of Applied Physiology 94: 2145-2150

Edmonds, C. 1993. *In-Water Oxygen Recompression: A potential field treatment option for technical divers.* AquaCorps, Number 5 (BENT):46-49.

Farm, F.P. Jr., E.M. Hayashi, and E.L. Beckman. 1986. *Diving and decompression sickness treatment practices among Hawaii's diving fishermen.* Sea Grant Technical Paper UNIHI-SEAGRANT-TP-86-01. University of Hawaii Sea Grant College Program, Honolulu, HI.

Flook V 2004. *Yo-Yo Diving and the risk of decompression Illness.* HSE Research Report 214

Gilliam, B. 1993. Chapter 10. Decompression management: Decompression sickness accident management. In: T. Mount and B. Gilliam (Eds.) *Mixed Gas Diving: The Ultimate Challange For Technical Diving.* Watersport Publishing, San Diego, CA, pp. 185-210.

Hill AB, Hill B 1968. "The life of Sir Leonard Erskine Hill FRS (1866-1952)". Proc. R. Soc. Med. 61 (3): 307–16. March 1968

Ikels KG. 1970 *Production of gas bubbles in fluids by tribonucleation.* J Appl Physiol 1970;28:524-7.

Jankowski LW, Nishi RY, Eaton DJ, et al. "Exercise during decompression reduces the amount of venous gas emboli." Undersea Hyperb Med (United States), Jun 1997, 24(2) p59-65

Kunkle, T.D. and E.L. Beckman. 1983. B*ubble dissolution physics and the treatment of decompression sickness.* Medical Physics 10(2):184-190.

Laden GDM and Grout P. 2004. *Aseptic bone necrosis in an amateur scuba diver.* Br J Sports Med. 2004:38

Lang, M.A. and C.E. Lehner (eds.). 2000. *Proceedings of the Reverse Dive Profiles Workshop.* October 29-30, 1999. Smithsonian Institution, Washington, D.C.

Lang, M.A. and R.D. Vann (eds.). 1991. *Proceedings of the AAUS Repetitive Diving Workshop.* Duke University, NC. 339 p.

Leffler CT. *Effect of ambient temperature on the risk of decompression sickness in surface decompression divers.* Aviat Space Environ Med (United States), May 2001, 72(5) p477-83

Meir B, Lock, JE. *Contemporary Management of Patent Foramen Ovale.* Circulation. 2003:107:5-9

Neumann, T. *Arterial Gas Embolism and Decompression Sickness,* News Physiol Sci 17: 77-81

Nishi RY. Doppler and Ultrasonic Bubble Detection in Bennett PB, Elliott DH, eds. *The Physiology and Medicine of Diving.* 4th ed. London: W B Saunders, 1993

Pyle R. "The case for in-water recompression". aquaCorps, No. 11:35-46.

Schwerzmann M, Seiler C. *Recreational scuba diving, patent foramen ovale and their associated risks.* Swiss Med Wkly (Switzerland), Jun 30 2001, 131(25-26) p365-74

Spencer, M. P. (1976). *Decompression limits for compressed air determined by ultrasonically determined blood bubbles.* J. Appl. Physiol., 40,227.

Spencer, M. P.; and S. D. Campbell (1968). *Development of bubbles in venous and arterial blood during hyperbaric decompression.* Bull. Mason Clinic., 22 (1), 26.

Spencer, M. P.; and D. C. Johanson (1974). *Investigations of New Principles for Decompression Schedules Using the Doppler Ultrasonic Blood Bubble Detector*. Technical Report. I.A.P.M., Seattle, Wa, 98122.

Wilmshurst P, Bryson P. *Relationship between the clinical features of neurological decompression illness and its causes*. Clin Sci (Lond) (England), Jul 2000, 99(1) p65-75

Wilmshurst P, Nightingale S. *Relationship between migraine and cardiac and pulmonary right-to-left shunts.* Clin Sci (Lond) (England), Feb 2001, 100(2) p215-220

Wisloff U, Brubakk AO. *Aerobic endurance training reduces bubble formation and increases survival in rats exposed to hyperbaric pressure*. J Physiol, 537 p607-611

Wisloff U, Richardson RS, Brubakk AO. *Exercise and nitric oxide prevent bubble formation: A novel approach to the prevention of decompression sickness?* J Physiol , 555 p825-829

Wisloff U, Richardson RS, Brubakk AO. *NOS inhibition increases bubble formation and reduces survival in sedentary but not exercised rats.* J Physiol , 546 p577-582

4 Saturation Diving

Comex 1996 *A Technological Breakthrough for Deep Diving Efficiency and Working Safety*

Eaton, B. *The Age of Discovery*

Pratt JA, Priest T, Castaneda CJ, 1997 *Offshore Pioneers: Brown & Root and the History of Offshore Oil and Gas.* Gulf Professional Publishing

U.S. Navy Diving Manual, Revision 4, 1999

Vorosmarti J. A 1997 *Very Short History of Saturation Diving,* Historical Diving Times Issue 20 (Winter 1997)

5 Nitrox

Behnke, AR. (1967) *The isobaric (oxygen window) principle of decompression.* In: The New Thrust Seaward. Trans. Third Marine Tech. Soc. Conf. 5-7 June, San Diego. Washington, DC: Marine Tech. Soc.

Berghage TE, McCraken TM. 1979. E*quivalent air depth: fact or fiction.* Undersea Biomed Res 1979 Dec:6(4):379-84

Hamilton RW 1992. *Evaluating Enriched Air (Nitrox) Diving Technology.* DEMA 1992 Nitrox Workshop Report

Harris RJ, Doolette DJ, Wilkinson DC, Williams DJ. "Undersea Hyperb Med. 2003 Winter; 30(4):285-91. Measurement of fatigue following 18 msw dry chamber dives breathing air or enriched air nitrox."

Martin, LM , 1999, *All You Really Need to Know to Interpret Arterial Blood Gases,* Lippincott Williams & Wilkins

Mount T and Gilliam G (Eds.) *Mixed Gas Diving: The Ultimate Challange For Technical Diving.* Watersport Publishing, San Diego, CA

Van Liew, HD, Conkin J, and Burkard ME. 1993 *The oxygen window and decompression bubbles: estimates and significance.* Aviat Space Environ Med 63: 859-865

6 Deep Stops and Bubble Models

Baker, E.C. 1998. *Understanding M-values.* Immersed. Vol. 3, No. 3, 23-27.

Baker, E.C. 1998. *Clearing up the confusion about deep stops.* Immersed. Vol. 3, No. 4, 23-31.

Bonuccelli C. *Calculating deco schedules with VPM*

Hennessy, T.R. and Hempleman H.V. 1977. *An examination of the critical released gas volume concept in decompression sickness.* Proc. R. Soc. Lond. B. 197:299-313.

Hills, B.A. 1966. *A thermodynamic and kinetic approach to decompression sickness.* Doctoral thesis, The university of Adelaide, Australia.

Hills, B.A. 1977. *Decompression Sickness.* John Wiley and Sons, Inc., New York.

Ikels KG. 1970 *Production of gas bubbles in fluids by tribonucleation.* J Appl Physiol 1970;28:524-7.

Imbert JP and Hugon J. 2003. *In search of models behind successful decompressions. Deep stops and modern decompression strategies workshop.* Tampa Florida 22-23 February 2003

Kaluza M. 2005. *VPM – The Inner Workings*

Lang, M.A. and C.E. Lehner (eds.). 2000. *Proceedings of the Reverse Dive Profiles Workshop.* October 29-30, 1999. Smithsonian Institution, Washington, D.C.

LeMessurier, D.H. and Hills, B.A. 1965. *Decompression Sickness: A Study of Diving Techniques in the Torres Strait.* Hvaldradets Skrifter 48:54-84.

Maiken, E.B. 1995. "Bubble Decompression Strategies." tek95 Diving Technology Conference.

Marroni A, Bennett P.B, Cronje F.J, Cali-Corleo R, Germonpre P, Pieri M, Bonucelli C, Balestra C. "A deep stop during decompression from 82 fsw (25m) significantly reduces bubbles and fast tissue gas tension" Undersea and Hyperbaric Medicine Journal, Volume 31 No 2.(2004)

Moon , R E. , A. A. Bove.2004 *Transcatheter occlusion of patent foramen ovale: A prevention for decompression illness?* Undersea and Hyperbaric Medicine Journal 2004, Vol., 31, No. 3

Pyle, RL. *The importance of Deep Safety Stops: Rethinking Ascent Patterns From Decompression Dives.* Deep Tech, Issue 5

Reinders D *The Varying Permeability Model – an explanation for the mathematically disinclined*

Weinke, B. 1995. *The reduced gradient bubble model and phase mechanics*. DeepTech, No. 3 (September 1995): 29-37.

Weinke, BR. *Basic Decompression. Theory & Application* 2nd Edition, Best Publishing Company. Flagstaff, Arizona ISBN: 1930536143

Weinke, BR. *Reduced Gradient Bubble Model,* Best Publishing Company. Flagstaff, Arizona ISBN: 1930536119

Yount, D.E. 1988. Chapter 6. Theoretical considerations of Safe Decompression. In: *Hyperbaric Medicine and Physiology* (Y-C Lin and A.K.C. Niu, eds.), Best Publishing Co., San Pedro, pp. 69-97.

Yount, D.E., Maiken, E.B., and Baker, E.C. 2000. Implications of the Varying Permeability Model for Reverse Dive Profiles. In: Lang, M.A. and Lehner, C.E. (eds.). *Proceedings of the Reverse Dive Profiles Workshop.* Smithsonian Institution, Washington, D.C. pp. 29-61.

7 Mixed Gas

Comex 1996 *A Technological Breakthrough for Deep Diving Efficiency and Working Safety*

D'Aoust, B.G., and C.J. Lambertsen. Isobaric gas exchange and supersaturation by counter diffusion. In: *The Physiology and Medicine of Diving and Compressed Air Work.* 3rd ed. Bennett, P.B. and D.H. Elliott. London: Balliere-Tindall: 383-403, 1983.

Doolette, D & Mitchell, S. 2003. *Biophysical basis for inner ear decompression sickness.* Journal of Applied Physiology 94: 2145-2150

Hamilton, R.W., Jr. M.R. Powell, D.J. Kenyon and M. Freitag. 1974. *Neon decompression.* Final report to Office of Nava: Research under Contract N00014-74-C-0424. Tarrytown: Union Carbide Corn.

Fife, W. P. (1979). "The use of Non-Explosive mixtures of hydrogen and oxygen for diving". Texas A&M University Sea Grant TAMU-SG-79-201.

Graves DJ, Idicula J, Lambertsen CJ, Quinn JA. *Bubble formation resulting from counterdiffusion supersaturation: a possible explanation for isobaric inert gas 'urticaria' and vertigo.* Phys Med Biol. 1973 Mar; 18(2): 256-64.

Lambertsen, C.J., and J. Idicula. *A new gas lesion syndrome in man induced by "isobaric gas counter diffusion".* J. Appl. Physiol. 39: 434-443, 1975.

Momsen, C. (1942). "Report on Use of Helium Oxygen Mixtures for Diving.". US Naval Experimental Diving Unit Technical Report (42-02).

Mount T and Gilliam B (Eds.) *Mixed Gas Diving: The Ultimate Challenge For Technical Diving.* Watersport Publishing, San Diego, CA

Strauss, R.H. and Kunkle, T.D. 1974. *Isobaric bubble growth: A consequence of altering atmospheric gas.* Science. 186:443-444.

Wienke BR, O'Leary TR. *Ins and Outs of Mixed Gas Counterdiffusion.* NAUI Technical Report 10144

Winstanley, F and Skorupka, R. *ISOBARIC COUNTER GAS TRANSPORT*, (The 'Vestibular Bend') http://www.cavedivinggroup.org.uk/Articles/ICGT.html

8 Other Decompression Models

Gerth WA and Vann RD. 1996. *Development of ISO-DCS Risk Air and Nitrox Decompression Tables Ising Statistical Bubble Dynamics Models.* NOAA Research Report

Hamilton, R. W., R. E. Rodgers, M. R. Powell, and R.D. Vann. *Development And Validation Of No-stop Decompression Procedures For Recreational Diving.* Diving Science and Technology. February 28, 1994, (pp. 78 + appendix).

Hempleman, HV. 1952. I*nvestigation into the decompression tables.* RNPL 4/52 Royal National Physiological Laboratory

Hennessy TR 1988 *Modelling human exposure to altered pressure environments. In: Environmental Ergonomics* (eds Mekjavik, IB, Banister, EW, Morrison, JB,). London: Taylor & Francis.

Hennessy TR, Hempleman HV. 1977 *An examination of the critical released gas volume concept in decompression sickness.* Proceedings of the Royal Society of London Series B - Biological Sciences 197(1128):299-313;

Lewis S. *Understanding the shape of the curve – a technique for demystifying decompression*

Lillo RS, Himm JF, Wethersby PK, Temple DJ, Gault KA, Dromsky DM. 2002 *Using animal data to improve prediction of human decompression risk following air-saturation dives.* J. Appl Physiol 93: 216-226

Nishi RY, Kuehn LA. 1973 *Digital computation of decompression profiles.* DCIEM Report No 884. Defence and Civil Institute of Environmental Medicine, Downsview, Ontario.

Nishi RY. 1982 DCIEM *Decompression tables for compressed air diving based on Kidd-Stubbs 1971 model.* DCIEM Report No 82-R-42 Defence and Civil Institute of Environmental Medicine, downsview, Ontario.

Nishi RY, Lauckner GR. 1984 *Development of the DCIEM 1983 decompression model for compressed air diving.* DCIEM Report No 44-R-44 Defence and Civil Institute of Environmental Medicine, downsview, Ontario.

Weathersby PK, Homer LD, Flynn ET. 1984 *On the likelihood of decompression sickness.* J Appl Physiol 57(3): 815-825

9 Decompression Calculations

Baker, E.C. 1998. *Understanding M-values.* Immersed. Vol. 3, No. 3, 23-27.

Baker, E.C. 1998. *Clearing up the confusion about deep stops.* Immersed. Vol. 3, No. 4, 23-31.

Braithwaite, WR. 1972. *Systematic Guide to Decompression Schedule Calculations.* Navy Experimental Diving Unit, Washington DC, AD0751027

Bühlmann, AA. 1984. *Decompression-Decompression Sickness.* Berlin: Springer-Verlag.

Bühlmann, AA. 1995. *Tauchmedizin.* Berlin: Springer-Verlag.

Hamilton RW, Muren A, Rockert H, Ornhagen H. 1988. *Proposed new Swedish air decompression tables.* In: Shields TG, ed. XIVth Annual Meeting of the EUBS. European Undersea Biomedical Society. Aberdeen: National Hyperbaric Center.

Hamilton RW, Rogers RE, Powell MR, Vann RD. 1994. *Development and validation of no-stop decompression procedures for recreational diving*: The DSAT Recreational Dive Planner. Santa Ana, CA: Diving Science and Technology Corp.

Hawkins J.A., Shilling C.W., and Hansen R.A., 1935, *A Suggested Change In Calculating Decompression Tables For Diving,* USN Med. Bull. 33, 327-338.

Van der Aue OE, Keller RJ, Brinton ES, et al. *Calculation and testing of decompression tables for air dives employing the procedure of surface decompression and the use of oxygen.* Research Report 13-51. Washington DC: US Navy EDU, 1951.

Weinke, BR. *Basic Decompression. Theory & Application* 2nd Edition, Best Publishing Company. ISBN: 1930536143

Weinke, BR. *Reduced Gradient Bubble Model,* Best Publishing Company. ISBN: 1930536119

Workman, R.D. 1965. *Calculation of decompression schedules for nitrogen-oxygen and helium-oxygen dives.* Research Report 6-65. U.S. Navy Experimental Diving Unit, Washington, D.C.

Yarborough O.D., 1937, *Calculations Of Decompression Tables,* USN Experimental Diving Unit Report, EDU 12-37, Washington DC

Index

U

V

W

X

Y

Z

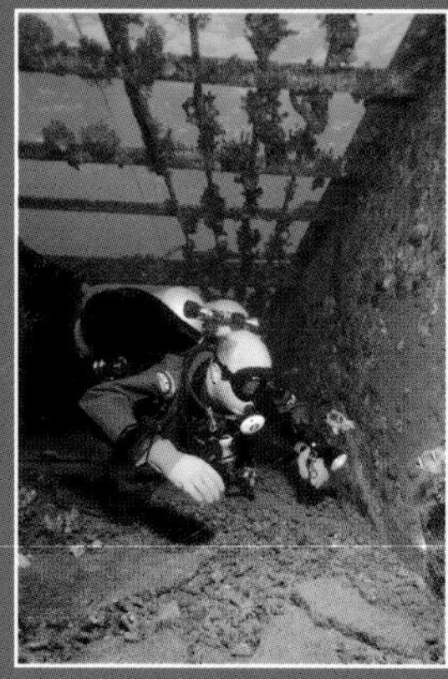

Deco for Divers provides a comprehensive overview of the principles underlying decompression theory and physiology. Mark Powell has written a book that for the first time allows the average diver to fully understand the principles behind this fascinating and critical aspect of diving. As well as a thorough examination of air decompression the book also addresses decompression using nitrox and mixed gases. It is completely up-to-date and includes information on the latest developments including deep stops and advanced bubble models. Deco for Divers bridges the gap between introductory books and specialist scientific journals and is suitable for new as well as highly experienced divers.

This is a truly remarkable book which covers all the various theories of decompression and ascents for divers in a most readable and understanding manner. There is no other comprehensive book on decompression to my knowledge which is so easy to read and understand by the average recreational or technical diver.

Peter B. Bennett, Ph.D., D.Sc. Executive Director, UHMS. Emeritus Professor of Anesthesiology, Duke University Medical Center. Founder & 1st President, DAN

This is the most comprehensive and well-written text I've seen that attempts to explain decompression theory to divers.

Dr Richard Vann Assistant Research Professor in Anesthesiology, Safety Officer and Director of Applied Research at the Duke Hyperbaric Center, and Vice President for Research at DAN.

This book is a "must read" for those who have ever wondered about decompression tables and how they are created. It is a straight forward book and devoid of technical jargon. It starts with the scientific giants who developed the physics of the gas laws and the physiology of diving and ends with M-values and tissue bubbles. For the curious diver – and all divers should be – it will be money well spent!

Michael R. Powell, MS, PhD. NASA (retired), Medical Sciences Division, Johnson Space Center, Texas

ISBN 1-905492-07-3
9 781905 492077

www.aquapress.co.uk